Pulmonary Disease

Editor

ALI I. MUSANI

MEDICAL CLINICS
OF NORTH AMERICA

www.medical.theclinics.com

Consulting Editor
BIMAL H. ASHAR

May 2019 • Volume 103 • Number 3

ELSEVIER

1600 John F. Kennedy Boulevard • Suite 1800 • Philadelphia, Pennsylvania, 19103-2899

http://www.theclinics.com

MEDICAL CLINICS OF NORTH AMERICA Volume 103, Number 3
May 2019 ISSN 0025-7125, ISBN-13: 978-0-323-67882-7

Editor: Jessica McCool
Developmental Editor: Kristen Helm

Medical Clinics of North America (ISSN 0025-7125) is published bimonthly by Elsevier Inc., 360 Park Avenue South, New York, NY 10010-1710. Months of publication are January, March, May, July, September, and November. Business and editorial offices: 1600 John F. Kennedy Boulevard, Suite 1800, Philadelphia, PA 19103-2899. Periodicals postage paid at New York, NY, and additional mailing offices. Subscription prices are USD $284.00 per year (US individuals), $611.00 per year (US institutions), $100.00 per year (US Students), $353.00 per year (Canadian individuals), $794.00 per year (Canadian institutions), $200.00 per year (Canadian and foreign students), $406.00 per year (foreign individuals), and $794.00 per year (foreign institutions). To receive student/resident rate, orders must be accompanied by name of affiliated institution, date of term, and the signature of program/residency coordinator on institution letterhead. Orders will be billed at individual rate until proof of status is received. Foreign air speed delivery is included in all Clinics' subscription prices. All prices are subject to change without notice. **POSTMASTER:** Send address changes to *Medical Clinics of North America*, Elsevier Health Sciences Division, Subscription Customer Service, 3251 Riverport Lane, Maryland Heights, MO 63043. **Customer Service: Telephone: 1-800-654-2452** (U.S. and Canada); **1-314-447-8871** (outside U.S. and Canada). **Fax: 314-447-8029. E-mail: journalscustomerserviceusa@elsevier.com** (for print support); **journalsonlinesupport-usa@elsevier.com** (for online support).

Reprints. For copies of 100 or more of articles in this publication, please contact the Commercial Reprints Department, Elsevier Inc., 360 Park Avenue South, New York, NY 10010-1710. Tel.: 212-633-3874; Fax: 212-633-3820; E-mail: reprints@elsevier.com.

Medical Clinics of North America is also published in Spanish by McGraw-Hill Interamericana Editores S. A., P.O. Box 5-237, 06500 Mexico, D.F., Mexico.

Medical Clinics of North America is covered in *MEDLINE/PubMed (Index Medicus), Current Contents, ASCA, Excerpta Medica, Science Citation Index,* and *ISI/BIOMED.*

PROGRAM OBJECTIVE
The goal of the *Medical Clinics of North America* is to keep practicing physicians up to date with current clinical practice by providing timely articles reviewing the state of the art in patient care.

TARGET AUDIENCE
All practicing physicians and other healthcare professionals.

LEARNING OBJECTIVES
Upon completion of this activity, participants will be able to:
1. Review treatment options and diagnosis for pulmonary hypertension.
2. Discuss the clinical presentation, diagnosis criteria, and treatment options for rare orphan lung diseases.
3. Recognize updates in the management of pleural effusions.

ACCREDITATION
The Elsevier Office of Continuing Medical Education (EOCME) is accredited by the Accreditation Council for Continuing Medical Education (ACCME) to provide continuing medical education for physicians.

The EOCME designates this enduring material for a maximum of 15 *AMA PRA Category 1 Credit*(s)™. Physicians should claim only the credit commensurate with the extent of their participation in the activity.

All other healthcare professionals requesting continuing education credit for this enduring material will be issued a certificate of participation.

DISCLOSURE OF CONFLICTS OF INTEREST
The EOCME assesses conflict of interest with its instructors, faculty, planners, and other individuals who are in a position to control the content of CME activities. All relevant conflicts of interest that are identified are thoroughly vetted by EOCME for fair balance, scientific objectivity, and patient care recommendations. EOCME is committed to providing its learners with CME activities that promote improvements or quality in healthcare and not a specific proprietary business or a commercial interest.

The planning committee, staff, authors and editors listed below have identified no financial relationships or relationships to products or devices they or their spouse/life partner have with commercial interest related to the content of this CME activity:
Matthew Aboudara, MD, FCCP; Vivek N. Ahya, MD, MBA; Muhammad Sajawal Ali, MD, MS; Bimal H. Ashar, MD, MBA, FACP; Emily P. Brigham, MD, MHS; Sean P. Duffy, MD; George A. Eapen, MD; Eno-Obong Essien, MD; Uzair Khan Ghori, MD; Nabeel Hamzeh, MD; Kristen Helm; David W. Hsia, MD; Alison Kemp; Sandhya Khurana, MD; Darlene Kim, MD; Christopher M. Kniese, MD; Katherine Krol, MD; Charles W. Lanks, MD; Oscar Llanos, MD; Lisa A. Maier, MD, MSPH; Stephen C. Mathai, MD, MHS; Jessica McCool; Mary Anne Morgan, MD; Ali I. Musani, MD; Faria Nasim, MD; Rodolfo M. Pascual, MD, FCCP; David M. Perlman, MD; Parth Rali, MD; Bruce F. Sabath, MD; Mona Sarkiss, MD, PhD; Angela Selzer, MD; Lubna Sorathia, MD; Jeyanthi Surendrakumar; Tianshi David Wu, MD, MHS.

The planning committee, staff, authors and editors listed below have identified financial relationships or relationships to products or devices they or their spouse/life partner have with commercial interest related to the content of this CME activity:
Sharon D. Cornelison, RCP, RRT-NPS: participates in a speakers bureau for Boehringer Ingelheim International GmbH and Mylan NV and is a consultant/advisor for Insight Therapeutics, LLC.
Gerard J. Criner, MD: is a consultant/advisor and receives research support from Boehringer Ingelheim International GmbH, AstraZeneca, Aries Pharmaceuticals, Inc, Novartis AG, IKARIA Canada Inc, BTG International Ltd, Pulmonx Corporation, GlaxoSmithKline plc, Koninklijke Philips NV, HGE Health Care Solutions, Inc, Almirall, SA, Actelion Pharmaceuticals US, Inc, Allergan, and Nuvaira Inc
Joshua M. Diamond, MD, MSCE: receives research funding from Merck Sharp & Dohme Corp.
M. Patricia George, MD: participates in a speakers bureau and is a consultant/advisor for Gilead Sciences, Inc. and Bayer AG; particpates in a speakers bureau, is a consultant/advisor, and receives research support from Actelion Pharmaceuticals US, Inc.
Fabien Maldonado, MD, FCCP: receives research support from Centurion Medical Products.
Meredith C. McCormack, MD, MHS: receives royalties from UpToDate, Inc.

UNAPPROVED/OFF-LABEL USE DISCLOSURE
The EOCME requires CME faculty to disclose to the participants;

1. When products or procedures being discussed are off-label, unlabelled, experimental, and/or investigational (not US Food and Drug Administration [FDA] approved); and
2. Any limitations on the information presented, such as data that are preliminary or that represent ongoing research, interim analyses, and/or unsupported opinions. Faculty may discuss information about pharmaceutical agents that is outside of FDA-approved labelling. This information is intended solely for CME and is not intended to promote off-label use of these medications. If you have any questions, contact the medical affairs department of the manufacturer for the most recent prescribing information.

TO ENROLL

To enroll in the *Medical Clinics of North America* Continuing Medical Education program, call customer service at 1-800-654-2452 or sign up online at http://www.theclinics.com/home/cme. The CME program is available to subscribers for an additional annual fee of USD $300.90.

METHOD OF PARTICIPATION

In order to claim credit, participants must complete the following;
1. Complete enrolment as indicated above.
2. Read the activity.
3. Complete the CME Test and Evaluation. Participants must achieve a score of 70% on the test. All CME Tests and Evaluations must be completed online.

CME INQUIRIES/SPECIAL NEEDS

For all CME inquiries or special needs, please contact elsevierCME@elsevier.com.

MEDICAL CLINICS OF NORTH AMERICA

FORTHCOMING ISSUES

July 2019
Women's Mental Health
Susan G. Kornstein and
Anita H. Clayton, *Editors*

September 2019
Cardiac Arrhythmias: A Compendium
Otto Costantini, *Editor*

November 2019
Genetics and Precision Medicine
Howard P. Levy, *Editor*

RECENT ISSUES

March 2019
Neurology for the Non-Neurologist
Tracey A. Milligan, *Editor*

January 2019
Gastroenterology for the Internist
Kerry B. Dunbar, *Editor*

November 2018
Otolaryngology
C. Matthew Stewart, *Editor*

SERIES OF RELATED INTEREST

Primary Care: Clinics in Office Practice
Physician Assistant Clinics
Clinics in Chest Medicine
Clinics in Geriatric Medicine

Contributors

CONSULTING EDITOR

BIMAL H. ASHAR, MD, MBA, FACP
Associate Professor of Medicine, Division of General Internal Medicine, Johns Hopkins
School of Medicine, Baltimore, Maryland

EDITOR

ALI I. MUSANI, MD, FCCP
Vice Chair, Global Health, Professor of Medicine and Surgery, Department of Medicine,
Director, Complex Airway Pillar of the Center for Lung and Breathing Director,
Interventional Pulmonology Program, Fellowship Director, Bronchoscopy Service,
University of Colorado Hospital, Division of Pulmonary Sciences and Critical Care
Medicine, University of Colorado School of Medicine, University of Colorado Denver,
University of Colorado Anschutz, Aurora, Colorado

AUTHORS

MATTHEW ABOUDARA, MD, FCCP
Division of Allergy, Pulmonary and Critical Care Medicine, Vanderbilt University Medical
Center, The Vanderbilt Clinic, Nashville, Tennessee

VIVEK N. AHYA, MD, MBA
Associate Professor of Medicine, Vice Chief, Clinical Affairs, Division of Pulmonary, Allergy
and Critical Care, Clinical Director, Paul F. Harron, Jr. Lung Center, Penn Medicine,
Perelman School of Medicine, University of Pennsylvania, Philadelphia, Pennsylvania

MUHAMMAD SAJAWAL ALI, MD, MS
Division of Pulmonary and Critical Care Medicine, Medical College of Wisconsin,
Milwaukee, Wisconsin

EMILY P. BRIGHAM, MD, MHS
Assistant Professor of Medicine, Division of Pulmonary and Critical Care Medicine, Johns
Hopkins School of Medicine, Baltimore, Maryland

SHARON D. CORNELISON, RCP, RRT-NPS
Department of Pulmonary and Cardiac Rehabilitation, J. Paul Sticht Center on Aging and
Rehabilitation, Wake Forest Baptist Medical Center, Winston-Salem, North Carolina

GERARD J. CRINER, MD
Professor, Department Chair, Department of Thoracic Medicine and Surgery, Lewis Katz
School of Medicine at Temple University, Philadelphia, Pennsylvania

JOSHUA M. DIAMOND, MD, MSCE
Associate Medical Director, Lung Transplantation Program, Assistant Professor of
Medicine, Division of Pulmonary, Allergy and Critical Care, Perelman School of Medicine,
University of Pennsylvania, Philadelphia, Pennsylvania

SEAN P. DUFFY, MD
Assistant Professor, Department of Thoracic Medicine and Surgery, Lewis Katz School of Medicine at Temple University, Philadelphia, Pennsylvania

GEORGE A. EAPEN, MD
Professor of Medicine, Department of Pulmonary Medicine, The University of Texas MD Anderson Cancer Center, Houston, Texas

ENO-OBONG ESSIEN, MD
Division of Internal Medicine Residency Program, Temple University Hospital, Philadelphia, Pennsylvania

M. PATRICIA GEORGE, MD
Associate Professor, Department of Medicine, National Jewish Health, Denver, Colorado

UZAIR KHAN GHORI, MD
Division of Pulmonary and Critical Care Medicine, College of Wisconsin, Milwaukee, Wisconsin

NABEEL HAMZEH, MD
Associate Professor, Division of Pulmonary, Critical Care and Occupational Medicine, University of Iowa College of Medicine, Iowa City, Iowa

DAVID W. HSIA, MD
Division of Respiratory and Critical Care Physiology and Medicine, Harbor-UCLA Medical Center, Torrance, California

SANDHYA KHURANA, MD
Associate Professor of Medicine, Co-Director, Pulmonary and Critical Care Medicine, Mary Parkes Center for Asthma and Pulmonary Care, University of Rochester School of Medicine, University of Rochester Medical Center, Rochester, New York

DARLENE KIM, MD
Associate Professor, Department of Medicine, National Jewish Health, Denver, Colorado

CHRISTOPHER M. KNIESE, MD
Fellow, Interventional Pulmonology, Division of Pulmonary Sciences and Critical Care Medicine, University of Colorado Denver, University of Colorado Anschutz, Aurora, Colorado

KATHERINE KROL, MD
Fellow, Pulmonary and Critical Care Medicine, University of Rochester School of Medicine, University of Rochester Medical Center, Rochester, New York

CHARLES W. LANKS, MD
Division of Respiratory and Critical Care Physiology and Medicine, Harbor-UCLA Medical Center, Torrance, California

OSCAR LLANOS, MD
Fellow, Division of Pulmonary, Critical Care and Occupational Medicine, University of Iowa College of Medicine, Iowa City, Iowa

LISA A. MAIER, MD, MSPH
Division of Environmental and Occupational Health Sciences, National Jewish Health, Division of Pulmonary and Critical Care Sciences, School of Medicine, Environmental Occupational Health Department, Colorado School of Public Health, University of Colorado, Denver, Colorado

FABIEN MALDONADO, MD, FCCP
Associate Professor of Medicine and Thoracic Surgery, Division of Allergy, Pulmonary and Critical Care Medicine, Vanderbilt University Medical Center, The Vanderbilt Clinic, Nashville, Tennessee

STEPHEN C. MATHAI, MD, MHS
Associate Professor of Medicine, The John Hopkins Hospital, Baltimore, Maryland

MEREDITH C. McCORMACK, MD, MHS
Associate Professor of Medicine, Division of Pulmonary and Critical Care Medicine, Johns Hopkins School of Medicine, Baltimore, Maryland

MARY ANNE MORGAN, MD
Associate Professor of Medicine, Associate Fellowship Program Director, Pulmonary and Critical Care Medicine, University of Rochester School of Medicine, University of Rochester Medical Center, Rochester, New York

ALI I. MUSANI, MD, FCCP
Vice Chair, Global Health, Professor of Medicine and Surgery, Department of Medicine, Director, Complex Airway Pillar of the Center for Lung and Breathing Director, Interventional Pulmonology Program, Fellowship Director, Bronchoscopy Service, University of Colorado Hospital, Division of Pulmonary Sciences and Critical Care Medicine, University of Colorado School of Medicine, University of Colorado Denver, University of Colorado Anschutz, Aurora, Colorado

FARIA NASIM, MD
Fellow, Department of Pulmonary Medicine, The University of Texas MD Anderson Cancer Center, Houston, Texas

RODOLFO M. PASCUAL, MD, FCCP
Department of Internal Medicine, Section on Pulmonary Medicine, Critical Care, Allergy and Immunologic Diseases, Wake Forest Baptist Medical Center, Winston-Salem, North Carolina

DAVID M. PERLMAN, MD
Division of Pulmonary and Critical Care Medicine, University of Minnesota, Minneapolis, Minnesota

PARTH RALI, MD
Assistant Professor, Division of Thoracic Surgery and Medicine, Director, Pulmonary Embolism Response Team (PERT), Temple University Hospital, Philadelphia, Pennsylvania

BRUCE F. SABATH, MD
Fellow, Department of Pulmonary Medicine, The University of Texas MD Anderson Cancer Center, Houston, Texas

MONA SARKISS, MD, PhD
Professor, Departments of Anesthesiology and Perioperative Medicine, and Pulmonary Medicine, The University of Texas MD Anderson Cancer Center, Houston, Texas

ANGELA SELZER, MD
Assistant Professor, Department of Anesthesiology, University of Colorado, Aurora, Colorado

LUBNA SORATHIA, MD
Assistant Medical Director, Innovage Greater CO PACE, Denver, Colorado

TIANSHI DAVID WU, MD, MHS
Postdoctoral Fellow, Division of Pulmonary and Critical Care Medicine, Johns Hopkins School of Medicine, Baltimore, Maryland

Contents

Foreword: Tom Brady's Lungs   xvii

Bimal H. Ashar

Preface: Pulmonary Disease   xix

Ali I. Musani

Interventional Pulmonology: A Focused Review for Primary Care Physicians   399

Christopher M. Kniese and Ali I. Musani

> Interventional pulmonology (IP) has evolved in recent decades, and recent advances have greatly expanded the services offered by IP physicians. IP is best defined as the use of advanced techniques for the evaluation and treatment of benign and malignant pulmonary disorders. The field has further advanced with the recent establishment of a board certification via the American Association of Bronchology and Interventional Pulmonology and the release in 2017 of accreditation standards for specialized fellowship training. This article provides a broad overview of the field to serve as a resource for primary care physicians.

Pulmonary Hypertension   413

Darlene Kim and M. Patricia George

> Pulmonary hypertension (PH) is a chronic and progressive disease that presents like many other lung diseases, often leading to a delay in diagnosis, and therefore a delay in optimal therapy. This article provides a review of PH for internists, covering clinical presentation, diagnostic algorithm, different types of PH, and overview of treatments. In addition, it emphasizes the importance of early referral to, and partnership between, PH specialists and physicians on the front lines to improve early diagnosis and optimize management of these complex patients.

Lung Transplantation   425

Vivek N. Ahya and Joshua M. Diamond

> Lung transplantation is an appropriate therapeutic option for select patients with end-stage lung diseases and offers the possibility of improved quality of life and longer survival. Unfortunately, the transplant recipient is at risk for numerous immunologic, infectious, and medical complications that threaten both of these goals. Median survival after lung transplantation is approximately 6 years. Optimizing outcomes requires close partnership between the patient, transplant center, and primary medical team. Early referral to a transplant center should be considered for patients with idiopathic pulmonary fibrosis and related interstitial lung diseases due to risk of acute exacerbation and accelerated development of respiratory failure.

Asthma in the Primary Care Setting   435

Tianshi David Wu, Emily P. Brigham, and Meredith C. McCormack

Asthma is one of the commonest respiratory diseases in the United States, affecting approximately 8% of adults. This article reviews the epidemiology, diagnosis, and treatment of asthma, with integration of recommendations from professional societies, with special attention to differential diagnosis. A framework for outpatient management of patients with asthma is presented, including indications for subspecialist referral. With integration of objective diagnostic information, systematic approach through modification of disease triggers and adjustment of controller medications, and patient empowerment to respond to varying symptoms using an asthma action plan, most individuals with asthma are successfully managed in the primary care setting.

Chronic Obstructive Pulmonary Disease: Evaluation and Management   453

Sean P. Duffy and Gerard J. Criner

Chronic obstructive pulmonary disease (COPD) is a leading cause of death nationally and worldwide. Cigarette smoking is the most common risk factor in the development of COPD. Disease course is variable with some patients having a high degree of obstruction and minimal symptoms, whereas others with better lung function have a greater symptoms burden. The goal of pharmacologic therapy is to minimize symptoms, improve exercise tolerance, and reduce exacerbation risk. No pharmacologic therapy has been shown to improve survival in COPD. Pulmonology referral is recommended for patients with COPD with symptoms despite first-line inhaled therapy, frequent exacerbations, any hospitalizations, or moderate-to-severe disease.

Lung Cancer   463

Faria Nasim, Bruce F. Sabath, and George A. Eapen

Lung cancer is the world's leading cause of cancer death. Screening for lung cancer by low-dose computed tomography improves mortality. Various modalities exist for diagnosis and staging. Treatment is determined by subtype and stage of cancer; there are several personalized therapies that did not exist just a few years ago. Caring for the patient with lung cancer is a complex task. This review provides a broad outline of this disease, helping clinicians identify such patients and familiarizing them with lung cancer care options, so they are better equipped to guide their patients along this challenging journey.

Update in the Management of Pleural Effusions   475

Matthew Aboudara and Fabien Maldonado

Pleural effusions are a common clinical problem for the primary care physician. Over the past 10 years, there has been a paradigm shift in the field due to emergence of new evidence, which includes the ubiquitous use of thoracic ultrasound, the reemergence of pleuroscopy as a diagnostic and therapeutic modality, the widespread use of indwelling pleural catheters for malignant pleural effusions, and the evidence-based approach to management of complex parapneumonic effusions. This review focuses on these advancements with an emphasis on practical clinical application.

Community-acquired Pneumonia and Hospital-acquired Pneumonia   487

Charles W. Lanks, Ali I. Musani, and David W. Hsia

Pneumonia is among the leading causes of morbidity and mortality worldwide. Although Streptococcus pneumoniae is the most likely cause in most cases, the variety of potential pathogens can make choosing a management strategy a complex endeavor. The setting in which pneumonia is acquired heavily influences diagnostic and therapeutic choices. Because the causative organism is typically unknown early on, timely administration of empiric antibiotics is a cornerstone of pneumonia management. Disease severity and rates of antibiotic resistance should be carefully considered when choosing an empiric regimen. When complications arise, further work-up and consultation with a pulmonary specialist may be necessary.

Orphan Lung Diseases   503

Muhammad Sajawal Ali, Uzair Khan Ghori, and Ali I. Musani

There are hundreds of rare orphan lung diseases. We have highlighted five of them, one from each of the five major categories of pulmonary disorders: pleuroparenchymal fibroelastosis (a rare diffuse parenchymal lung disease), pulmonary alveolar proteinosis (a rare autoimmune and diffuse parenchymal lung disease), lymphangioleiomyomatosis (a rare cystic lung disease), yellow nail syndrome (a rare pleural disease), and Mounier–Kuhn syndrome (a rare airway disorder). The pathogenesis, clinical presentation, diagnostic criteria, treatment options, and prognosis of each disorder is discussed. This review is by no means exhaustive and further research is needed to improve our understanding of these disorders.

Palliative Care in Chronic Obstructive Pulmonary Disease   517

Lubna Sorathia

Advanced chronic obstructive pulmonary disease (COPD), is characterized by high morbidity and mortality. Patients with COPD and their families experience a range of stresses and suffering from a variety of sources throughout the disease's progression. COPD is the fourth leading cause of death in the world. It exists as a significant contributor to global morbidity and mortality, and it results in substantial economic and social burden. This review provides some key facts regarding disease burden and encourages clinician to familiarize themselves and use both conventional and palliative approach early in the disease progression for a better quality of life.

Sarcoidosis   527

Oscar Llanos and Nabeel Hamzeh

Sarcoidosis is a multisystemic granulomatous disease that affects individuals worldwide. The lungs are most commonly involved but any organ can be involved. It has variable manifestations and clinical course. Diagnosis of sarcoidosis is based on clinicopathologic findings and the exclusion of other causes of granulomatous disease. Its hallmark is the formation of granulomas in affected organs. Immunosuppressive therapy is the cornerstone of the management of sarcoidosis and is indicated when there is evidence of symptomatic or progressive disease or when critical organs (ocular, cardiac, nervous system) are involved.

Occupational Lung Disease   535

David M. Perlman and Lisa A. Maier

Occupational exposures are a major cause of lung disease and disability worldwide. This article reviews the broad range of types of occupational lung diseases, including airways disease, pneumoconioses, and cancer. Common causes of occupational lung disease are reviewed with specific examples and clinical features. Emphasis on the importance of a detailed history to make an accurate diagnosis of an occupational lung disease is discussed.

Pulmonary Embolism   549

Eno-Obong Essien, Parth Rali, and Stephen C. Mathai

Venous thromboembolism (VTE) includes pulmonary embolism (PE) and deep vein thrombosis. PE is the third most common cause of cardiovascular death worldwide after stroke and heart attack. Management of PE has evolved recently with the availability of local thrombolysis; mechanical extraction devices; hemodynamic support devices, like extracorporeal membrane oxygenation; and surgical embolectomy. There has been development of multidisciplinary PE response teams nationwide to optimize the care of patients with VTE. This review describes the epidemiology of PE, discusses diagnostic strategies and current and emerging treatments for VTE, and considers post-PE follow-up care.

Pulmonary Function Testing and Cardiopulmonary Exercise Testing: An Overview   565

Katherine Krol, Mary Anne Morgan, and Sandhya Khurana

Respiratory symptoms are common reasons for patients to seek care and contribute significantly to use of health care resources. Identifying the underlying etiology of a respiratory symptom is key to management; yet, pinpointing the cause can be a challenge. Familiarity with the tools available to help discern between the various contributing etiologies is crucial in guiding management. Assessment and quantification of pulmonary function can provide an objective measure to guide diagnosis and therapy. We review key points of pulmonary function evaluation, highlighting indications and contraindications, fundamentals of interpretation, and the limitations of each individual component.

Pulmonary Rehabilitation in the Management of Chronic Lung Disease   577

Sharon D. Cornelison and Rodolfo M. Pascual

Pulmonary rehabilitation is a core component of management of patients with chronic lung disease that have exercise or functional limitations.

Causes of these limitations are manifold but include loss of skeletal muscle mass, power and endurance, diminished respiratory capacity owing to respiratory muscle weakness, inefficient gas exchange, and increased work of breathing, and impaired cardiovascular functioning. Besides physical limitations, patients with chronic lung disease have high rates of depression and anxiety leading to social isolation and increased health care use. Pulmonary rehabilitation uses a comprehensive and holistic approach that has been shown to ameliorate most effects of chronic lung disease.

Preoperative Pulmonary Evaluation 585

Angela Selzer and Mona Sarkiss

The preanesthesia evaluation is an opportunity to elucidate a patient's underlying medical disease, determine if the patient is optimized, treat modifiable conditions, screen for potentially unrecognized disorders, and present the clear picture of the patient's overall risk for perioperative complications. This article presents the preoperative assessment of pulmonary patients in 2 sections. First, the components of a thorough assessment of patients presenting for preanesthesia evaluation, which should occur for all patients, regardless of the presence of pulmonary pathology, are discussed. Then, the considerations unique to patients with pulmonary diseases commonly encountered are described.

Foreword
Tom Brady's Lungs

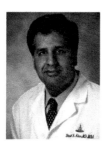

Bimal H. Ashar, MD, MBA, FACP
Consulting Editor

It's Super Bowl Sunday. I am watching the game, in awe of the athletic prowess and cardiopulmonary stamina of these men. Not only football players but all professional athletes amaze me with their ability to perform physical feats with ease and grace. Despite bursts of speed and agility, they seem to rarely be out of breath. Although some athletes (eg, Jackee Joyner-Kersee, Emmett Smith) have noted lung disease (asthma), most athletes would not be able to do what they do if they had significant pulmonary disease.

Chronic respiratory disease is the fourth leading cause of death in the United States (after heart disease, cancer, and accidents), accounting for over 150,000 deaths yearly. Over the last three and one-half decades, the mortality from respiratory disease has increased by almost 30%. This has occurred despite advances in diagnosis and treatment.

In this issue of the *Medical Clinics of North America*, Dr Musani and colleagues discuss the impact, diagnosis, and advances in treatments of pulmonary diseases, such as asthma, chronic obstructive pulmonary disease, pulmonary hypertension, and interstitial lung diseases. Utilizing the information presented will not necessarily turn our patients into Tom Brady, but it is hoped will help them breathe easier.

Bimal H. Ashar, MD, MBA, FACP
Division of General Internal Medicine
Johns Hopkins University School of Medicine
601 North Caroline Street
#7143
Baltimore, MD 21287, USA

E-mail address:
Bashar1@jhmi.edu

Med Clin N Am 103 (2019) xvii
https://doi.org/10.1016/j.mcna.2019.02.002
0025-7125/19/© 2019 Published by Elsevier Inc.

medical.theclinics.com

Preface

Pulmonary Disease

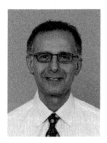

Ali I. Musani, MD, FCCP
Editor

Amazing growth is evident in a number of different areas of pulmonary medicine, including the screening, diagnosis, and staging of lung cancer and the introduction of personalized treatments for chronic obstructive pulmonary disease, pulmonary hypertension, and asthma. Advances in interventional pulmonology have contributed significantly to changes in lung cancer management. This issue brings you up to speed with concise reviews that will enhance your knowledge and allow you to better serve your patients.

I would like to express how extremely grateful I am to all of the authors who contributed to this issue of *Medical Clinics of North America* focusing on pulmonary diseases. Their altruism, dedication, and expertise are what truly allows this issue to be a succinct collection of the latest information in a rapidly changing field. Their work helps us to stay abreast of the most recent and evidence-based developments in pulmonary medicine and to be able to offer our patients the best treatments available. Subject matter experts from all over the country were invited to write articles for this issue, and you will no doubt recognize many names in the table of contents. It's been an honor to work with such a distinguished group of authors and to serve as an editor, reviewer, and contributor for this issue.

Med Clin N Am 103 (2019) xix–xx
https://doi.org/10.1016/j.mcna.2019.02.001
0025-7125/19/© 2019 Published by Elsevier Inc.

Finally, I can't thank my wife, Lubna, and our wonderful children, Sara and Sef, enough for allowing me to participate in extracurricular activities like editing this issue in addition to my very busy day job.

Ali I. Musani, MD, FCCP
Global Health
Department of Medicine
Interventional Pulmonology Program
Bronchoscopy Service
University of Colorado Hospital
Division of Pulmonary Sciences & Critical Care Medicine
University of Colorado School of Medicine
Research Complex 2
12631 E 17TH Avenue, Room # 9119
Aurora, CO 80045, USA

E-mail address:
Ali.Musani@ucdenver.edu

Interventional Pulmonology

A Focused Review for Primary Care Physicians

Christopher M. Kniese, MD*, Ali I. Musani, MD

KEYWORDS

- Interventional pulmonology • Pleural disease • Lung cancer • Bronchoscopy

KEY POINTS

- Interventional pulmonology is a fairly new field that encompasses advanced diagnostic and therapeutic bronchoscopic and pleural procedures.
- New diagnostic modalities include endobronchial ultrasonography for mediastinal staging of lung cancer and navigation bronchoscopy for diagnosis of peripheral pulmonary nodules.
- Therapeutic modalities include rigid bronchoscopy for foreign body or tumor removal, laser and other forms of thermal ablation, airway stenting for benign and malignant obstructions, and bronchial thermoplasty for severe asthma.
- Thoracentesis, indwelling pleural catheters, and medical thoracoscopy can be used for the evaluation and treatment of various pleural diseases.

INTRODUCTION

Interventional pulmonology (IP) has rapidly expanded over the past 2 decades. However, its roots go back much further in history, to the late 1800s. Many view Gustav Killian, a German otolaryngologist, as the father of bronchoscopy, a technique he pioneered when he famously removed a pork bone from the airway of a farmer using an esophagoscope in 1876[1]. This incident led to further innovations, including the development of the first rigid bronchoscopes by the American otolaryngologist Chevalier Jackson in the early twentieth century,[1] which was followed in the second half of the twentieth century by the development of the fiberoptic (flexible) bronchoscope by the famed Japanese physician Shigeto Ikeda.[1] Nowadays, IP encompasses a broad field within the larger realm of pulmonary medicine that focuses on advanced diagnostic and therapeutic modalities to manage a complex array of pulmonary conditions. Seijo and Sterman[2] aptly referred to IP as "a new field within pulmonary medicine focused on the use of advanced bronchoscopic and pleuroscopic

Disclosure: C.K. Kniese has no relevant disclosures to make.
Interventional Pulmonology, Division of Pulmonary Sciences and Critical Care Medicine, University of Colorado-Denver, University of Colorado Anschutz, 12700 East 19th Avenue, Research Complex 2, C272, Aurora, CO 80045, USA
* Corresponding author.
E-mail address: christopher.kniese@ucdenver.edu

Med Clin N Am 103 (2019) 399–412
https://doi.org/10.1016/j.mcna.2018.12.001
0025-7125/19/© 2019 Elsevier Inc. All rights reserved.

medical.theclinics.com

techniques for the treatment of a spectrum of thoracic disorders ranging from tracheo-bronchial stenosis to pleural effusions associated with malignant tumors."

Formalized training in IP took shape in the early 2000s, with a rapid growth in the number of training programs across the United States and Canada.[3] Trainees in IP have received prior training in pulmonary medicine, most commonly through American Board of Internal Medicine (ABIM)–accredited fellowships in pulmonary and critical care medicine. The IP fellowship is an additional 1 to 2 years of subspecialty training in addition to general pulmonology training. Professional guidelines outlining standards for training in interventional pulmonology were published in 2017 in a joint statement between the American College of Chest Physicians (ACCP), American Thoracic Society (ATS), American Association of Bronchology and Interventional Pulmonology (AABIP), and the Association of Interventional Pulmonology Program Directors (AAPID).[4] Likewise, as of 2016, the AABIP began offering board certification in IP for those physicians who have met established criteria based on training and procedural experience, in addition to a standardized examination.[5]

This article provides an overview of IP to guide clinicians, particularly those in primary care, on the breadth of subspecialty services that such physicians can offer. It outlines various conditions that may be addressed by interventional pulmonologists, with particular focus on the specific expertise provided by IP physicians, as well as an emphasis on recent advances in evidence-based practice.

DIAGNOSTIC BRONCHOSCOPY

Chest medicine took a giant leap forward in 1968 when the first fiberoptic broncho-scope, developed by Shigeto Ikeda, became commercially available.[1] This broncho-scope gave pulmonary physicians a new tool in the diagnosis and treatment of lung ailments and opened the door for subsequent innovations in the field. Current training in pulmonary medicine includes standard bronchoscopic procedures such as bron-choalveolar lavage, transbronchial biopsy, and endobronchial biopsies.[6] The focus here is on more advanced diagnostic modalities, including the use of endobronchial ultrasonography and newer technologies such as navigation bronchoscopy.

Flexible Bronchoscopy

Flexible bronchoscopy is considered a core procedure in training programs for pulmo-nary medicine. In recent years, there has been increased focus on improving proce-dural competency among trainees, with attempts to establish training standards that would ensure a basic level of expertise with performance of bronchoscopy.[6] Many centers now use simulation models to help achieve this goal.[7] Bronchoalveolar lavage, transbronchial biopsy, and endobronchial biopsy all remain integral proced-ures in the evaluation of lung disease. However, techniques such as blind transbron-chial needle aspiration of lymph nodes have now been largely replaced by newer, advanced diagnostic procedures that allow image guidance during biopsy.[1] As such, training programs have been forced to adapt and provide training in these newer techniques. However, as expected, there is a substantial learning curve with new tech-nologies, including endobronchial ultrasonography, and not all fellows achieve competence by the end of their fellowship training.[8] Therefore, advanced procedural training is recommended for those performing this procedure in clinical practice.

Endobronchial Ultrasonography

Endobronchial ultrasonography (EBUS) refers to a specialized bronchoscope that has a built-in ultrasonography probe to allow real-time ultrasonography imaging during bronchoscopy. EBUS has gained widespread adoption since the early 2000s, with numerous publications describing its utility in the evaluation of structures in and around the airways. One of the largest series was published in 2000 by Becker and Herth[9] from Germany, who described their experience using EBUS to evaluate centrally located lung tumors.[9,10] There are 2 commercially available EBUS designs: the radial EBUS probe, which is deployed through the working channel of a therapeutic bronchoscope and provides a 360° view of the airway and surrounding structures, and the convex EBUS probe, which is built into a specially designed bronchoscope (**Figs. 1**and **2**).[9] The first applications of EBUS were described with the radial probe, which was used to evaluate central and peripheral airway lesions.[9] Although radial EBUS provided excellent imaging of target lesions, a major limitation was that the probe had to be removed to allow tools such as aspiration needles or biopsy forceps to be deployed through the scope, thus it could not provide real-time imaging during tissue sampling.[1]

The next evolution of EBUS came with the development of the convex EBUS probe (see **Figs. 1** and **2**). This probe provides a 30° forward oblique view of the airway wall and adjacent structures, as opposed to the 360° view provided by radial EBUS. The working channel of the scope is adjacent to the ultrasonography probe, allowing transbronchial needle aspiration (TBNA) during real-time ultrasonography guidance. In the past 2 decades, EBUS has gained an integral role in the evaluation and diagnosis of mediastinal lymphadenopathy, particularly with regard to mediastinal staging of lung cancer.[11] Historically, this was accomplished via surgical mediastinoscopy. However, recent data have suggested that EBUS can provide equivalent diagnostic yield in less invasive fashion.[12] There is currently a large, prospective, multicenter trial ongoing to better compare the two.[13] There are some differences in the mediastinal lymph nodes that can be accessed via EBUS as opposed to mediastinoscopy, summarized in **Table 1**. A large systematic review pooling multiple studies concluded EBUS-guided TBNA (EBUS-TBNA) to be a safe and effective procedure, with no reported major complications.[14] Based on this, the 2013 guidelines from the ACCP recommend EBUS-TBNA as part of the initial evaluation of patients with known or suspected lung cancer.[15]

Use of EBUS has expanded rapidly in the past 2 decades. A recent survey of training programs in pulmonary and critical care medicine showed that 89% of institutions had EBUS equipment available, with more EBUS procedures performed in institutions that had specialists in IP.[16] A study assessing the learning curve of EBUS in trainees

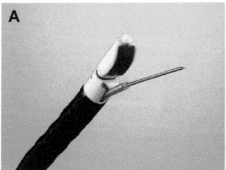
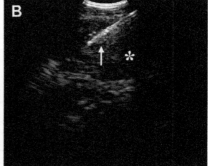

Fig. 1. Endobronchial ultrasonography. (*A*) Convex-probe endobronchial ultrasonography scope (Olympus BF-UC180F). (*B*) Real-time imaging of needle aspiration (*white arrow*) of a lymph node (*asterisk*). (*Courtesy of* [*A*] Olympus America, Inc., Center Valley, PA.)

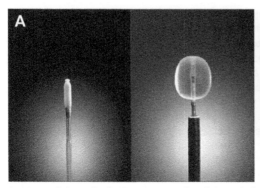
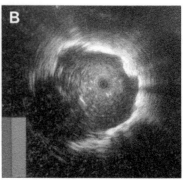

Fig. 2. Endobronchial ultrasonography. (*A*) Radial ultrasonography with balloon in the working channel of the bronchoscope, with (*B*) 360° image of airway with surrounding tumor. ([*A*] *From* Kurimoto N, Fielding D, Musani A. Endobronchial Ultrasonography. Hoboken(NJ): John Wiley & Sons; 2011. p. 36–51; with permission; and [*B*] *Courtesy of* C.M. Kniese, MD, Aurora, CO and A. Musani, MD, Aurora, CO.)

suggested that more than 200 procedures were needed to achieve expert-level proficiency.[8] In addition, data from the ACCP Quality Improvement Registry, Evaluation, and Education (AQuIRE) database, a large multicenter database tracking outcomes of EBUS, suggest that higher-volume centers have demonstrably higher diagnostic yield with this technology.[17] This finding suggests that EBUS should be performed at experienced centers with specialized training.

Navigation Bronchoscopy

The publication of the National Lung Screening Trial, which showed reduced mortality with screening for lung cancer in selected patients (aged 55–74 years, at least 30 packs per year smoking history, and quit smoking within 15 years), led to a marked increase in the use of chest computed tomography (CT) scanning and subsequently the detection of peripheral pulmonary nodules.[18,19] As such, new technologies, including navigation bronchoscopy, have emerged to allow pulmonologists to biopsy lesions that were not previously accessible via conventional flexible bronchoscopy.

Table 1
Mediastinal lymph node stations

Mode of Sampling	Stations Accessible
Mediastinoscopy	Superior mediastinal, paratracheal, subcarinal (stations 1, 2, 3, 4, and 7)
VATS	Superior mediastinal, subcarinal, para-aortic, and subaortic (stations 1, 2R, 3, 4R, 5, 6, and 7)
c-TBNA	Superior mediastinal, paratracheal, subcarinal, hilar, interlobar, lobar (stations 1, 2, 4, 7, 10, 11, and 12)
EUS-FNA	Left lower paratracheal, subaortic, subcarinal, inferior mediastinal (stations 4L, 7, 8, and 9)
EBUS-TBNA	Superior mediastinal, paratracheal, subcarinal, hilar, interlobar, lobar (stations 1, 2, 4, 7, 10, 11, and 12)

Abbreviations: c-TBNA, conventional TBNA; EUS-FNA, endoscopic ultrasonography-guided fine-needle aspiration; VATS, video-assisted thoracoscopic surgery.

Historically, these lesions were biopsied via transthoracic needle aspiration (TTNA). However, this procedure has risks, with reported rates of pneumothorax as high as 25%.[20] In this article, the term navigation bronchoscopy is used to refer to newer image-guided bronchoscopy techniques that include virtual bronchoscopy and electromagnetic navigation bronchoscopy.

Navigation bronchoscopy generally refers to techniques, including electromagnetic navigation (EMN) bronchoscopy and virtual bronchoscopy, whereby virtual mapping of the airway is created from CT imaging through the use of specialized software and a route to the target lesion is developed. Sensors placed on the patient help sync the virtual map to the patient's airway, and a specialized probe and sheath is directed to the distal airways to the target. Tools, such as needles, brushes, and biopsy forceps, are then deployed to sample the lesion. Navigation bronchoscopy, used in conjunction with radial EBUS, has shown demonstrably better diagnostic yield (80%) compared with radial EBUS and standard transbronchial biopsies alone (67%).[21] A recent meta-analysis combining all studies on navigation bronchoscopy showed a pooled diagnostic yield of 70%, which is much higher than prior studies of traditional transbronchial biopsies that reported yields ranging from 14% to 63%.[20] In addition, the rate of pneumothorax was 1.5%, much lower than that of TTNA. Thus, the most recent guidelines from ACCP regarding pulmonary nodules include the use of navigation bronchoscopy for peripheral pulmonary nodules in experienced centers.[22] As with other advanced diagnostic modalities discussed here, the use of this technology requires specialized training.

THERAPEUTIC BRONCHOSCOPY

The roots of IP go back to some of the original therapeutic applications of rigid and flexible bronchoscopy. As previously mentioned, the first reported bronchoscopy was used for removal of a foreign body, which remains a common indication for this procedure. Some of the therapeutic applications for both rigid and flexible bronchoscopy are briefly summarized here to provide readers with an understanding of common procedures in interventional pulmonology.

Rigid Bronchoscopy

Rigid bronchoscopy, unlike flexible bronchoscopy, involves the use of a rigid metal scope that is inserted directly into the airway via the oropharynx, with the scope functioning as both tool and mechanism of ventilation. Generally performed under general anesthesia, rigid bronchoscopy allows much larger working channels, as well as direct visualization of the airway, and at the same time provides a conduit for mechanical ventilation of anesthetized patients.[23] Although rigid bronchoscopy is at times used for procedures such as foreign body removal, the most common indication is central airway obstruction.[23] In this case, the rigid bronchoscope allows passage of various tools, including laser, coagulation, and cautery probes; debridement tools; and even the flexible bronchoscope.[24] In some cases, the rigid scope can be used as a coring tool to remove tumor from the airway lumen. In addition, rigid bronchoscopy is required for the placement of silicone airway stents.[23] Some of these modalities are discussed further later in this article.

Rigid bronchoscopy is not routinely taught in general pulmonary fellowship training, and thus is performed by a minority of pulmonologists in the United States.[1] However, it is considered a core skill for those training in IP, and, given its resurgence in recent years, programs have attempted to develop standardized competency-based training programs for learners to ensure baseline skill level with the procedure.[4,25]

Endobronchial Ablative Therapies

Ablative therapies generally refer to the techniques applied to relieve airway obstruction. These techniques include forms of heat and cold energy that can be applied to lesions in the airway, including malignant lesions and benign bronchial strictures. A few examples of the therapies available include electrocautery tools, which use high-frequency electric current to generate heat that is applied to the lesion; laser, which uses light to apply heat in a noncontact fashion; argon plasma coagulation, which uses concentrated gas to generate heat; and cryotherapy, which uses the cytotoxic effects of cold temperature to destroy tissue.[26] All of these therapies have been adapted into tools that be used through either the flexible bronchoscope or the rigid bronchoscope. They have applications that range from destruction of endobronchial tumors to opening of strictures caused by inflammation.[26] In addition to heat and cold energy, balloons can also be used via the bronchoscope to achieve airway dilation. There are no head-to-head trials comparing effectiveness of one modality versus the others, although there many published series of the individual tools. Thus, the choice of which modality to use for a particular situation is often left to the preference of the operator. A good summary of endobronchial ablative therapies for those interested to learn more was provided in the review by Wahidi and colleagues[27] in 2007.

Two additional techniques that deserve mention are photodynamic therapy (PDT) and brachytherapy. These techniques offer local treatment of lung cancer, particularly in patients who may not be candidates for standard therapies such as surgery, radiation, or chemotherapy. PDT is a form of nonionizing radiation that uses a photosynthesizing drug combined with light activation to produce singlet oxygen and induce cell death.[28] The patient is first administered the drug, a photosynthesizing agent, and then undergoes bronchoscopy, whereby light is applied to the lesion, causing a reaction that leads to tumor destruction. In contrast, brachytherapy refers to the localized application of radiation to endobronchial tumors, accomplished via bronchoscopy.[29] At this point, brachytherapy has largely been used in palliative fashion for patients who are not good candidates for external beam radiation. The roles of both of these modalities in the treatment of lung cancer are yet to be determined and investigations are ongoing.

Airway Stenting

As with elsewhere in this article, the topic of airway stenting has been the subject of dedicated reviews. Stents are prosthetic devices placed in the airways for conditions causing airway obstruction, both benign and malignant, and come in a variety of forms. This article focuses on 2 types of stents: silicone stents and metallic stents. J.F. Dumon revolutionized bronchoscopy with his introduction of silicone stents that could be used to hold open airways in cases of obstruction.[1] Central airway obstruction is a significant cause of morbidity and mortality in patients with advanced malignancy, particularly lung and esophageal cancers, thus stents are often considered when airway patency is reduced to 50% or less of normal area.[23] Metallic stents, covered and uncovered, can also be used for this purpose. A key difference is that metallic stents can be deployed via flexible bronchoscopy, whereas silicone stents require the use of rigid bronchoscopy.[1]

At present, metallic stents are mostly reserved for obstructions caused by malignant conditions. This trend results from metallic stents, compared with silicone stents, inducing more granulation tissue growth in the airway, which can make them harder to remove, thus they are often avoided in benign conditions, with the exception of bronchial dehiscence after lung transplant.[1] Airway stenting has been shown to be effective at palliating respiratory symptoms in patients with malignant central airway obstruction and is now often used in conjunction with other modalities, such as radiation therapy.[30] In addition, recent data have shown that airway stenting may facilitate extubation in critically ill patients who present with respiratory failure caused by malignant central airway obstruction.[31]

Although stents are sometimes used for various benign conditions, this is largely up to the discretion of the interventional pulmonologist. One unique condition is tracheobronchomalacia, a condition in which weakening of the cartilaginous structures of the airways leads to excessive dynamic airway collapse during expiration. Although alternative modalities, including continuous positive airway pressure, are often used in these patients, stents can be used as a temporizing measure to assess for improvement in dyspnea.[32] Silicone stents are predominantly used in this setting. In some centers, stenting trials are performed and, if patients achieve symptomatic improvement, they are referred for consideration of surgical therapy such as tracheoplasty.

Endoscopic Lung Volume Reduction

Surgical lung volume reduction, whereby a thoracic surgeon removes emphysematous portions of the lung to allow reexpansion of less damaged lung tissue, has been shown to improve symptoms and even mortality in selected patients with chronic obstructive pulmonary disease.[33] However, not all patients are considered surgical candidates. Therefore, in recent years there has been interest in the possibility of bronchoscopic lung volume reduction, whereby select portions of the lung are occluded with devices such as endobronchial valves that then lead to atelectasis of the target segments, and thereby achieve similar physiology effects of lung volume reduction surgery.[34] The rationale is that a minimally invasive approach may be preferred in patients with advanced lung disease. Thus far, endoscopic lung volume reduction has shown improvement in symptoms as well as health-related quality of life at 6 months in patients with heterogeneous emphysema.[34] In addition, the procedure seems to be safe. Other modalities, including endobronchial blockers, coils, and sclerosants, have been trialed, but thus far the endobronchial valves have shown the best results.[35] Long-term studies are needed to better assess the outcomes and effectiveness of this strategy, although endobronchial valves have now been granted US Food and Drug Administration approval for this indication.

Endobronchial valves have been applied in other situations as well, such as persistent air leak caused by alveolar-pleural or bronchopleural fistula (BPF).[36] Although they are now approved for use in patients with persistent air leaks after lung surgery, such as lobectomy, their effectiveness for situations such as BPF caused by spontaneous pneumothorax is still under investigation.[36]

Bronchial Thermoplasty

Bronchial thermoplasty (BT) refers to the application of thermal energy to the airway walls to reduce the mass of airway smooth muscle with the intent of improving asthma control in patients who are refractory to medical management.[37] BT is performed via sequential bronchoscopy procedures, generally spaced a 2 weeks apart. BT is first performed on the right lower lobe, then the left lower lobe, and lastly the upper lobes. The Asthma Intervention Research (AIR2) trial showed reductions in asthma exacerbations and improvements in asthma-related quality of life compared with sham bronchoscopy.[38] Follow-up data at 5 years have shown sustained reductions in asthma exacerbations and emergency room visits for respiratory symptoms.[39] However, BT has risks, with reports of respiratory complications in up to 11% of patients during the periprocedural period, including asthma exacerbations.[40] At present, BT is reserved for patients with severe asthma refractory to medical management, including those on chronic corticosteroids. Investigations are ongoing to better define the safety, efficacy, and long-term effectiveness of this procedure.

PLEURAL DISEASE

Pleural effusions affect in excess of 1.5 million people annually in the United States alone, thus they are commonly encountered, both in inpatient and outpatient visits.[41] Pleural effusions can be caused by a wide array of conditions, both benign and malignant, with common causes including congestive heart failure, liver disease, pneumonia, and malignancy.[42] Therefore, it is imperative that patients with effusions receive care from physicians who are comfortable and experienced in their evaluation and management. In recent years there have been substantial new developments regarding evidence-based practice for management of both benign and malignant pleural diseases, thus this article primarily focuses on these. Other conditions, including pneumothorax, are not discussed here given that they frequently present in emergent settings.

Thoracentesis

Thoracentesis has long been the mainstay of evaluation and treatment of pleural effusion. Chemical analysis of pleural fluid has been an essential part of the diagnostic work-up of pleural effusion for decades, and use of Richard Light's criteria for distinguishing between transudates and exudates remains ubiquitous today.[43] Recent developments in pleural disease management include the use of ultrasonography imaging to aid in the performance of thoracentesis. Bedside ultrasonography increases success rates while simultaneously reducing complications from thoracentesis, thus its use when performing the procedure is recommended by expert society guidelines.[44]

Pleural effusions are gaining increasing recognition as prognostic indicators in systemic disease. Studies have showed that both malignant and benign pleural effusions are associated with high mortality, likely because they generally develop in advanced states of disease, highlighting the need for timely diagnostic and therapeutic interventions.[45,46] Based on this need, current guidelines on the management of pleural disease from the British Thoracic Society recommend early referral to a specialist in lung disease when pleural effusion of unknown cause is encountered.[47]

Concurrent with this recognition that pleural effusions indicate significant disease processes is a notable decline in competency among medical trainees in the performance of pleural procedures. A recent survey of medical school graduates in their first year of postgraduate training sought to evaluate comfort level with the performance of various procedures deemed common in medical practice. They found that, among this population, thoracentesis was among the least-performed (and therefore lowest level of competency) procedures.[48] Furthermore, other recent studies have shown high rates of iatrogenic complications when thoracentesis was performed by nonexperienced providers compared with colleagues in radiology who routinely perform the procedure.[49] Importantly, in this same study, a standardized training intervention that included use of ultrasonography in all thoracentesis procedures led to a significant reduction in complication rates.[49]

The recent trends in subspecialization, along with declining comfort among recent medical graduates in the performance of thoracentesis, has led to a shift toward a more evidence-based procedural approach.[50] Providers performing the procedure should be comfortable and experienced with the use of lung ultrasonography. Although studies assessing ultrasonography training are heterogeneous, a structured clinical training program is likely of benefit for those aiming to gain or maintain competence in this procedure.[51] To adapt to this changing landscape in the management of pleural disease, some centers, both in the United States and abroad, have developed specialized pleural service teams who specifically focus on diagnosis and management of pleural disease.[52]

Indwelling Pleural Catheters

Indwelling pleural catheters (IPCs) are small, flexible catheters designed for tunneled insertion into the pleural space to allow drainage of recurrent pleural effusions. They were originally designed for use in patients with malignant pleural effusions (MPEs) who were not candidates for alternative treatment modalities such as surgery or pleurodesis.[53,54] However, their use has become much more widespread in recent years after studies showed symptomatic improvement, low complication rates, and decreased length of hospital stay in patients with MPE.[55,56] IPCs are frequently placed by interventional pulmonologists, often in an outpatient setting using light to moderate sedation or simply local anesthetic. Once placed, the IPC allows the patient to drain the effusion at home using specially designed drainage kits on an as-needed basis. In addition, recent data suggest that more aggressive drainage strategies may yield higher rates of pleurodesis in patients with malignant effusions.[57] In addition, the combination of IPCs with other means of pleurodesis, such as talc, is an area of great interest in current medical literature.[58,59]

Recent attention has been placed on using IPCs for nonmalignant pleural effusions that have proven refractory to medical management,[60] including effusions caused by congestive heart failure, chronic kidney disease, and hepatic hydrothorax.[61–63] Although using IPCs for these indications is largely experimental, it is becoming increasingly common, particularly as evidence mounts that some patients achieve spontaneous pleurodesis simply by having the IPC in place for a period of time, without requiring further therapeutic interventions.[60] **Table 2** provides a concise listing of pleural conditions that have reported favorable outcomes with IPCs in the literature.

Complicated Pleural Effusion/Empyema

Tube thoracostomy (ie, chest tube drainage) and antibiotics remain the mainstays of treatment of complicated parapneumonic effusions and empyema.[46] Historically, surgical decortication was performed in patients with severe disease or those who failed medical management. However, one of the major breakthroughs in pleural disease came with the publication of the Second Multicenter Intrapleural Sepsis (MIST II) trial in 2011, which outlined the use of intrapleural fibrinolytic therapy in patients with pleural infection.[64] Although there were prior reports of using intrapleural fibrinolytic therapies such as streptokinase, this trial, which used tissue plasminogen activate and dornase alfa, was the first randomized controlled trial that showed significant reductions in hospital stay and need for surgery. Note that only the combination of the 2 agents showed benefit, whereas neither agent alone did. Coupled with more recent trends in the use of smaller-bore chest tubes, this has led to an increased role for IP physicians in the management of pleural space infections. Compared with large-bore, surgically placed chest tubes, these smaller percutaneously placed tubes offer similar rates of successful drainage, with less patient discomfort.[65] Surgical therapy remains the definitive treatment of those failing medical management.

Table 2 Indications for indwelling pleural catheters	
Cause of Effusion	**Indwelling Pleural Catheter**
Benign	
CHF	Yes
Hepatic hydrothorax	Yes
Chronic kidney disease	Unclear
Parapneumonic/empyema	Unclear
Malignant	
Lung primary	Yes
Metastatic disease	Yes
Mesothelioma	Yes
Trapped/entrapped lung[a]	Yes

Abbreviation: CHF, congestive heart failure
[a] Can be either benign or malignant.

Pleuroscopy/Medical Thoracoscopy

Medical thoracoscopy, also termed pleuroscopy, is a procedure in which a rigid or semirigid scope is inserted through a small incision in the posterior or lateral chest wall for diagnostic or therapeutic purposes.[66] Unlike video-assisted thoracoscopic surgery (VATS), which is performed by thoracic surgeons under general anesthesia, pleuroscopy is less invasive and can often be performed in an ambulatory setting under local anesthesia with or without moderate sedation by trained interventional pulmonologists.[66] The most common indication for medical thoracoscopy is in the evaluation of an exudative effusion of unclear cause.[67] In this case, thoracoscopy is used to aid in biopsy of the parietal pleural, which can provide valuable diagnostic information that cannot be obtained solely from pleural fluid analysis. Compared with closed pleural biopsy, which has fallen out of favor among practicing pulmonologists in recent years, medical thoracoscopy shows improved yield with comparable complication rates.[66] A recent survey of interventional pulmonologists across the United States revealed this to be the procedure of choice in such patients.[67] In some cases, providers choose to place IPCs at the time of pleuroscopy to allow continued drainage as the underlying condition is addressed.

An additional application of pleuroscopy is to aid in pleurodesis. In many cases, surgical pleurodesis remains the best choice for patients. However, in patients who are not surgical candidates, pleuroscopy may be considered. Practices in pleurodesis vary widely among providers,[68] but pleurodesis remains a common indication for the procedure. Medical thoracoscopy combined with instillation of talc poudrage likely confers benefit compared with talc slurry administration via chest tube.[66,69] However, in patients who are surgical candidates, pleuroscopy has not been proved superior to VATS.

SUMMARY

IP is a broad field that encompasses advanced diagnostic and therapeutic modalities that can be applied to a wide array of conditions affecting the lung. The recent advents of board certification and standardized fellowship training have helped to advance the field. Ongoing technological breakthroughs continue to advance the field, and in many ways interventional pulmonologists are on the cutting edge of medical technology. IP physicians are thus well suited to address a variety of pathologic conditions, both benign and malignant. As more prospective, multicenter trials emerge, further breakthroughs in evidence-based management are expected.

REFERENCES

1. Panchabhai TS, Mehta AC. Historical perspectives of bronchoscopy. Connecting the dots. Ann Am Thorac Soc 2015;12(5):631–41.
2. Seijo LM, Sterman DH. Interventional pulmonology. N Engl J Med 2001;344:740–9.
3. Bolliger CT, Mathur PN, Beamis JF, et al. ERS/ATS statement on interventional pulmonology. Eur Respir J 2002;19:356–73.
4. Mullon JJ, Burkart KM, Silvestri G, et al. Interventional pulmonology fellowship accreditation standards: executive summary of the Multisociety Interventional Pulmonology Fellowship Accreditation Committee. Chest 2017;151(5):1114–21.
5. American Association of Bronchology and Interventional Pulmonology. Board certification. 2017. Available at: https://aabronchology.org/board-certification/. Accessed September 21, 2018.
6. Ernst A, Wahidi MM, Read CA, et al. Adult bronchoscopy training. current state and suggestions for the future: CHEST expert panel report. Chest 2015;148(2):321–32.
7. Fielding DI, Maldonado F, Murgu S. Achieving competency in bronchoscopy: challenges and opportunities. Respirology 2014;19(4):471–82.
8. Stather DR, Chee A, MacEachem P, et al. Endobronchial ultrasound learning curve in interventional pulmonary fellows. Respirology 2015;20(2):333–9.
9. Becker HD, Herth F. Endobronchial ultrasound of the airways and the mediastinum. In: Bolliger CT, Mathur PN, editors. Progress in respiratory research, vol. 30. Basel-Freiburg (France): Interventional Bronchoscopy. S. Karger; 2000. p. 80–93.
10. Figueiredo VR, Jacomelli M, Rodrigues AJ, et al. Current status and clinical applicability of endobronchial ultrasound-guided transbronchial needle aspiration. J Bras Pneumol 2013;39:226–37.
11. Kinsey CM, Arenberg DA. Endobronchial ultrasound-guided transbronchial needle aspiration for non-small cell lung cancer staging. Am J Respir Crit Care Med 2014;189(6):640–9.
12. Um SW, Kim HK, Jung SH, et al. Endobronchial ultrasound versus mediastinoscopy for mediastinal nodal staging of non-small cell lung cancer. J Thorac Oncol 2015;10:331–7.
13. Bousema JE, Dijkgraaf MGW, Papen-Botterhuis NE, et al. MEDIASTinal staging of non-small cell lung cancer by endobronchial and endoscopic ultrasonography with or without additional surgical mediastinoscopy (MEDIASTrial): study protocol of a multicenter randomised controlled trial. BMC Surg 2018;18(1):27.
14. Varela-Lema L, Fernandez-Villar A, Ruano-Ravina A. Effectiveness and safety of endobronchial ultrasound-guided transbronchial needle aspiration: a systematic review. Eur Respir J 2009;33:1156–64.
15. Detterbeck FC, Lewis SZ, Diekemper R, et al. Executive summary: diagnosis and management of lung cancer, 3rd ed: American College of Chest Physicians Evidence-Based Clinical Practice Guidelines. Chest 2013;143(5 Suppl):7S–37S.
16. Tanner NT, Pastis NJ, Silvestri G. Training for linear endobronchial ultrasound among us pulmonary/critical care fellowships: a survey of fellowship directors. Chest 2013;143(2):423–8.

17. Ost DE, Ernst A, Lei X, et al. Diagnostic yield of endobronchial ultrasound-guided transbronchial needle aspiration: results of the AQuIRE bronchoscopy registry. Chest 2011;140(6):1557–66.
18. Aberle DR, Adams AM, Berg CD, et al. Reduced lung-cancer mortality with low-dose computed tomographic screening. N Engl J Med 2011;365:395–409.
19. Spira A, Halmos B, Powell CA. Update in lung cancer 2015. Am J Respir Crit Care Med 2016;194(6):661–71.
20. Wang Memoli JS, Nietert PJ, Silvestri GA. Meta-analysis of guided bronchoscopy for the evaluation of the pulmonary nodule. Chest 2012;142(2):385–93.
21. Ishida T, Asano F, Yamazaki K, et al. Virtual bronchoscopic navigation combined with endobronchial ultrasound to diagnose small peripheral pulmonary lesions: a randomised trial. Thorax 2011;66(12):1072–7.
22. Gould MK, Donington J, Lynch WR, et al. Evaluation of individuals with pulmonary nodules: when is it lung cancer? Diagnosis and management of lung cancer, 3rd ed: American College of Chest Physicians Evidence-Based Clinical Practice Guidelines. Chest 2013;143(5 Suppl):e93S–120S.
23. Semaan R, Yarmus L. Rigid bronchoscopy and silicone stents in the management of central airway obstruction. J Thorac Dis 2015;7(S4):S352–62.
24. Ost DE, Sterman DH. Interventional bronchoscopy in 2015: removing endoluminal and methodological obstructions. Ann Am Thorac Soc 2015;12(9):1265–6.
25. Mahmood K, Wahidi MM, Osann KE, et al. Development of a tool to assess basic competency in the performance of rigid bronchoscopy. Ann Am Thorac Soc 2016;13(4):502–11.
26. Sachdeva A, Pickering EM, Lee HJ. From electrocautery, balloon dilation, neodymium-doped:yttrium-aluminum-garnet (Nd:YAG) laser to argon plasma coagulation and cryotherapy. J Thorac Dis 2015;7(S4):S363–79.
27. Wahidi MM, Herth FJF, Ernst A. State of the art: interventional pulmonology. Chest 2007;131:261–74.
28. Simone CB, Cengel KA. Photodynamic therapy for lung cancer and malignant pleural mesothelioma. Semin Oncol 2014;41(6):820–30.
29. Youroukou A, Gkiozos I, Kalaitzi Z, et al. The potential role of brachytherapy in the irradiation of patients with lung cancer: a systematic review. Clin Transl Oncol 2017;19(8):945–50.
30. Razi SS, Lebovics RS, Schwartz G, et al. Timely airway stenting improves survival in patients with malignant central airway obstruction. Ann Thorac Surg 2010;90:1088–93.
31. Oki M, Saka H, Hori K. Airway stenting in patients requiring intubation due to malignant airway stenosis: a 10-year experience. J Thorac Dis 2017;9(9):3154–60.
32. Murgu SD. Pneumatic stenting for tracheobronchomalacia. J Bronchology Interv Pulmonol 2014;21(2):109–12.
33. Gordon M, Duffy S, Criner GJ. Lung volume reduction surgery or bronchoscopic lung volume reduction: is there an algorithm for allocation? J Thorac Dis 2018;10(Suppl 23):S2816–23.
34. Sterman DH, Mehta AC, Wood DE, et al. A multicenter pilot study of a bronchial valve for the treatment of severe emphysema. Respiration 2010;79:222–3.
35. Zhang JJ, Yin Y, Hou G. The bronchoscopic interventions for chronic obstructive pulmonary disease according to different phenotypes. J Thorac Dis 2017;9(5):1361–5.
36. Dugan KC, Laxmana B, Murgu S, et al. Management of persistent air leaks. Chest 2017;152(2):417–23.

37. Cox PG, Miller J, Mitzner W, et al. Radiofrequency ablation of airway smooth muscle for sustained treatment of asthma: preliminary investigations. Eur Respir J 2004;24:659–63.
38. Castro M, Rubin AS, Laviolette M, et al. Effectiveness and safety of bronchial thermoplasty in the treatment of severe asthma: a multicenter, randomized, double-blind, sham-controlled clinical trial. Am J Respir Crit Care Med 2010;181:116–24.
39. Wechsler ME, Laviolette M, Rubin AS, et al. Bronchial thermoplasty – long term safety and effectiveness in severe persistent asthma. J Allergy Clin Immunol 2013;132(6):1295–302.
40. Burn J, Sims AJ, Keltie K, et al. Procedural and short-term safety of bronchial thermoplasty in clinical practice: evidence from a national registry and hospital episode statistics. J Asthma 2017;54(8):872–9.
41. Light RW. Pleural effusions. Med Clin North Am 2011;95:1055–107.
42. Kinasewitz GT. Transudative effusions. Eur Respir J 1997;10:714–8.
43. Light RW, Macgregor MI, Luchsinger PC, et al. Pleural effusions: the diagnostic separation of transudates and exudates. Ann Intern Med 1972;77:507–13.
44. Havelock T, Teoh R, Laws D, et al. Pleural procedures and thoracic ultrasound: British Thoracic Society Pleural Disease Guideline 2010. Thorax 2010;65(Suppl 2):ii61–76.
45. DeBiasi E, Puchalski J. Pleural effusions as markers of mortality and disease severity: a state-of-the-art review. Curr Opin Pulm Med 2016;22:386–91.
46. Feller-Kopman D, Light R. Pleural disease. N Engl J Med 2018;378:740–51.
47. Hooper C, Lee YC, Maskell N. Investigation of a unilateral pleural effusion in adults: British Thoracic Society Pleural Disease Guideline 2010. Thorax 2010; 65(Suppl 2):ii4–17.
48. Promes SB, Chudgar SM, Grochowski CO, et al. Gaps in procedural experience and competency in medical school graduates. Acad Emerg Med 2009;16(Suppl 2):S58–62.
49. Duncan DR, Morgenthaler TI, Ryu JH, et al. Reducing iatrogenic risk in thoracentesis: establishing best practice via experiential training in a zero-risk environment. Chest 2009;135:1315–20.
50. Schildhouse R, Lai A, Barsuk JH, et al. Safe and effective bedside thoracentesis: a review of the evidence for practicing clinicians. J Hosp Med 2017;12:266–76.
51. Pietersen PI, Madsen KR, Graumann O, et al. Lung ultrasound training: a systematic review of published literature in clinical lung ultrasound training. Crit Ultrasound J 2018;10:23.
52. Evison M, Blyth KG, Bhatnagar R, et al. Providing safe and effective pleural medicine services in the UK: an aspirational statement from UK pleural physicians. BMJ Open Respir Res 2018;5:e000307.
53. Spector M, Pollak JS. Management of malignant pleural effusions. Semin Respir Crit Care Med 2008;29:405–13.
54. Gompelmann D, Eberhardt R, Herth FJ. Advanced malignant lung disease: what the specialist can offer. Respiration 2011;82:111–23.
55. Tremblay A, Michaud G. Single-center experience with 250 tunnelled pleural catheter insertions for malignant pleural effusion. Chest 2006;129:362–8.
56. Suzuki K, Servais EL, Rizk NP, et al. Palliation and pleurodesis in malignant pleural effusion: the role for tunneled pleural catheters. J Thorac Oncol 2011;6: 762–7.
57. Wahidi MM, Reddy C, Yarmus L, et al. Randomized trial of pleural fluid drainage frequency in patients with malignant pleural effusions. The ASAP trial. Am J Respir Crit Care Med 2017;195:1050–7.

58. Thomas R, Fysh ETH, Smith NA, et al. Effect of an indwelling pleural catheter vs talc pleurodesis on hospitalization days in patients with malignant pleural effusion: the AMPLE randomized clinical trial. JAMA 2017;318:1903–12.

59. Bhatnagar R, Keenan EK, Morley AJ, et al. Outpatient talc administration by indwelling pleural catheter for malignant effusion. N Engl J Med 2018;378: 1313–22.

60. Patil M, Dhillon SS, Attwood K, et al. Management of benign pleural effusions using indwelling pleural catheters: a systematic review and meta-analysis. Chest 2017;151(3):626–35.

61. Chen A, Massoni J, Jung D, et al. Indwelling tunneled pleural catheters for the management of hepatic hydrothorax. A pilot study. Ann Am Thorac Soc 2016; 13:862–6.

62. Kniese C, Diab K, Ghabril M, et al. Indwelling pleural catheters in hepatic hydrothorax: a single-center series of outcomes and complications. Chest 2018; S0012-3692(18):31053–5.

63. Shojaee S, Rahman N, Haas K, et al. Indwelling tunneled pleural catheters for refractory hepatic hydrothorax in patients with cirrhosis: a multicenter study. Chest 2018. https://doi.org/10.1016/j.chest.2018.08.1034.

64. Rahman NM, Maskell NA, West A, et al. Intrapleural use of tissue plasminogen activator and DNase in pleural infection. N Engl J Med 2011;365:518–26.

65. Light RW. Pleural controversy: optimal chest tube size for drainage. Respirology 2011;16:244–8.

66. Murthy V, Bessich JL. Medical thoracoscopy and its evolving role in the diagnosis and treatment of pleural disease. J Thorac Dis 2017;9:S1011–21.

67. Raman T, McClelland S, Bartter T, et al. Current practice in management of exudative pleural effusions–a survey of American Association of Bronchology and Interventional Pulmonology (AABIP). J Thorac Dis 2018;10:3874–8.

68. Lee YC, Baumann MH, Maskell NA, et al. Pleurodesis practice for malignant pleural effusions in five English-speaking countries: survey of pulmonologists. Chest 2003;124:2229–38.

69. Lee P, Mathur PN, Colt HG. Advances in thoracoscopy: 100 years since Jacobaeus. Respiration 2010;79:177–86.

Pulmonary Hypertension

Darlene Kim, MD, M. Patricia George, MD*

KEYWORDS

- Pulmonary hypertension • Pulmonary arterial hypertension • Clinical presentation
- Diagnostic algorithm • Treatment

KEY POINTS

- Pulmonary hypertension (PH) is a chronic and progressive disease that often goes misdiagnosed for years.
- Early diagnosis and treatment of PH is critical to ensure optimal outcomes.
- Referral to a PH specialist should be considered when a patient presents with signs and symptoms of PH and echocardiographic evidence of PH and/or right ventricular dysfunction.

Pulmonary hypertension (PH) is a chronic and progressive disease that presents like many other lung diseases, often leading to a delay in diagnosis, and therefore a delay in optimal therapy.[1–5] This article provides a review of PH for internists, covering clinical presentation, diagnostic algorithm, different types of PH, and overview of treatments. In addition, it emphasizes the importance of early referral to, and partnership between, PH specialists and physicians on the front lines to improve early diagnosis and optimize management of these complex patients.

DEFINITIONS

At the Sixth World Symposium on Pulmonary Hypertension a change to this definition was recently proposed, with a mean pulmonary artery pressure of greater than 20 mm Hg.[1] Increased pulmonary pressures overwork the right heart and lead to progressive right heart dysfunction, the major cause of morbidity and mortality in this population. PH is organized into 5 broad categories roughly based on pathophysiology and thus common treatment pathways, called World Health Organization (WHO) groups (**Box 1**). Pulmonary arterial hypertension (PAH) is a term that specifically refers to WHO group 1.

Disclosure: M.P. George has served in an advisory and/or speaking role for Actelion, Gilead, and Bayer. The author has research projects that are supported by an Actelion investigator-initiated grant.
Department of Medicine, National Jewish Health, 1400 Jackson Street, Denver CO 80206, USA
* Corresponding author. Department of Medicine, National Jewish Health, 1400 Jackson Street, J231, Denver CO 80206.
E-mail address: georgem@njhealth.org

Med Clin N Am 103 (2019) 413–423
https://doi.org/10.1016/j.mcna.2018.12.002
0025-7125/19/© 2019 Elsevier Inc. All rights reserved.

Box 1
World Health Organization clinical classification of pulmonary hypertension

WHO group 1: PAH
  Idiopathic PAH
  Heritable PAH (BMPR2, ALK1)
  Drug and toxin induced
  Associated with:
    Connective tissue disease
    Congenital heart disease
    Portal hypertension
    Human immunodeficiency virus infection
    Schistosomiasis

WHO group 1: pulmonary veno-occlusive disease/pulmonary capillary hemangiomatosis

WHO group 2: PH caused by/because of left heart disease
  Heart failure with reduced ejection fraction
  Heart failure with preserved ejection fraction
  Valvular heart disease

WHO group 3: PH caused by lung diseases/hypoxemia
  Chronic obstructive pulmonary disease
  Interstitial lung disease
  Sleep disordered breathing
  Developmental abnormalities

WHO group 4: chronic thromboembolic pulmonary hypertension

WHO group 5: PH of miscellaneous or uncertain causes
  PH with unclear multifactorial mechanisms
  Hematologic disorders: myeloproliferative disorders, splenectomy
  Systemic disorders: sarcoidosis, pulmonary Langerhans cell histiocytosis,
  lymphangioleiomyomatosis, neurofibromatosis, vasculitis
  Metabolic disorders: glycogen storage disease, Gaucher disease, thyroid disorders
  Others: tumoral obstruction, fibrosing mediastinitis, chronic renal failure on dialysis with
  arteriovenous fistula

Fifth World Symposium on Pulmonary Hypertension, Nice, France, 2013.

Abbreviation: BMPR2, Bone Morphogenetic Protein Receptor Type 2.
  Adapted from Simonneau G, Gatzoulis MA, Adatia I, et al. Updated clinical classification of pulmonary hypertension. J Am Coll Cardiol 2013;62(25 Suppl):D36; with permission.

WHO group 1 PH encompasses multiple disease processes that share a similar common final histopathology, with proliferative vasculopathy and unfavorable remodeling in the distal pulmonary arterial bed.[6] It is a rare disease, affecting approximately 15 people per million. Because early symptoms can mirror symptoms seen in other respiratory conditions, it often goes misdiagnosed for several years.[2,3] Misdiagnosis has serious consequences, because the median survival in patients with PAH without therapy is approximately 2.8 years.[4] The most common form of PAH is idiopathic PAH, followed by connective tissue disease–associated PAH.[7] Patients with certain predisposing conditions are at higher risk for developing PAH.[3,8] The prevalence of PAH in patients with systemic sclerosis ranges from 5% to 18% of patients without interstitial lung disease (ILD), and even higher in those with ILD.[9,10] One in 200 patients with human immunodeficiency virus (HIV) develop PAH, even in the era of highly active antiretroviral therapy.[11] The recent methamphetamine epidemic has also been associated with increased PAH, although the exact prevalence among methamphetamine users is unknown.[12] The remaining WHO groups 2 to 5 are referred to as PH and refer to PH associated with left heart disease (LHD), chronic lung disease or hypoxia, chronic thromboembolic disease, and miscellaneous systemic or multifactorial disorders (see **Box 1**).

Outcomes in PAH depend on severity of disease at time of diagnosis, and response to treatment. With modern medical therapy, outcomes have improved dramatically. Data from the REVEAL Registry (Registry to Evaluate Early and Long-term PAH Disease Management) between 2006 and 2009 reported a 1-year survival rate of 86.3% and 5-year survival of 61% for newly diagnosed patients. The Pulmonary Hypertension Connection registry confirmed similar survival rates of 86% at 1 year and 61% at 5 years.[13,14] Of note, these data predate our 3 most recent landmark, event-driven trials, which showed significant advantages in combination therapy since being adopted in clinical practice, so the survival rates may now be better.[15–17] Progress made in the last 20 years in medical therapies has greatly improved outcomes in PAH. However, early diagnosis and early referral to a PH specialist are critical to enable the greatest chance at clinical improvement and survival (**Box 2**).

In the past, a dichotomous distinction between pulmonary arterial versus pulmonary venous disease has been made. They have also been called precapillary and postcapillary disease and is defined hemodynamically as having a pulmonary capillary wedge pressure as greater than 15 mm Hg. WHO group 2, or LHD-PH has been known as postcapillary PH, and WHO groups 1, 3, 4, and 5 are largely recognized as precapillary, defined as a pulmonary capillary wedge pressure of 15 mm Hg or less. However, there is increasing recognition based on histopathologic data that considerable overlap within pulmonary vascular disease exists, and that pulmonary arterial and pulmonary venous disorders may coexist to varying degrees.[18] Although the predominant characterization may be principally pulmonary arterial (as in idiopathic PAH), or pulmonary venous (as in WHO group 2), almost all forms of PH may involve both arterial and venous pathologic remodeling, contributing with varying weights to the end result of an increase in pulmonary vascular pressures.[18] Not only does overlap exist but patients may also migrate across the spectrum and between categories, unmasking diastolic dysfunction or arterial vascular remodeling.

PRESENTATION

The principal presenting symptom of PH is dyspnea on exertion. Often progressive, it is sometimes accompanied by fatigue and symptoms of venous congestion (ie, peripheral edema or ascites). In severe cases, exertional syncope is a particularly ominous clinical presentation, the result of inadequate cardiac output from right heart failure. Physical examination may reveal distended neck veins or pitting lower extremity edema, a prominent pulmonic component of the second heart sound (P2), and a murmur consistent with tricuspid insufficiency, or less frequently a right-sided S3 or right ventricular heave. Exertional or nocturnal hypoxia may also be present, and note that often only resting pulse oximetry is routinely measured.

Box 2
When to consult a PH specialist

- Signs or symptoms consistent with PH
- Echocardiographic findings concerning for PH (RVSP >/= 40 mm Hg and/or signs of right ventricular dysfunction

Diagnostic Algorithm

When patients present with signs or symptoms concerning for PH, the guidelines recommend a screening echocardiogram. The echocardiogram is critical in cases in which a diagnosis of PH is suspected, because an estimation of right ventricular systolic pressure (RVSP), and thereby the pulmonary artery systolic pressure (PASP), may be obtained. When the image quality is adequate and this measure is performed with appropriate expertise, increased RVSP is associated with high sensitivity and specificity for detecting PH.[19,20] However, the echo estimation can both overestimate and underestimate the actual PASP, especially if a patient has underlying lung disease, and so should be interpreted in context.[21,22] Many centers regard an RVSP or PASP of greater than 40 mm Hg as a threshold for concern. Findings of right ventricular (RV) enlargement, interventricular septal flattening consistent with RV volume or pressure overload, and certain RV outflow tract Doppler patterns are also worrisome for PH. As such, these abnormal findings should not be dismissed if a high estimated PASP is absent. In addition, an increased PASP in the presence of echocardiographic findings of left ventricular (LV) abnormalities (eg, reduced LV ejection fraction, diastolic dysfunction, LV hypertrophy, left atrial enlargement, mitral or aortic valve disease) may indicate possible PH caused by LHD.[20] If echocardiographic probability of PH is assessed as high or intermediate, further evaluation is recommended.[23]

The next steps should be to evaluate for underlying heart or lung diseases.[22] If a diagnosis of heart or lung disease is made with no signs of severe PH or RV dysfunction, then it is recommended to treat the underlying heart or lung disease. The authors recommend a follow-up echocardiographic assessment after initiating therapy as well. However, if there is no significant underlying for the patient's heart or lung disease, or if there are signs of severe PH and/or RV dysfunction on echocardiogram, we recommend patient referral to a PH expert for definitive diagnosis and treatment.[24]

At present, a diagnosis of PH is only accepted as confirmed (or excluded) by right heart catheterization (RHC). PH is defined as a mean PAP greater than or equal to 20 mm Hg at rest. PAH is defined as precapillary PH with mean PAP greater than or equal to 20 mm Hg, pulmonary artery wedge pressure (PAWP) less than or equal to 15 mm Hg, and pulmonary vascular resistance (PVR) greater than 3 Wood units.[1]

RHC is a low-risk outpatient procedure that, when performed at expert centers, has a mortality of less than 0.1%.[18] Given that the diagnosis of PH is determined by the hemodynamic measurements obtained during RHC, the quality and accuracy of the measurements are of utmost importance. Once a diagnosis of PH is confirmed on RHC, and PAH is suspected based on cardiac and pulmonary evaluation, a PH expert will evaluate for cause of PAH: connective tissue disease, HIV, liver disease, and use of illicit drugs. A ventilation/perfusion (V/Q) scan is also critical to screen for chronic thromboembolic disease.[23]

WORLD HEALTH ORGANIZATION GROUPS 2 TO 5
WHO Group 2: Pulmonary Hypertension Caused by Left Heart Disease

PH-LHD is an increase in pulmonary pressures caused by passive congestion from pulmonary venous hypertension, or postcapillary PH, as shown by an increased mean PAP greater than or equal to 25 mm Hg with a PAWP greater than 15 mm Hg. These patients include patients with heart failure with reduced ejection fraction (HFrEF) or heart failure with preserved ejection fraction (HFpEF), and valvular disease. The increased pressures arise from LV dysfunction and left atrial stiffness.[25] There is a subset of patients who have combined postcapillary and precapillary PH, and this phenotype has been associated with poorer prognosis.[26] Patients with WHO group 2 PH, compared with patients with PAH, tend to be older, female, and have systemic hypertension and features of metabolic syndrome.[13,27,28]

Treatment of WHO group 2 PH is targeted at treating the underlying left-sided heart disease: HFrEF, HFpEF, and valvular disease. Optimal medical therapy for systolic dysfunction, ischemia, hypertension, atrial fibrillation, and metabolic syndrome are key. Diuretics are often a mainstay of treatment. There are no recommendations currently for the use of pulmonary vasodilator therapy because of inadequate evidence that pulmonary vasodilator therapy is beneficial in HFpEF, and it may possibly be harmful.[14]

World Health Organization Group 3: Pulmonary Hypertension Associated with Underlying Lung Disease, Hypoxemia, or Sleep Disordered Breathing

WHO group 3 PH is defined as precapillary PH with underlying chronic lung disease, hypoxemia, and/or sleep disordered breathing. Mild PH in the setting of lung disease is common; however, severe PH (mean PAP $\geq$35 mm Hg) is variable.

In patients with chronic obstructive pulmonary disease (COPD), PH is more commonly found in severe disease. In patients with Global Initiative for Chronic Obstructive Lung Disease (GOLD) stage 4 COPD, approximately 90% of patients have mild to moderate PH, but only 3% to 5% have severe PH.[29–31] COPD with PH is associated with decreased survival.[29,32,33] Most patients with idiopathic pulmonary fibrosis (IPF) develop PH at some point; however, in most cases it is mild. Unlike COPD, the degree of PH is not strongly associated with the degree of disease severity by restrictive physiology.[34] However, like COPD, even mild PH in IPF is associated with worse outcomes.

Current guidelines recommend treating the underlying lung disease and against treatment of WHO group 3 PH with pulmonary vasodilator therapy because of inadequate evidence and concern for possible harm from vasodilator therapies in IPF.[35,36] However, because of the worse prognosis associated with PH in patients with lung disease, there is active ongoing interest in looking for effective therapies in these diseases. In patients with lung disease and findings suspicious for severe PH, the authors recommend referral to a PH specialist for further diagnostic evaluation.

Sleep disordered breathing is also associated with PH and is a common comorbidity of restrictive lung disease and LV diastolic dysfunction. Approximately 30% of patients with obstructive sleep apnea without other lung disease or LV diastolic dysfunction have PH.[37]

World Health Organization Group 4: Chronic Thromboembolic Pulmonary Hypertension

Chronic thromboembolic pulmonary hypertension (CTEPH) is a disease of pulmonary artery obstruction from pulmonary emboli (PEs) that have remodeled rather than resolved after acute PE.[38] CTEPH has been reported to occur in between 0.1% and 9.1% of patients within 2 years after an acute PH.[23] Pengo and colleagues[39] reported that 3.8% of patients treated for symptomatic PE went on to develop CTEPH. Patients with PAH may also be found to have CTEPH despite no known history of symptomatic PE, and, because treatment of CTEPH targets removal or surgical decrease in the chronic thromboembolic burden with pulmonary thromboendarterectomy or balloon pulmonary angioplasty, screening for CTEPH is recommended in every patient with PH using a V/Q scan.[40]

World Health Organization Group 5: Pulmonary Hypertension Caused by Unclear or Multifactorial Mechanisms

WHO group 5 PH is a category of diseases in which the exact mechanism of disease is not known, and therefore optimal treatment is unclear. This category includes sarcoidosis, sickle cell disease, and rare lung diseases. There are no randomized controlled trials to guide treatment in these disorders, therefore treatment of the underlying lung disease is emphasized.[35]

TREATMENT IN PULMONARY ARTERIAL HYPERTENSION
Risk Assessment

Newer treatment options and changes in treatment strategies have made a significant impact on outcomes, leading to the adjustment of guidelines to incorporate more aggressive, upfront oral combination therapy. The focus has also shifted to the concept of goal-directed therapy based on risk stratification. There are 2 commonly implemented risk stratification systems.

The most recent consensus-based guidelines advocate assessing several criteria that have been identified by experts as important in predicting survival.[23] Guidelines support the use of initial and serial risk assessments with treatments designed to shift patients to as many of the low-risk criteria as possible to improve survival, and the number of low-risk factors has been found to be predictive of improved 1-year and 5-year survival.[41–43]

Another risk stratification method was developed in the United States through data from the REVEAL cohort, which was a predictive formula derived from risk factors identified though statistical analysis, and has been validated in multiple studies (Table 1).[44,45] Improvement in serial assessments of the REVEAL score was also associated with improved 1-year survival.[46]

Medical therapies

There are now 14 US Food and Drug Administration–approved medications for PAH that exploit 3 key vasodilatory pathways and are available in oral, inhaled, intravenous (IV), and subcutaneous (SC) forms (Table 2). Determining which initial treatment should be chosen for each patient is largely based on functional class (Table 3) and risk assessment at presentation, as per guidelines. In patients who are WHO functional class IV, IV epoprostenol is recommended.[23] Epoprostenol is the only medication that has been shown to improve mortality in PH in randomized placebo-controlled trials.[47,48] In patients who are WHO functional class II or III, there are a variety of treatment options. In general, based on recent evidence, many PH physicians are using more aggressive treatment strategies, with combined treatment strategies targeting 2 or even 3 pathways, early in the treatment of disease.[15–17] Because of the rapidly evolving therapeutic strategies, complexity of medications, and need to manage their side effects, it is crucial that patients are treated by a PH specialist.[23]

Once initiated on PH-specific medications, it is imperative that patients continue these medications. Patients should not have their vasodilator medications altered without the directive of their PH specialist. Abrupt discontinuation of medications (especially continuous infusion medications) can be life threatening because of rebound PH. If IV access is lost, the medication may be given through a peripheral IV and this must be done immediately. Because oral medications have become more potent as well, discontinuation will likewise be uncomfortable for the patient.

Table 1 REVEAL risk calculator		
	Risk Factors	
WHO Group I Subgroup	APAH-CTD +1	APAH-PoPH +2
Demographics and Comorbidities	Renal insufficiency +1	Male age >60 y +2
NYHA/WHO Functional Class	I −2	III +1
Vital Signs	SBP <110 mm Hg +1	HR >92 mm Hg +1
6-Minute Walk Test	≥440 m −1	<165 m +1
BNP	<50 pg/mL −2	>180 pg/mL +1
Echocardiogram	Pericardial effusion +1	—
Pulmonary Function Tests	% pred DLCO ≥80 −1	% pred DLCO <32 +1
RHC	mRAP >20 mm Hg within 1 y +1	PVR >32 Wood units +2
Sum of Above		
(Starting Score)		
REVEAL Risk Score		

	Low Risk	Average Risk	Moderate High Risk	High Risk	Very High Risk
Risk Score	1–7	8	9	10	≥12
Predicted 1-y Survival (%)	95–100	90 to <95	85 to <90	70 to <85	<70

Abbreviations: % pred, percentage predicted; APAH, associated PAH; CTD, connective tissue disease; HPAH, heritable PAH; HR, heart rate; mRAP, mean right atrial pressure; NYHA, New York Heart Association; PoPH, portopulmonary PH; SBP, systolic blood pressure.

Modified from Benza RL, Gomberg-Maitland M, Miller DP et al. The REVEAL registry risk score calculator in patients newly diagnosed with pulmonary arterial hypertension. Chest 2012;141(2):356; with permission.

Table 2 Medical treatments for pulmonary arterial hypertension		
Nitric Oxide–Soluble Guanylate Cyclase	Endothelin Pathway	Prostacyclin Pathway
Sildenafil Tadalafil Riociguat	Bosentan Ambrisentan Macitentan	IV epoprostenol Room-temperature stable epoprostenol IV treprostinil subcutaneous treprostinil Inhaled iloprost Inhaled treprostinil Oral treprostinil Selexipag

Abbreviations: cAMP, cyclic adenosine monophosphate; cGMP, cyclic guanine monophosphate; ERA, endothelin receptor antagonist.

Table 3
World Health Organization functional classification

WHO Functional Class	Symptoms
I	Patients with PH but without limitations of physical activity. Ordinary activity does not cause dyspnea or presyncope
II	Patients with PH with slight limitation in ordinary activity. They are comfortable at rest. Ordinary activity causes dyspnea, fatigue, or presyncope
III	Patients with PH with marked limitation in ordinary activity. They are comfortable at rest. Less than ordinary activity causes dyspnea, fatigue, or presyncope
IV	Patients PH with an inability to perform any physical activity without symptoms. These patients have signs of right heart failure and dyspnea and/or fatigue may be present at rest. Discomfort is increased with any activity. Exertional syncope, an ominous sign, also pertains to this functional class

Data from Galiè N, Humbert M, Vachiery JL, et al. 2015 ESC/ERS guidelines for the diagnosis and treatment of pulmonary hypertension: the Joint Task Force for the Diagnosis and Treatment of Pulmonary Hypertension of the European Society of Cardiology (ESC) and the European Respiratory Society (ERS): endorsed by: Association for European Paediatric and Congenital Cardiology (AEPC), International Society for Heart and Lung Transplantation (ISHLT). Eur Respir J 2015;46(4):903–75.

Surgical therapies

When medical therapies are ineffective, or in a patient has severe WHO group 3 PH, lung transplant should be considered. In general, the authors advocate early referral to a transplant center when patients are progressing despite parenteral therapy, or if there is a poorer prognosis because of underlying lung disease. This referral is important to allow adequate time for evaluation, and it is preferable to do it when the patient is ambulatory rather than during a hospitalization for acute respiratory failure.

Another surgical procedure sometimes performed when patients have severe RV failure is atrial septostomy. It relieves the RV from pressure overload and can help treat the failing RV. In selected patients, atrial septostomy and continued medical therapy can lengthen survival, especially as a bridge to lung transplant or for palliative measures.[49]

As mentioned, pulmonary thromboendarterectomy and balloon pulmonary angioplasty are treatments used in patients with CTEPH, and all patients should be evaluated for surgical candidacy at a CTEPH center.[23]

SUMMARY

This article discusses PH, and the basic diagnostic and treatment algorithms, and shows that although survival has improved with progress, patients with PH still often experience misdiagnosis or delay in diagnosis, which delays treatment and, given the progressive nature of this disease, may have serious consequences. This overview emphasizes the complexity of this disease and encourages early referral to a PH specialist for accurate diagnosis and treatment. Our hope is that, through good communication, PH specialists may work with internists or local pulmonologists or cardiologists to help each patient achieve the best outcome.

REFERENCES

1. Simonneau G, Montani D, Celermajer DS, et al. Haemodynamic definitions and updated clinical classification of pulmonary hypertension. Eur Resp J 2018. [Epub ahead of print].
2. Strange G, Gabbay E, Kermeen F, et al. Time from symptoms to definitive diagnosis of idiopathic pulmonary arterial hypertension: the DELAY study. Pulm Circ 2013;3(1):89–94.
3. Humbert M, Sitbon O, Chaouat A, et al. Pulmonary arterial hypertension in France: results from a national registry. Am J Respir Crit Care Med 2006; 173(9):1023–30.
4. D'Alonzo GE, Barst RJ, Ayres SM, et al. Survival in patients with primary pulmonary hypertension. Results from a national prospective registry. Ann Intern Med 1991;115(5):343–9.
5. Deaño RC, Glassner-Kolmin C, Rubenfire M, et al. Referral of patients with pulmonary hypertension diagnoses to tertiary pulmonary hypertension centers. JAMA Intern Med 2013;173(10):887–93.
6. Wilkins MR. Pulmonary hypertension: the science behind the disease spectrum. Eur Respir Rev 2012;21(123):19–26.
7. Badesch DB, Raskob GE, Elliott CG, et al. Pulmonary arterial hypertension: baseline characteristics from the REVEAL registry. Chest 2010;137(2):376–87.
8. Badesch DB, Champion HC, Sanchez MA, et al. Diagnosis and assessment of pulmonary arterial hypertension. J Am Coll Cardiol 2009;54(1 Suppl):S55–66.
9. Launay D, Mouthon L, Hachulla E, et al. Prevalence and characteristics of moderate to severe pulmonary hypertension in systemic sclerosis with and without interstitial lung disease. J Rheumatol 2007;34(5):1005–11.
10. Avouac J, Airò P, Meune C, et al. Prevalence of pulmonary hypertension in systemic sclerosis in European Caucasians and metaanalysis of 5 studies. J Rheumatol 2010;37(11):2290–8.
11. Sitbon O, Lascoux-Combe C, Delfraissy JF, et al. Prevalence of HIV-related pulmonary arterial hypertension in the current antiretroviral therapy era. Am J Respir Crit Care Med 2008;177(1):108–13.
12. Ramirez RL 3rd, Perez VJ, Zamanian RT. Methamphetamine and the risk of pulmonary arterial hypertension. Curr Opin Pulm Med 2018;24(5):416–24.
13. Robbins IM, Newman JH, Johnson RF, et al. Association of the metabolic syndrome with pulmonary venous hypertension. Chest 2009;136(1):31–6.
14. Cao JY, Wales KM, Cordina R, et al. Pulmonary vasodilator therapies are of no benefit in pulmonary hypertension due to left heart disease: a meta-analysis. Int J Cardiol 2018;273:213–20.
15. Galie N, Barberà JA, Frost AE, et al. Initial use of ambrisentan plus tadalafil in pulmonary arterial hypertension. N Engl J Med 2015;373(9):834–44.
16. Sitbon O, Channick R, Chin KM, et al. Selexipag for the treatment of pulmonary arterial hypertension. N Engl J Med 2015;373(26):2522–33.
17. Pulido T, Adzerikho I, Channick RN, et al. Macitentan and morbidity and mortality in pulmonary arterial hypertension. N Engl J Med 2013;369(9):809–18.
18. Dorfmuller P, Humbert M, Perros F, et al. Fibrous remodeling of the pulmonary venous system in pulmonary arterial hypertension associated with connective tissue diseases. Hum Pathol 2007;38(6):893–902.
19. Lafitte S, Pillois X, Reant P, et al. Estimation of pulmonary pressures and diagnosis of pulmonary hypertension by Doppler echocardiography: a retrospective

comparison of routine echocardiography and invasive hemodynamics. J Am Soc Echocardiogr 2013;26(5):457–63.

20. Hammerstingl C, Schueler R, Bors L, et al. Diagnostic value of echocardiography in the diagnosis of pulmonary hypertension. PLoS One 2012;7(6):e38519.

21. Arcasoy SM, Christie JD, Ferrari VA, et al. Echocardiographic assessment of pulmonary hypertension in patients with advanced lung disease. Am J Respir Crit Care Med 2003;167(5):735–40.

22. Fisher MR, Forfia PR, Chamera E, et al. Accuracy of Doppler echocardiography in the hemodynamic assessment of pulmonary hypertension. Am J Respir Crit Care Med 2009;179(7):615–21.

23. Galie N, Humbert M, Vachiery JL, et al, ESC Scientific Document Group. 2015 ESC/ERS guidelines for the diagnosis and treatment of pulmonary hypertension: the Joint Task Force for the Diagnosis and Treatment of Pulmonary Hypertension of the European Society of Cardiology (ESC) and the European Respiratory Society (ERS): endorsed by: Association for European Paediatric and Congenital Cardiology (AEPC), International Society for Heart and Lung Transplantation (ISHLT). Eur Respir J 2015;46(4):903–75.

24. Benza RL, Miller DP, Gomberg-Maitland M, et al. Predicting survival in pulmonary arterial hypertension: insights from the registry to evaluate early and long-term pulmonary arterial hypertension disease management (REVEAL). Circulation 2010;122(2):164–72.

25. Vachiéry JL, Adir Y, Barberà JA, et al. Pulmonary hypertension due to left heart diseases. J Am Coll Cardiol 2013;62(25 Suppl):D100–8.

26. Gerges C, Gerges M, Lang MB, et al. Diastolic pulmonary vascular pressure gradient: a predictor of prognosis in "out-of-proportion" pulmonary hypertension. Chest 2013;143(3):758–66.

27. Zhang L, Liebelt JJ, Madan N, et al. Comparison of predictors of heart failure with preserved versus reduced ejection fraction in a multiracial cohort of preclinical left ventricular diastolic dysfunction. Am J Cardiol 2017;119(11):1815–20.

28. Lam CSP, Chandramouli C. Fat, female, fatigued: features of the obese HFpEF phenotype. JACC Heart Fail 2018;6(8):710–3.

29. Seeger W, Adir Y, Barberà JA, et al. Pulmonary hypertension in chronic lung diseases. J Am Coll Cardiol 2013;62(25 Suppl):D109–16.

30. Andersen KH, Iversen M, Kjaergaard J, et al. Prevalence, predictors, and survival in pulmonary hypertension related to end-stage chronic obstructive pulmonary disease. J Heart Lung Transplant 2012;31(4):373–80.

31. Chaouat A, Bugnet AS, Kadaoui N, et al. Severe pulmonary hypertension and chronic obstructive pulmonary disease. Am J Respir Crit Care Med 2005;172(2):189–94.

32. Wells JM, Washko GR, Han MK, et al. Pulmonary arterial enlargement and acute exacerbations of COPD. N Engl J Med 2012;367(10):913–21.

33. Oswald-Mammosser M, Weitzenblum E, Quoix E, et al. Prognostic factors in COPD patients receiving long-term oxygen therapy. Importance of pulmonary artery pressure. Chest 1995;107(5):1193–8.

34. Olschewski H, Behr J, Bremer H, et al. Pulmonary hypertension due to lung diseases: updated recommendations from the Cologne Consensus Conference 2018. Int J Cardiol 2018;272S:63–8.

35. Galie N, Humbert M, Vachiery JL, et al. 2015 ESC/ERS guidelines for the diagnosis and treatment of pulmonary hypertension: the Joint Task Force for the Diagnosis and Treatment of Pulmonary Hypertension of the European Society of Cardiology (ESC) and the European Respiratory Society (ERS): endorsed by:

Association for European Paediatric and Congenital Cardiology (AEPC), International Society for Heart and Lung Transplantation (ISHLT). Eur Heart J 2016;37(1): 67–119.

36. Raghu G, Behr J, Brown KK, et al. Treatment of idiopathic pulmonary fibrosis with ambrisentan: a parallel, randomized trial. Ann Intern Med 2013;158(9):641–9.

37. Kholdani C, Fares WH, Mohsenin V. Pulmonary hypertension in obstructive sleep apnea: is it clinically significant? A critical analysis of the association and pathophysiology. Pulm Circ 2015;5(2):220–7.

38. Simonneau G, Torbicki A, Dorfmüller P, et al. The pathophysiology of chronic thromboembolic pulmonary hypertension. Eur Respir Rev 2017;26(143):1–14.

39. Pengo V, Lensing AW, Prins MH, et al. Incidence of chronic thromboembolic pulmonary hypertension after pulmonary embolism. N Engl J Med 2004;350(22): 2257–64.

40. Tunariu N, Gibbs SJ, Win Z, et al. Ventilation-perfusion scintigraphy is more sensitive than multidetector CTPA in detecting chronic thromboembolic pulmonary disease as a treatable cause of pulmonary hypertension. J Nucl Med 2007; 48(5):680–4.

41. Kylhammar D, Kjellström B, Hjalmarsson C, et al. A comprehensive risk stratification at early follow-up determines prognosis in pulmonary arterial hypertension. Eur Heart J 2017;39(47):4175–81.

42. Gall H, Felix JF, Schneck FK, et al. The Giessen pulmonary hypertension registry: survival in pulmonary hypertension subgroups. J Heart Lung Transplant 2017; 36(9):957–67.

43. Boucly A, Weatherald J, Savale L, et al. Risk assessment, prognosis and guideline implementation in pulmonary arterial hypertension. Eur Respir J 2017;50(2) [pii:1700889].

44. Sitbon O, Benza RL, Badesch DB, et al. Validation of two predictive models for survival in pulmonary arterial hypertension. Eur Respir J 2015;46(1):152–64.

45. Benza RL, Gomberg-Maitland M, Miller DP, et al. The REVEAL registry risk score calculator in patients newly diagnosed with pulmonary arterial hypertension. Chest 2012;141(2):354–62.

46. Benza RL, Miller DP, Foreman AJ, et al. Prognostic implications of serial risk score assessments in patients with pulmonary arterial hypertension: a registry to evaluate early and long-term pulmonary arterial hypertension disease management (REVEAL) analysis. J Heart Lung Transplant 2015;34(3):356–61.

47. Barst RJ, Rubin LJ, Long WA, et al. A comparison of continuous intravenous epoprostenol (prostacyclin) with conventional therapy for primary pulmonary hypertension. N Engl J Med 1996;334(5):296–301.

48. Barst RJ, Rubin LJ, McGoon MD, et al. Survival in primary pulmonary hypertension with long-term continuous intravenous prostacyclin. Ann Intern Med 1994; 121(6):409–15.

49. Sandoval J, Gaspar J, Peña H, et al. Effect of atrial septostomy on the survival of patients with severe pulmonary arterial hypertension. Eur Respir J 2011;38(6): 1343–8.

Lung Transplantation

Vivek N. Ahya, MD, MBA[a],*, Joshua M. Diamond, MD, MSCE[b]

KEYWORDS

- Lung transplantation • Outcomes • Allocation • Complications

KEY POINTS

- Lung transplantation is an option for select patients with advanced lung diseases.
- Demand for organs exceeds supply.
- The most common indications for lung transplantation are pulmonary fibrosis, chronic obstructive pulmonary disease, cystic fibrosis, and pulmonary vascular diseases.
- The clinician should be aware that the lung transplant recipient is at risk for immunologic, infections, and numerous medical complications.
- Early referral to ta transplant center should be considered, especially for patients with interstitial lung diseases.

INTRODUCTION

The first lung transplant procedure was performed by Dr James Hardy and colleagues[1] at the University of Mississippi in 1963. The recipient had chronic obstructive pulmonary disease (COPD) but was a suboptimal candidate for several reasons, including the presence of advanced lung cancer and renal insufficiency. Furthermore, the patient was incarcerated on death row and had in part agreed to the experimental procedure with the knowledge that his prison sentence may be commuted in exchange—an agreement that would be prohibited on ethical grounds today. Nevertheless, the patient survived 18 days before succumbing to complications related to renal failure.[1] On autopsy, pathologic evaluation of the graft did not show evidence for allograft rejection, offering hope that the feared immunologic barriers to transplantation were not insurmountable.

Disclosures: V.N. Ahya: None. J.M. Diamond: receives research funding from Merck & Co. (USA) to conduct a clinical trial to evaluate and treat lung transplant recipients who have received organs from donors exposed to hepatitis C.
[a] Division of Pulmonary, Allergy and Critical Care Division, Paul F. Harron Jr. Lung Center, Penn Medicine, Perelman School of Medicine, University of Pennsylvania, 9035 Gates Building, 3400 Spruce Street, Philadelphia, PA 19104, USA; [b] Lung Transplantation Program, Division of Pulmonary, Allergy and Critical Care, Perelman School of Medicine, University of Pennsylvania, 9039 Gates Building, 3400 Spruce Street, Philadelphia, PA 19104, USA
* Corresponding author.
E-mail address: Vivek.Ahya@uphs.upenn.edu

OUTCOMES

Survival has improved significantly since Dr Hardy's first transplant. Optimization of surgical techniques and the introduction of the novel immunosuppressive agent, cyclosporine, in the early 1980s led to dramatic improvement in outcomes after solid organ transplantation. It was in this era that the first combined heart-lung transplant procedure was performed at Stanford Medical Center in a patient with idiopathic pulmonary arterial hypertension.[2] Two years later, in 1983, the Toronto Lung Transplant Group performed the first successful isolated lung transplant procedure. The patient was transplanted for idiopathic pulmonary fibrosis (IPF) and survived more than 7 years.[3] Unfortunately, over the past 2 decades, outcomes have improved only modestly, with chronic lung allograft dysfunction (CLAD), infections, and other medical complications remaining as the primary obstacles to long-term survival. Data from the most recent annual report of the US Organ Procurement and Transplantation Network (OPTN) and the Scientific Registry of Transplant Recipients (SRTR) reported survival rates of 85% at 1 year, 68% at 3 years, and 55% at 5 years.[4]

INDICATIONS

Since the 1980s, approximately 65,000 adult lung transplant procedures have been reported to the registry of the International Society for Heart and Lung Transplantation (ISHLT), with 4554 performed in 2016, the highest number reported in a single year.[5] More than half of these cases were performed in the United States.[4] The primary indications for lung transplantation are fibrotic lung disorders, now accounting for more than 57% of cases in the United States.[4] COPD, cystic fibrosis, and pulmonary vascular disorders comprise the other primary indications for lung transplantation.

WAITLIST MORTALITY

Although the number of lung transplants performed annually has steadily increased, more patients are waitlisted each year than transplanted. With this imbalance between demand for donor organs and supply, waitlist mortality remains significant. Annually, approximately 20% of waitlisted patients die on the lung transplantation waiting list or are removed because they become too sick to transplant.[4] Multiple approaches are required to reduce waitlist mortality. These include

1. Expanding the organ donor pool through efforts to enhance donor authorization rates[6]
2. Increasing utilization of organs previously deemed high risk (eg, hepatitis C(+) donors[7] and organs from donors with circulatory determination of death)[8]
3. Optimizing donor management to increase organ yield from the existing donor pool[9]
4. Rehabilitation of organs deemed poor quality through novel approaches (eg, ex vivo lung perfusion)[10]
5. Intensive support of patients with lung failure (eg, use of extracorporeal life support) to extend waitlist survival[11]
6. Establishment of clear rules to ethically prioritize organs for distribution to waitlisted patients[12]

LUNG ALLOCATION

When a donor is identified, lung allocation follows an established algorithm based initially on donor age (pediatric vs adult) and location of donor hospital (organs are prioritized based on geographic proximity to donor hospital—currently, a radius of 250 nautical miles from the donor hospital encompasses the initial area for allocation priority). If lungs are not used within the initial geographic region, only then are they allocated to transplant centers in more distant areas. These fixed geographic boundaries are controversial and are currently being reexamined in the face of legal scrutiny.[13]

Within a geographic area, donor lungs are then restricted to candidates with the appropriate blood type and size. In this subgroup of waitlisted patients, the donor organ is then allocated to the patient with the highest lung allocation score (LAS). The LAS prioritizes patients based on medical urgency and likelihood of benefiting from the transplant procedure. A complex multivariable model that includes more than 13 clinical and demographic variables is used to calculate the LAS.[14]

REFERRAL TO TRANSPLANT CENTER AND PATIENT SELECTION

In general, patients with advanced lung diseases should be considered for lung transplantation if they have progressive disease not responsive to other treatments, are predicted to have reduced short-term survival (ie, high likelihood for death in the next 1 year to 2 years), have a poor quality of life, and are deemed likely to survive the rigorous transplantation procedure and tolerate the necessary administration of immunosuppressive agents, multiple antimicrobial drugs, and other medications. For additional information on patient selection criteria, the reader is referred to the ISHLT consensus guidelines from 2014.[15] Stated absolute contraindications include presence of active malignancy (other than nonmelanoma skin cancer) or insufficient disease-free survival to predict low recurrence risk; untreatable significant extrapulmonary organ dysfunction, unless the patient is a candidate for multiorgan transplant; infection with highly resistant infectious pathogens that pose major risk for poor posttransplant outcome; extremes of age and weight; unreliable social support system; poorly controlled psychiatric disorders; and impaired functional status with poor rehabilitation potential.[15] Patient selection criteria, however, are evolving and differ among transplant centers based on center-specific experience, volume, outcomes, and level of risk aversion.[16] Thus, if a patient is deemed to be not an appropriate candidate at one center, it may be worthwhile contacting another center for a second opinion.

Although it is beyond the scope of this article to delve deeply into disease-specific recommendations for timing of patient referral (**Fig. 1**), the group that should be considered for early referral to a transplant center is patients who have IPF or other similar fibrotic disorders (eg, fibrotic nonspecific interstitial pneumonia [NSIP]) due to risk for acute exacerbations during which stable patients progress rapidly to respiratory failure.[15,17] Early referral also facilitates patient and family education and allows time to address potential medical and social contraindications.

POST-TRANSPLANT MANAGEMENT AND COMPLICATIONS

Primary graft dysfunction, acute lung rejection, CLAD, and infectious complications remain the main obstacles to early and long-term survival after transplantation. Additionally, organ recipients frequently develop numerous other medical comorbidities, such as hypertension, hyperlipidemia, cancer, chronic kidney disease (CKD), osteoporosis, and diabetes mellitus.

IMMUNOSUPPRESSION

The advent of potent immunosuppressive drugs that inhibit alloimmune responses and prevent and treat graft rejection has been critical to improving outcomes after

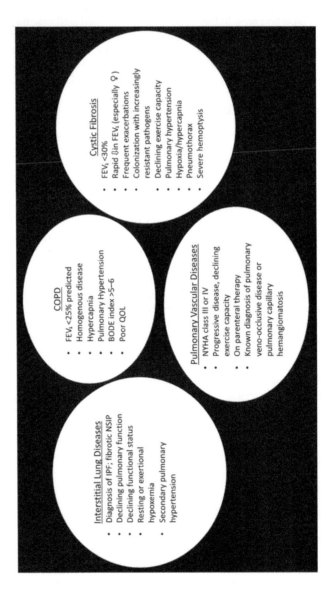

Fig. 1. General guidelines for timing of referral to a transplant center. BODE index, body mass index, airway obstruction, dyspnea, and exercise capacity[40]; NYHA, New York Heart Association; QOL, quality of life.

solid organ transplantation. Post–lung transplant immunosuppression typically consists of triple therapy with glucocorticosteroids, calcineurin inhibitors (CNIs) (tacrolimus or cyclosporine), and an antiproliferative agent (eg, mycophenolate mofetil and azathioprine). Other classes of medication that may be used are mammalian target of rapamycin inhibitors (eg, sirolimus and everolimus), cytotoxic T-lymphocyte–associated protein 4 inhibitors (eg, belatacept), and induction agents (eg, thymoglobulin and basiliximab). Many of the medical complications seen after transplantation are a direct result of these medications.[18]

ACUTE CELLULAR REJECTION AND ANTIBODY-MEDIATED REJECTION

Antibody cellular rejection (ACR), a common complication after lung transplantation, occurring in 10% to 45% of patients, is an important risk factor for CLAD development. Its diagnosis requires pathologic evaluation with diagnostic tissue typically obtained with transbronchial biopsies. The presence and severity of rejection is based on the extent of perivascular mononuclear cell infiltrate and is graded on a scale from A0 to A4. Treatment depends on severity of ACR and may range from observation with short-term re-evaluation or augmentation of immunosuppression with high doses of corticosteroids or lymphocyte-depleting agents.[19]

Antibody-mediated rejection (AMR) is a distinct form of graft injury mediated by the humoral immune system and occurs in the presence of complement-activating donor-specific anti-HLA antibodies (DSAs). At present, there are insufficient data regarding optimal surveillance protocols for DSA monitoring or AMR treatment. Treatment of severe AMR may involve plasmapheresis, administration of high doses of immunosuppressive agents, and intravenous immunoglobulin.[19–21]

CHRONIC LUNG ALLOGRAFT DYSFUNCTION

CLAD is the leading cause of death after lung transplantation. Current guidelines for CLAD phenotyping split the entity into obstructive CLAD (also called bronchiolitis obliterans syndrome) and restrictive CLAD. CLAD onset and severity are defined by a decline in forced expiratory volume in first second of expiration (FEV_1) from a peak post-transplant baseline with the exclusion of reversible etiologies (ie, acute rejection, infection, and airway complications). Important risk factors for CLAD include previous episodes (especially high grade) of ACR, respiratory infections, gastroesophageal reflux disease, presence of DSAs, and postoperative primary graft dysfunction. To date, no medical therapy reliably treats or prevents CLAD, although azithromycin, a macrolide antibiotic with anti-inflammatory properties, has shown efficacy in several studies.[22]

INFECTIONS

Infections are a leading cause of mortality throughout the post-transplant period and are the primary cause of death from 1 month to 1 year post-transplant.[23] Bacterial, viral, fungal, and mycobacterial pathogens can be present in the pretransplant period or acquired in the community or health care setting after transplantation. Community-acquired respiratory viruses are an especially common cause of upper and lower respiratory tract infections and have been linked to an increased risk of both ACR and CLAD.[24] *Aspergillus*, the most common fungal pathogen detected after lung transplantation, is associated with early ischemic airways injury and may increase CLAD risk and mortality.[25] Infection with nontuberculous mycobacteria, such as

Mycobacterium abscessus, are increasingly recognized, difficult to treat, and associated with poor outcomes.[26]

With the widespread use of potent prophylactic antimicrobial agents, the medical community needs to be vigilant for the emergence of new, dangerous pathogens that are highly resistant to currently available therapies.

MEDICAL COMPLICATIONS
Post-transplant Hypertension

Systemic hypertension is frequently seen after lung transplantation and may be due in part to use of CNIs.[27] Clinicians should be aware of two important but less common syndromes that may present with systemic hypertension. These conditions are associated with CNI administration.

Posterior reversible encephalopathy syndrome is characterized by endothelial damage, platelet aggregation, and enhanced vasoconstriction, leading to impaired cerebral autoregulation and brain vasogenic edema; this syndrome can present clinically with severe hypertension, headaches, seizures, mental status change, and intracerebral bleeding. In addition to emergent blood pressure control, prompt discontinuation of the CNI is crucial to disease management.[28]

CNI therapy may also be associated with thrombotic microangiopathy presenting with hypertension, schistocytosis, intravascular hemolysis, and acute kidney injury. In addition to medical management, prompt cessation of the offending CNI is essential, although subsequent reintroduction of an alternative CNI is possible.[29]

Hyperlipidemia

Hyperlipidemia has been reported in 22.2% of lung recipients within the first year and more than half develop it by the fifth post-transplant year. Immunosuppressive agents have been implicated in causing hyperlipidemia. CNIs (cyclosporine more than tacrolimus) lead to increased low-density lipoprotein (LDL) production and decreased LDL clearance. Corticosteroid administration promotes insulin resistance and elevated cholesterol and triglycerides levels. Half of all patients treated with sirolimus develop dyslipidemia in the setting of reduced LDL clearance.[30] Appropriate lipid management after transplant improves patient survival and decreases the risk of CKD development.[31] Although statins are likely beneficial, initial doses should be low, with close monitoring for toxicity.

Malignancy

Lung transplant recipients are at significantly increased risk for developing cancer, representing the third most commonly reported cause of death in this population.[32] Key risk factors include inhibition of immune system tumor surveillance with administration of immunosuppression, older age, and high rates of tobacco exposure.[33] The 2 most frequently encountered malignancies are nonmelanoma skin cancers, lung cancer, and post-transplant lymphoproliferative disorder.[33,34]

Chronic Kidney Disease

Multiple studies have documented the extremely high rate of CKD after lung transplantation, due in significant part to the nephrotoxic effects of CNIs.[35–37] There is strong interplay between the mechanisms causing hypertension and those leading to CKD. In a recent study of 113 lung transplant recipients, CKD developed in 80% of recipients by 2 years after transplant.[37] Close monitoring of renal function; minimization or elimination of other potentially nephrotoxic medications, including nonsteroidal anti-inflammatory drugs; and close monitoring of CNI blood levels are key to minimizing risk of CKD.

Osteoporosis

Osteoporosis or osteopenia is often present prior to transplant due to chronic medical illness, extended periods of limited mobility, malnutrition, and treatment with glucocorticoid medications. After transplantation, patients are treated with CNIs, which also have been implicated in bone loss. Furthermore, transplant recipients receive varying doses of glucocorticoids lifelong.[38] Potential lung transplant candidates should be screened for osteoporosis prior to lung transplantation, and treatment, including bisphosphonates, calcium, and vitamin D, should be started to mitigate fracture risk.

Diabetes

High rates of diabetes have been reported after lung transplantation. In a recently published study, more than half of all transplant recipients developed diabetes, with the prevalence approaching 100% in patients with cystic fibrosis.[39] Engagement with endocrinology early is important to help develop a treatment plan to limit complications associated with poorly controlled diabetes.

SUMMARY

Lung transplantation has evolved from being a rare extreme surgical treatment of advanced lung diseases to one that is now an accepted therapeutic option for select patients with advanced lung diseases. Lung transplantation offers these patients the hope for longer survival and better quality of life. Unfortunately, numerous complications threaten this objective. The patient, family, medical, and surgical teams must be aware of the potential for these complications and work closely to prevent and treat them.

REFERENCES

1. Hardy JD, Webb WR, Dalton ML Jr, et al. Lung homotransplantation in man. JAMA 1963;186:1065–74.
2. Reitz BA. The first successful combined heart-lung transplantation. J Thorac Cardiovasc Surg 2011;141(4):867–9.
3. Toronto Lung Transplant Group. Unilateral lung transplantation for pulmonary fibrosis. N Engl J Med 1986;314(18):1140–5.
4. Valapour M, Lehr CJ, Skeans MA, et al. OPTN/SRTR 2016 annual data report: lung. Am J Transplant 2018;18(Suppl 1):363–433.
5. Chambers DC, Cherikh WS, Goldfarb SB, et al. The international thoracic organ transplant registry of the international society for heart and lung transplantation: thirty-fifth adult lung and heart-lung transplant report-2018; focus theme: multiorgan transplantation. J Heart Lung Transplant 2018;37(10):1169–83.
6. Goldberg DS, French B, Abt PL, et al. Increasing the number of organ transplants in the United States by Optimizing Donor Authorization Rates. Am J Transplant 2015;15(8):2117–25.
7. Abdelbasit A, Hirji A, Halloran K, et al. Lung transplantation from hepatitis c viremic donors to uninfected recipients. Am J Respir Crit Care Med 2018; 197(11):1492–6.

8. Villavicencio MA, Axtell AL, Spencer PJ, et al. Lung transplantation from donation after circulatory death: United States and single center experience. Ann Thorac Surg 2018;106(6):1619–27.

9. Kotloff RM, Blosser S, Fulda GJ, et al. Management of the potential organ donor in the ICU: Society of Critical Care Medicine/American College of Chest Physicians/Association of Organ Procurement Organizations Consensus Statement. Crit Care Med 2015;43(6):1291–325.

10. Cypel M, Yeung JC, Liu M, et al. Normothermic ex vivo lung perfusion in clinical lung transplantation. N Engl J Med 2011;364(15):1431–40.

11. Hakim AH, Ahmad U, McCurry KR, et al. Contemporary outcomes of extracorporeal membrane oxygenation used as bridge to lung transplantation. Ann Thorac Surg 2018;106(1):192–8.

12. Organ procurement and transplantation network: final rule. Available at: https://optn.transplant.hrsa.gov/governance/about-the-optn/final-rule/. Accessed October 14, 2018.

13. Public Comment Proposal: Frameworks for Organ Distribution; OPTN/UNOS Ad Hoc Geography Committee. Available at: https://optn.transplant.hrsa.gov/media/2565/geography_publiccomment_201808.pdf. Accessed October 14, 2018.

14. Egan TM. How should lungs be allocated for transplant? Semin Respir Crit Care Med 2018;39(2):126–37.

15. Weill D, Benden C, Corris PA, et al. A consensus document for the selection of lung transplant candidates: 2014–an update from the Pulmonary Transplantation Council of the International Society for Heart and Lung Transplantation. J Heart Lung Transplant 2015;34(1):1–15.

16. Jay C, Schold JD. Measuring transplant center performance: The goals are not controversial but the methods and consequences can be. Curr Transplant Rep 2017;4(1):52–8.

17. Lederer DJ, Martinez FJ. Idiopathic pulmonary fibrosis. N Engl J Med 2018;378(19):1811–23.

18. Scheffert JL, Raza K. Immunosuppression in lung transplantation. J Thorac Dis 2014;6(8):1039–53.

19. Hachem RR. Acute rejection and antibody-mediated rejection in lung transplantation. Clin Chest Med 2017;38(4):667–75.

20. Levine DJ, Glanville AR, Aboyoun C, et al. Antibody-mediated rejection of the lung: a consensus report of the International Society for Heart and Lung Transplantation. J Heart Lung Transplant 2016;35(4):397–406.

21. Tambur AR, Campbell P, Claas FH, et al. Sensitization in transplantation: assessment of risk (STAR) 2017 working group meeting report. Am J Transplant 2018;18(7):1604–14.

22. Shah RJ, Diamond JM. Update in chronic lung allograft dysfunction. Clin Chest Med 2017;38(4):677–92.

23. Yusen RD, Edwards LB, Dipchand AI, et al. The registry of the international society for heart and lung transplantation: thirty-third adult lung and heart-lung transplant report-2016; focus theme: primary diagnostic indications for transplant. J Heart Lung Transplant 2016;35(10):1170–84.

24. Paulsen GC, Danziger-Isakov L. Respiratory viral infections in solid organ and hematopoietic stem cell transplantation. Clin Chest Med 2017;38(4):707–26.

25. De La Cruz O, Silveira FP. Respiratory fungal infections in solid organ and hematopoietic stem cell transplantation. Clin Chest Med 2017;38(4):727–39.

26. Chandrashekaran S, Escalante P, Kennedy CC. Mycobacterium abscessus disease in lung transplant recipients: diagnosis and management. J Clin Tuberc Other Mycobact Dis 2017;9:10–8.
27. Hoskova L, Malek I, Kopkan L, et al. Pathophysiological mechanisms of calcineurin inhibitor-induced nephrotoxicity and arterial hypertension. Physiol Res 2017;66(2):167–80.
28. Liman TG, Bohner G, Heuschmann PU, et al. The clinical and radiological spectrum of posterior reversible encephalopathy syndrome: the retrospective Berlin PRES study. J Neurol 2012;259(1):155–64.
29. Verbiest A, Pirenne J, Dierickx D. De novo thrombotic microangiopathy after nonrenal solid organ transplantation. Blood Rev 2014;28(6):269–79.
30. Tannock LR, Reynolds LR. Management of dyslipidemia in patients after solid organ transplantation. Postgrad Med 2008;120(1):43–9.
31. Stephany BR, Alao B, Budev M, et al. Hyperlipidemia is associated with accelerated chronic kidney disease progression after lung transplantation. Am J Transplant 2007;7(11):2553–60.
32. Yusen RD, Edwards LB, Kucheryavaya AY, et al. The registry of the international society for heart and lung transplantation: thirty-second official adult lung and heart-lung transplantation report–2015; focus theme: early graft failure. J Heart Lung Transplant 2015;34(10):1264–77.
33. Olland A, Falcoz PE, Massard G. Malignancies after lung transplantation. J Thorac Dis 2018;10(5):3132–40.
34. Magruder JT, Crawford TC, Grimm JC, et al. Risk factors for de novo malignancy following lung transplantation. Am J Transplant 2017;17(1):227–38.
35. Cardinal H, Poirier C, Fugere JA, et al. The evolution of kidney function after lung transplantation: a retrospective cohort study. Transplant Proc 2009;41(8):3342–4.
36. Paradela de la Morena M, De La Torre Bravos M, Prado RF, et al. Chronic kidney disease after lung transplantation: incidence, risk factors, and treatment. Transplant Proc 2010;42(8):3217–9.
37. Sole A, Zurbano F, Borro JM, et al. Prevalence and diagnosis of chronic kidney disease in maintenance lung transplant patients: ICEBERG Study. Transplant Proc 2015;47(6):1966–71.
38. Yu TM, Lin CL, Chang SN, et al. Osteoporosis and fractures after solid organ transplantation: a nationwide population-based cohort study. Mayo Clin Proc 2014;89(7):888–95.
39. Fazekas-Lavu M, Reyes M, Malouf M, et al. High prevalence of diabetes before and after lung transplantation: target for improving outcome? Intern Med J 2018;48(8):916–24.
40. Celli BR, Cote CG, Marin JM, et al. The body-mass index, airflow obstruction, dyspnea, and exercise capacity index in chronic obstructive pulmonary disease. N Engl J Med 2004;350(10):1005–12.

Asthma in the Primary Care Setting

Tianshi David Wu, MD, MHS, Emily P. Brigham, MD, MHS,
Meredith C. McCormack, MD, MHS*

KEYWORDS

- Asthma • Review • Outpatient • Ambulatory • Treatment • Diagnosis

KEY POINTS

- Asthma may become clinically apparent at any age, but exclusion of diseases that mimic asthma is especially important in older individuals.
- A confident diagnosis of asthma can be made with demonstration of reversible obstruction on spirometry, and the risk of misdiagnosis is higher in the absence of this objective information.
- Inhaled corticosteroids are the cornerstone of pharmacologic asthma treatment of persistent disease, with additional therapies added on the basis of inadequate disease control.
- Patients should be empowered to respond to changing symptoms through use of an asthma action plan.
- Specialist referral is indicated for individuals with severe or difficult-to-control asthma; however, most individuals with asthma are successfully managed in the primary care setting.

Asthma is a chronic disease principally characterized by episodic wheeze, cough, and breathlessness resulting from airway hyperresponsiveness and inflammation. It is one of the most common chronic lung diseases in the United States, affecting approximately 8% of adults, or about 20 million individuals.[1,2]

Consequently, asthma is frequently encountered in the primary care setting. In the vast majority of cases, asthma is successfully managed by the generalist, and most individuals with asthma are expected to achieve good control. This article summarizes the epidemiology, diagnosis, and chronic and acute management of asthma from the primary care perspective.

Disclosure Statement: This article was supported by NIH grants F32ES028578 (D. Wu), KL2TR001077 (E. Brigham) and M.C. McCormack receives royalties for authorship for UpToDate.
Division of Pulmonary and Critical Care Medicine, Johns Hopkins University School of Medicine, 1830 East Monument Street, 5th Floor, Baltimore, MD 21205, USA
* Corresponding author.
E-mail address: mmccor16@jhmi.edu

EPIDEMIOLOGY

Asthma is significantly more prevalent in women (10.4%) than in men (6.2%), those below the poverty line (11.8%), and in those who report being an ethnic or racial minority, especially black race (10.2%) and Puerto Rican Hispanic ethnicity (14.9%). Geographic prevalence also ranges widely, from 4.9% to 12.7% by state. Despite a wide array of treatment options, almost half of adults with asthma report having one or more attacks in the previous year, highlighting the importance of symptom management and disease control.[3]

Asthma is classically thought of as a disease that begins in youth. Although it is true that asthma is most commonly first diagnosed in childhood, it can become clinically apparent at any age. Indeed, a national survey suggests that the rate of first asthma diagnosis for those older than 65 (3.1% per year) is not substantially different than those between 18 and 34 (4.0% per year).[4] The estimated prevalence of asthma among adults over 65 years of age is 7%, which is similar to the overall prevalence. History of prematurity, early lung infections, rhinitis, smoking, and obesity are all risk factors for adult-onset asthma.[5-7] Therefore, the onset of chronic cough in an older patient should not dissuade the clinician from considering asthma.

DIAGNOSIS

The confident diagnosis of asthma requires an integration of patient-reported symptoms and pulmonary function testing. Because the symptoms of asthma are often nonspecific and can be precipitated by other disease processes, the exclusion of diseases that mimic asthma is important, especially in older individuals, who may be more likely to have alternate conditions. A suggested diagnostic model of asthma is included (**Fig. 1**).

History

Common symptoms of asthma are wheeze, chest tightness, and cough. These symptoms are often episodic and may vary in intensity. The variability in symptoms often corresponds to changes in exposures, such as allergens, airway irritants, or respiratory infections. Some patients experience bronchoconstriction in response to exercise, and this can result in asthma symptoms. Individuals with uncontrolled disease may present with chronic symptoms at rest. Chest tightness is rarely the sole presenting complaint and should increase suspicion for cardiac disease.[8] Individuals with asthma often have concurrent rhinitis and sinusitis, and allergic rhinitis is a risk factor for incident asthma.[9] The presence of upper airway symptoms, which are thought to represent different manifestations of a common allergic pathophysiology, should be elicited.

Providers should inquire about potential exposures that worsen the patient's respiratory complaints. Identifiable triggers increase the probability of underlying asthma.[10] Allergens are commonly recognized triggers and may be seasonal (typically outdoor) or perennial (typically indoor). The distribution and timing of outdoor allergen exposure are highly variable across the United States. Outdoor allergens typically consist of forms of pollen and can be from trees, grass, and weeds, which are detectable at various times throughout the year. Perennial allergens include sources such as dust mites, mice, cockroaches, molds, and animal dander from pets. Other nonallergic triggers include cigarette use, secondhand smoke exposure, irritants, perfumes or strong odors, extremes of temperature, exercise, or psychosocial distress. Occupational exposures can lead to the onset of asthma (occupational asthma) or worsening of existing asthma (work-exacerbated asthma).[11,12] It is important to inquire about workplace

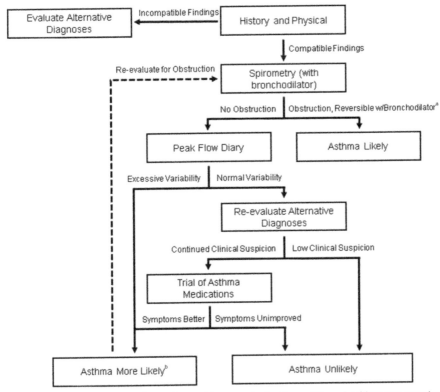

Fig. 1. Iterative evaluation of a patient with suspected asthma. [a]Bronchodilator responsiveness is defined as an improvement in FEV_1 or FVC by greater than 12% and greater than 200 mL. Patients may have improvement that does not meet this threshold and still benefit from bronchodilator therapy. Reversibility implies that spirometry improves to normal after bronchodilator. If only partially reversible, consider possibility of COPD, asthma-COPD overlap, or severe asthma. [b]Probability of asthma is substantially increased with the finding of obstruction at least one time on spirometry; reevaluation should occur at regular intervals. The likelihood of identifying obstruction while already on asthma medications is lower.

exposures in relationship to asthma diagnosis and fluctuation in symptoms (eg, differences in symptoms between weekdays and weekends[13] or during time away from work). Changes in respiratory symptoms during travel are suggestive of environmental sensitivity and support a potential diagnosis of asthma.

   Table 1 lists common asthma mimics and associated symptoms. Depending on the patient, additional history evaluating these conditions may be obtained. In particular, for the adult patient presenting with asthmalike symptoms, "cardiac asthma," wheezing as the result of unrecognized heart failure and consequent volume overload, and chronic obstructive pulmonary disease (COPD) should be considered. It is additionally possible for these conditions to coexist with asthma.

Physical Examination

The physical examination is most useful in assessing for the presence of comorbid or mimicking conditions. A pulmonary examination in a patient with asthma is often normal. Expiratory wheezing may be present, but is neither sensitive nor specific for

Table 1
Differential diagnoses in a patient presenting with asthmalike symptoms

Condition	Associated Signs and Symptoms
Allergic bronchopulmonary aspergillosis	Infiltrates, mucus plugging, bronchiectasis, elevated serum total IgE, and sensitization to *Aspergillus* (either skin testing or by specific IgE)
Bronchiectasis	Productive cough, history of recurrent pulmonary infections
Carcinoid syndrome	Episodic flushing, diarrhea, emesis
COPD	History of smoking or biomass exposure (especially in those residing in rural areas), irreversible obstruction on spirometry
Congestive heart failure	Pulmonary crackles, lower extremity edema, jugular venous distension, family or personal history of cardiovascular disease
Eosinophilic bronchitis	Chronic cough, upper airway symptoms, no hyperresponsiveness
Eosinophilic granulomatosis with polyangiitis	Migratory pulmonary infiltrates, concurrent sinus disease, antineutrophil cytoplasmic antibodies
Foreign body aspiration	Localized area of wheeze, segmental atelectasis on computed tomography (CT) scan
Interstitial lung disease (ILD)	Infiltrates, reticulation, or frank fibrosis on CT scan; signs and symptoms vary with ILD type; hypersensitivity pneumonitis and cryptogenic organizing pneumonia are types of ILD with atopic association
Postnasal drip	History of rhinitis and sinusitis, but no variable airflow obstruction
Tracheal stenosis/ tracheomalacia	Tracheal narrowing on CT scan, history of intubations
VCD	Sudden onset of dyspnea, prominent inspiratory wheezing, blunting of the inspiratory limb of the flow-volume loop

this condition. Inspiratory wheezing is not typical and may suggest an additional or alternate diagnosis. Similarly, crackles should elicit consideration of alternative diagnoses. Patients may have signs of concurrent rhinitis or postnasal drip. A skin examination may reveal eczema. Finally, a cardiac examination should be performed to evaluate for signs of heart failure.

Diagnostic Testing

If the history and physical examination suggest asthma as a likely diagnosis, the next step is to perform spirometry before and after bronchodilator administration to evaluate for the 2 key criteria central to asthma diagnosis: expiratory airflow obstruction and variability in airflow limitation. Spirometry demonstrating both expiratory airflow obstruction and full reversal of airflow obstruction following bronchodilator administration supports a diagnosis of asthma. However, because variability in symptoms and airflow limitation is a key feature of asthma, spirometry is frequently normal when asthma is well controlled. Furthermore, some patients with asthma who present with expiratory airflow obstruction may not fully reverse after bronchodilator administration, because of a greater disease severity at presentation or because of airway remodeling in chronically uncontrolled asthma. As partial reversibility is also a feature of COPD or asthma-COPD overlap, these other conditions should be considered. In such situations, spirometry cannot reliability distinguish between asthma and COPD.

The presence of airflow obstruction is defined by a ratio of fractional exhaled volume in the first second (FEV_1) to the total volume forcefully exhaled (FVC) less than the lower limit of normal (LLN). The LLN is based on distributions from healthy normal populations and is preferred to using a fixed cutoff (eg, 70%) because the LLN accounts for the expected decline in FEV_1/FVC that occurs with aging. Postbronchodilator responsiveness is defined by an increase in FEV_1 or FVC by greater than 12% and greater than 200 mL after bronchodilator.[14] These thresholds are provided by guidelines,[15,16] which acknowledge clinical context should be taken into account when interpreting test results. For example, a patient who has a 10% improvement in FEV_1 after bronchodilator and who demonstrates improvement in prebronchodilator FEV_1 after a trial of inhaled corticosteroids (ICS) would have had a clinically significant response that is highly consistent with a diagnosis of asthma, despite falling short of the 12% and 200-mL threshold.

If spirometry is normal, but clinical suspicion for asthma remains, repetition of spirometry at another time point is essential, because at least one episode of obstruction should be documented to support the diagnosis of asthma. Variability in airflow limitation, if not identifiable by reversibility on spirometry, may also be documented by serial testing with a peak flow meter. The patient is instructed to record the best of 3 attempted peak flows twice daily (generally morning and evening) over a 2-week period or more often during periods of respiratory symptoms. Excessive variability in peak flows in the setting of normal spirometry can also diagnose variable airflow limitation; this is defined by a 1-week average of each day's highest to lowest recorded measurement, divided by the day's average, greater than 10%.[15]

Bronchoprovocation testing for airway hyperresponsiveness, such as a methacholine challenge, has a low specificity for asthma. Airway hyperresponsiveness is present in other pulmonary conditions, including COPD, and in the normal population, where the prevalence has ranged from 4% to 37%.[17] This test has consequently become less used in the confirmation of asthma but retains a role in select populations to rule out asthma given its high negative predictive value, which has been reported to approach 100%.[18,19]

Unless the patient is highly symptomatic at initial presentation, the preferred approach is a stepwise diagnostic process that involves spirometry or peak flow testing to establish both obstruction and variable airflow limitation. Identifying asthma-related obstruction is challenging when patients are already on asthma medications. A recent Canadian study suggested that as many as one-third of individuals with a physician diagnosis of asthma did not truly have it. These patients were less likely to have had formal testing for airflow limitation, and study findings reinforce the value of objective testing to support the diagnosis of asthma.[20]

Radiographic studies and blood tests are generally unnecessary in the diagnostic process unless there is suspicion for an alternative diagnosis. Elevations in eosinophils, immunoglobulin E (IgE), or allergen-specific IgE, although helpful in diagnosing allergic disease or when considering advanced therapies, is neither sensitive nor specific for the initial diagnosis of asthma. Fractional exhaled nitric oxide (FeNO) is a marker of eosinophilic airway inflammation but is typically unnecessary in the diagnosis of asthma.

Variants of Asthma

Individuals with cough-variant asthma manifest cough as their primary symptom.[21,22] It is thought that the cough is a neural response to bronchoconstriction rather than from mucus secretion, but the exact mechanism is unknown.[23] These individuals typically do not complain of wheeze, and the differential necessarily revolves around other causes of chronic cough.

Exercise-induced asthma occurs in individuals who experience symptoms after vigorous physical activity due to excessive airway sensitivity to cold or dry air that occurs during exercise-associated hyperventilation.[24] These individuals complain of typical asthma symptoms shortly after finishing exercise that lasts for up to 1 hour afterward.

Aspirin-exacerbated respiratory disease (AERD) is asthma that is precipitated or worsened by medications that inhibit cyclo-oxygenase 1, an enzyme involved in degradation of proinflammatory leukotrienes. It is also known as Samter's triad, which describes the combination of asthma, aspirin sensitivity, and sinus disease with nasal polyposis. The condition is somewhat of a misnomer, in that all nonsteroidal anti-inflammatory drugs, not only aspirin, can precipitate worsening. AERD is typically more severe and uncontrolled than other forms of asthma; it is present in approximately 14% of patients with severe asthma and 7% of all comers with asthma.[25]

Vocal cord dysfunction (VCD) is not a variant of asthma but deserves special mention, because it is a classic mimic of asthma that may also be a comorbid condition. In VCD, there is paradoxic closure of the vocal cords mainly during inspiration, causing wheezing and dyspnea.[26] VCD should be considered in patients who have sudden onset wheezing, occurring predominantly during inspiration, which is short in duration with limited or no response to asthma medications. For those with VCD, including those with coexisting asthma, speech therapy by a therapist knowledgeable about VCD can be very beneficial, and it is important to recognize this condition in order to provide treatment.

MANAGEMENT

Because asthma by definition demonstrates variability in symptoms and airflow limitation, its successful management involves continual reassessment over time to optimize disease control and treat underlying inflammation while minimizing side effects from prescribed medications. At each visit, the clinician should assess symptoms, risk of worsening, medication tolerance and adherence, and comorbidities. **Fig. 2** lists a typical stepwise approach for a patient with established or newly diagnosed asthma. With optimal treatment, the vast majority of patients can expect to be well controlled.

Assessment of Asthma Control Versus Asthma Severity

Asthma severity may be assessed before the initiation of medical therapy, based on lung function, symptom frequency, and history of exacerbations. Severity is helpful in guiding initial therapeutic decisions and is classified as intermittent, mild persistent, moderate persistent, or severe persistent. The classification of mild intermittent is no longer recommended because it implies that other severities cannot also be intermittently symptomatic. Importantly, asthma severity is not a static property and should be reassessed at each visit with reclassification based on the magnitude of treatment needed to control, or alleviate the symptoms of, asthma. Asthma severity reflects the intensity of the overall disease process, and changes in asthma severity may indicate new environmental exposures, comorbidities, or advancing disease.

At each visit, a patient's asthma control, the frequency of a patient's asthma symptoms and their associated effects, should be assessed. Both EPR-3 and GINA suggest assessing control by 4 frequency questions over a 2- to 4-week recall: days with asthma symptoms, days with nocturnal awakening, days of activity limitation due to asthma, and days of rescue inhaler use outside of those taken before exercise.[15,16]

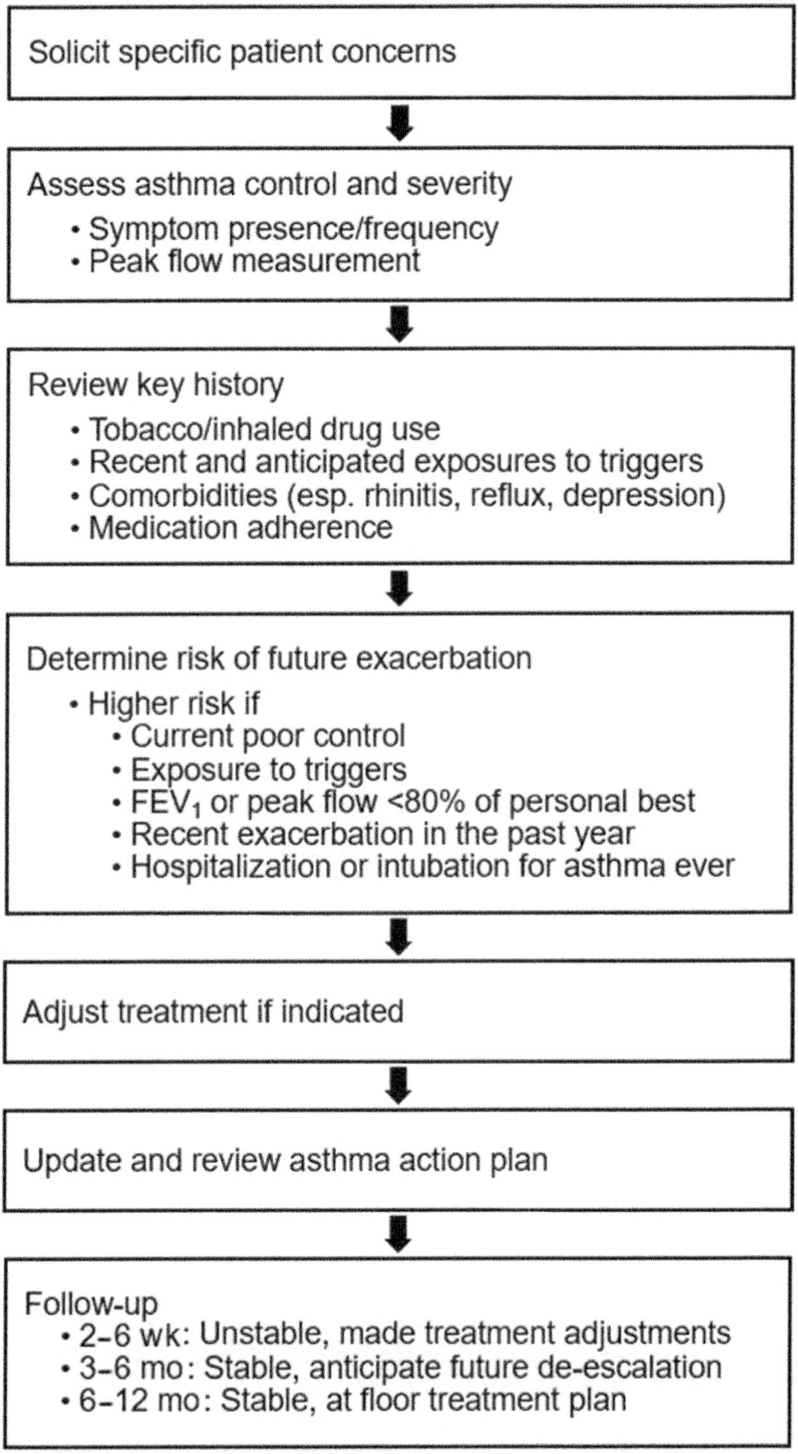

Solicit specific patient concerns

Assess asthma control and severity
- Symptom presence/frequency
- Peak flow measurement

Review key history
- Tobacco/inhaled drug use
- Recent and anticipated exposures to triggers
- Comorbidities (esp. rhinitis, reflux, depression)
- Medication adherence

Determine risk of future exacerbation

- Higher risk if
    - Current poor control
    - Exposure to triggers
    - FEV_1 or peak flow <80% of personal best
    - Recent exacerbation in the past year
    - Hospitalization or intubation for asthma ever

Adjust treatment if indicated

Update and review asthma action plan

Follow-up
- 2–6 wk: Unstable, made treatment adjustments
- 3–6 mo: Stable, anticipate future de-escalation
- 6–12 mo: Stable, at floor treatment plan

Fig. 2. Progression of an outpatient visit for asthma.

Asthma is considered well controlled if there are 2 or less days of symptoms, 2 or less days of rescue inhaler use, and no days nocturnal awakening or activity limitation due to asthma, over the prior 2 weeks. The use of patient-completed questionnaires that assess asthma control, such as the Asthma Control Test or Asthma Control Question-naire, can be applied in clinical settings and provides improved sensitivity to detect changes in control over time.[27,28]

Although both control and severity may be expected to change over time, they are distinct concepts: a patient with uncontrolled asthma does not necessarily have se-vere asthma. Furthermore, several factors may confound assessment, including improper inhaler technique, barriers to adherence, ongoing exposure to triggers, and contributing comorbidities, all of which should be queried in the setting of poor control. Importantly, asthma control is more relevant than asthma severity for predict-ing risk of future exacerbation.[29]

Finally, prebronchodilator spirometry, with attention to FEV_1, should be routinely performed. Individuals with prebronchodilator FEV_1 below the LLN likely represent un-controlled disease and are at increased risk for subsequent exacerbation.[30,31] Tailoring asthma therapy based on sputum eosinophilia or FeNO has been associated with reduced exacerbations, but there is insufficient evidence to support implement-ing this in clinical practice.[32]

Nonpharmacologic Interventions

Avoidance of triggers is a cornerstone of asthma management. Common triggers and strategies to address them are included in **Table 2**. In those with seasonal allergies or sensitivity to air pollution, patients are advised to stay indoors and close windows

Table 2
Common asthma triggers and suggested remediation strategies

Trigger[a]	Strategies
Ambient air pollution	Remain indoors during poor air quality days
Certain foods	Test for food-specific allergies, avoidance
Cigarette smoke	Smoking cessation assistance, home smoking ban
Cockroaches	Sweep and vacuum regularly, use roach traps
Combustion smoke	Avoid use of wood-burning fireplaces
Dust mites	Use mattress and pillowcase covers, avoid down-filled pillows and blankets, wash bedding regularly
Emotional distress	Address comorbid depression, involve behavioral specialists
Fragrances	Avoidance
Indoor air pollution	Reduce source exposure (eg, perform maintenance to reduce NO_2 from appliances, such as gas stoves and gas heaters); routinely change central air filters; portable air purifiers
Molds	Address leaks, reduce home humidity
Pets	Remove or keep pets outdoors
Pollens	Remain indoors during morning through midday when specific agent is pollinating
Weather events (eg, rain, heat)	Remain indoors during weather events

[a] Trigger-specific strategies should only be suggested if patient is sensitive to that trigger; each pa-tient will have different patterns of asthma triggers.

during periods of high pollen counts or poor outdoor air quality, respectively. Importantly, the timing of pollen avoidance is specific to each patient's aeroallergen sensitization profile, which should be determined if there is a strong history of seasonal allergies and requires referral to an allergist. Avoidance of secondhand smoke and smoking cessation are emphasized.[33] Avoidance of indoor allergens, targeting specific allergens to which the patient is sensitized, is recommended but is difficult to implement because of difficulties in achieving total allergen remediation and cost of interventions.[34,35]

A common option is to treat symptomatic gastroesophageal reflux disease, under the premise that acid reflux may precipitate bronchoconstriction. However, objective evidence of efficacy in improving asthma control or severity in adults is inconsistent.[36] Similarly, treatment of allergic rhinitis may also be attempted, although benefit in asthma for those who are already on ICS may be small.[37]

Adults with asthma should receive an early dose of the PPSV23 vaccine before age 65.[38] Recommendations are otherwise not different from healthy adults.

As part of overall health maintenance, overweight or obese patients should be counseled on weight reduction, and all patients should be encouraged to consume a healthy diet. Interventional studies have demonstrated improvement in asthma severity and control with weight reduction, with magnitude in the order of 10 to 15 kgs.[39]

Pharmacologic Therapy

Pharmacologic therapy is broadly divided into controller medications and rescue medications. Asthma treatment guidelines organize drug treatment for asthma into therapeutic steps, with higher steps reflecting more intense controller treatment. A diagram of recommended medications adapted from GINA is included in **Fig. 3**. More

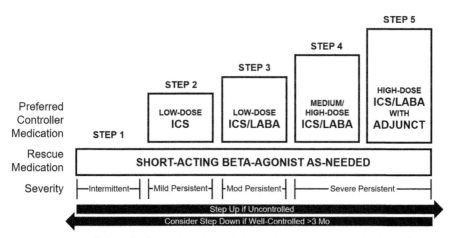

Fig. 3. Steps of asthma pharmacologic treatment. Adjunct therapies include a long-acting muscarinic antagonist or biologic therapies in selected populations. Immune therapy may be considered for persistent asthma (steps 2–5). Leukotriene modifiers may be considered as an alternative to LABA but are generally less effective. Mod., moderate. (*Adapted from* Bateman ED, Hurd SS, Barnes PJ, et al. Global strategy for asthma management and prevention: GINA executive summary. Eur Respir J 2008;31(1):157; and National Asthma Education and Prevention Program. Expert panel report 3: guidelines for the diagnosis and management of asthma. Washington (DC): US Department of Health and Human Services, National Heart, Lung, and Blood Institute; 2007. p. 343; with permission.)

detailed charts that include alternative options are available from the source publications.[15,16]

Controller Medications

The general goal of controller therapy is to intervene in the inflammatory process underlying asthma and to prevent the development of irreversible airway remodeling. To this end, controller therapies are offered to all individuals with persistent asthma, even those with mild disease. Patients should be counseled that asthma is a chronic condition, and that the absence of asthma symptoms is the result of effective controller use. The conceptualization of "no symptoms, no asthma" is strongly associated with worse outcomes.[40]

ICS form the backbone of controller therapy. Common side effects include oral thrush, which may be ameliorated through the use of a spacer device and rinsing the mouth after ICS use, and dysphonia, which may be anecdotally improved by switching to a different delivery device. Long-acting beta agonists (LABA) or leukotriene modifiers may be added to ICS if control is suboptimal, with the former option more effective than the latter.[41,42] Long-acting muscarinic antagonists, which are commonly used in COPD, do not appear to be superior to LABA as add-on therapy in asthma and are typically reserved for severe disease.[43,44] Importantly, there is an absolute contraindication to LABA monotherapy (ie, without concurrent ICS) because of a consistent association with increased asthma-related mortality; LABA monotherapy is inappropriate and should never be prescribed for a patient with asthma.

Rescue Medications

A rescue inhaler in the form of albuterol should be offered to all patients. This short-acting medication provides immediate bronchodilation in patients with acute symptoms and may be performed up to 4 times a day. To an adult patient with appropriate instruction, albuterol delivered by metered-dose inhaler (MDI) without spacer, MDI with spacer, or nebulizer is equally effective. However, in practice, spacers and nebulizers can deliver medication more reliably.[45,46] Patients with intermittent asthma may achieve control with a short-acting beta-agonist alone; those with persistent asthma (ie, use their albuterol inhaler more than twice weekly to resolve symptoms) necessitate addition of ICS.

The importance of verifying inhaler technique and adherence cannot be overstated. As many as two-thirds of patients have errors in MDI use, leading to suboptimal delivery of medication and worse asthma control.[47,48] Videos demonstrating the proper use of an MDI and other devices are available from the US Centers for Disease Control and Prevention (CDC)[49] and the American Lung Association.[50] Verification of inhaler technique will only become more important as manufacturers develop increasingly specialized delivery devices.

Similarly, medication adherence, the proportion of scheduled doses that are actually taken, should also be queried. Dose counters and pharmacy data, if logistically possible, are valuable objective sources of adherence information. Studies estimate average adult ICS adherence in the range of 22% to 63%, suggesting that true corticosteroid doses may be as much as half the amount on a patient's medication list.[51] Aside from older age and belief in medication necessity, there are no consistent factors that are associated with nonadherence.[52] Unfortunately, very few adherence interventions have shown improvement in asthma outcomes, highlighting the complexity of this important aspect of asthma care.[51,53]

Initiating and Modifying Treatment

For the patient who is beginning therapy, professional recommendations provide guidance regarding medication initiation based on severity assessment.[15,16]

For the well-controlled patient who is already on therapy, symptom free over the past 3 months, deescalation may be considered. The goal is to decrease risk of adverse effects associated with inappropriately intensive treatment and to find the therapeutic "floor," allowing adequate ascertainment of disease severity. The patient should be counseled to return to the higher treatment step if there is evidence of worsening control, including decreased peak flow or increased symptoms.

For the uncontrolled patient who is already on therapy, a recurrent search for precipitating factors may reveal environmental changes (providing an opportunity for environmental counseling) or a lapse in inhaler adherence (providing an opportunity to reinforce inhaler need and adherence). Temporary or permanent escalation of therapy by 1 to 2 steps may be necessary to regain or establish control. Symptoms that continue to worsen and are unresponsive to escalation in therapy should prompt a search for an alternative or overlapping diagnosis (see **Table 1**).

In selected cases, if a patient is thought to have uncontrolled disease because of technical (cannot reliably coordinate the actuation with inspiration, necessary for MDI) or physiologic reasons (inability to take in a rapid breath, necessary for dry powder inhalers), he or she may be switched to a different delivery device of the same equivalent dose of medication. Overall, there is no delivery device that is clearly superior to another among all patients.

Self-Management and the Asthma Action Plan

Asthma self-management involves empowerment of the patient to avoid triggers and modify his or her treatment regimen in response to changes in symptoms or in lung function.

The foundation of asthma self-management is an asthma action plan. Patients are provided with a peak flow meter, and a personal best measurement *for that device* is determined during a period of good control; the use of prediction equations for peak flows do not perform well, likely due to variation in accuracy between devices and patients.[54] Patients then check their peak flows daily or when experiencing worsened symptoms, and depending on the value are classified as in the green ($\geq$80% of personal best), yellow (50%–79% of personal best), or red zone (<50% of personal best). Alternatively, patients may be classified based solely on symptoms, whereby experiencing any wheezing, cough, or nocturnal awakening classifies a patient in the yellow zone, and experiencing severe symptoms, including inability to perform any of their usual activities or disabling shortness of breath, classifies a patient in the red zone. A combination of both approaches is encouraged, particularly in patients with poor recognition of symptoms progression.

Options for yellow zone interventions vary, but generally involve rescue inhaler use, notification of the physician and possible step-up in controller medication, and initiation of an oral corticosteroid if symptoms and peak flow do not normalize within a specific time period. Doubling of ICS in the yellow zone does not appear to be effective, but quadrupling of ICS has been shown to reduce risk of progressing to oral corticosteroids or having an acute asthma visit by 20%, at the expense of increased dysphonia and oral thrush.[55] Patients in the red zone should immediately use their rescue inhaler and contact the physician or present to an emergency department.

Physicians may consider a step-up in controller regimen relative to preexacerbation regimen.

Self-management strategies have been shown to prevent exacerbations, decrease asthma-related health care utilization, and improve quality of life.[56] Using peak flow measurement or symptoms to guide management appears to be generally equivalent.[57] Asthma action plan forms are available from the CDC, the National Institutes of Health, and the American Lung Association.[58–60]

Other Treatment Options in Severe Asthma

Additional therapeutic options may be warranted in severe asthma, and consideration of advanced therapies should trigger referral to a pulmonologist and/or an allergist-immunologist.[61]

Recent advances in biologic therapies have resulted in several new medications available for severe asthma with emerging treatments in the pipeline. The indications for these are based on individual patient characteristics, and such medications are typically administered in consultation with a subspecialist.

The allergic inflammatory pathway is a common target. Omalizumab is an antibody against serum IgE, an immunoglobulin that interfaces with mast cells, eosinophils, and basophils in the allergic cascade.[62] It is approved in patients with moderate to severe asthma with documented allergen sensitivity that is not controlled with ICS and is administered every 2 to 4 weeks. Mepolizumab, reslizumab, and benralizumab are antibodies targeting the interleukin-5 pathway, involved in recruitment and activation of eosinophils.[63–65] They are approved in the United States for patients with severe asthma and persistent eosinophilia despite adequate ICS therapy and are administered every 4 to 8 weeks in health care settings, subcutaneously for mepolizumab and benralizumab, and intravenously for reslizumab. For patients with difficult-to-control asthma and prominent allergies, subcutaneous immunotherapy has been shown to reduce asthma severity, need for systemic corticosteroids, and need for rescue inhaler use.[66] There is a small risk of anaphylaxis, but literature is insufficient to comment on its magnitude and severity.

Bronchial thermoplasty (BT) is an endoscopic procedure whereby radiofrequency heat energy is applied to the airways, ablating airway smooth muscle and reducing its ability to cause bronchoconstriction.[67] Evidence suggests that BT reduces exacerbations, reduces asthma-related health care utilization, and improves quality of life in individuals with severe asthma.[68] This procedure is typically performed by experienced centers only and is associated with transient increase in exacerbation risk during the treatment course.

Risk Assessment and Follow-Up

At the conclusion of the visit, the risk of future asthma exacerbation or poor outcomes is assessed. Major factors that are currently considered are uncontrolled disease, abnormal FEV_1, unmitigated recent exposure to a known personal trigger, and history of exacerbations requiring hospitalization or intubation. Patients who display one or more of these features, including those who had therapy modification in the present visit, should have a short interval follow-up, generally within 2 to 6 weeks. Patients at lower risk can be seen every 3 months, and these visits may be spaced further to every 6 months or annually pending optimization of therapy and disease stability. The optimal interval for repeat lung function testing is unknown, but is recommended by consensus opinion to be every 1 to 2 years in those with stable disease, with attention to development of fixed obstruction, which is suggestive of chronically inadequate control.

ACUTE OUTPATIENT EXACERBATIONS OF ASTHMA

For the outpatient presenting with acute worsening of asthma symptoms, a focused history and physical examination will readily guide management. On history, recent sick contacts, abrupt discontinuation of controller therapies, and exposure to personal asthma triggers should be inquired about. Most acute exacerbations are precipitated by viral respiratory infections, in particular, rhinovirus.[69] The pace of symptom worsening should be documented. On examination, signs of infection and overall respiratory status should be evaluated. Hypoxemia, use of accessory muscles, inspiratory and expiratory wheezing, and absence of wheezing associated with respiratory discomfort are worrisome symptoms. If the patient is able to safely perform respiratory maneuvers and does not require immediate emergency referral, serial peak flow determinations should be performed before and after in-office albuterol. Radiographic abnormalities are rare in an uncomplicated exacerbation, and chest imaging is not routinely performed.

Nebulizers and MDIs (with spacers) are equivalent when used in the acute setting and are dependent on preference.[70] The optimal dosing of albuterol appears to be 2.5-mg aliquots every 20 minutes (for nebulizer) or 3 to 5 puffs (for MDI) every 10 minutes, up to 3 times.[71,72] In addition to removal from exposure to triggers, oral corticosteroids are the mainstay treatment of asthma exacerbation and intervention in the underlying inflammatory response. Doses higher than 40 to 100 mg of prednisone daily or longer than 5 to 10 days do not appear to be superior.[73] In general, tapering is unnecessary. If symptoms and peak flow have returned to baseline on completion of corticosteroids and the inciting factor can be avoided, patients may resume their green zone treatment regimen. Otherwise, maintenance treatment may need to be escalated to the next step of the treatment ladder pending reevaluation, or in selected cases, oral corticosteroids may be extended.

Despite progress made in the protocolization of asthma treatment, decision for referral to the emergency department remains a clinical one, combining consideration of disease trajectory, potential ongoing exposure to trigger, and ability of patient to manage necessary therapies on an outpatient basis. Patients should be seen within 2 weeks after an exacerbation to reassess symptoms, lung function, and appropriateness of current controller therapy. Asthma exacerbations, especially those associated with hospitalization or emergency department treatment, have been associated with long-term declines in lung function,[74,75] and prevention should be emphasized.

Box 1
Common indications for specialist referral

Alternative pulmonary diagnosis suspected

Asthma diagnosis suspected, but confirmation elusive

Possible occupational asthma

Persistently uncontrolled disease

More than 1 exacerbation in past year

History of life-threatening exacerbation

Difficulty with medication selection

Difficulty managing asthma due to comorbidities

Severe disease requiring specialized therapy

INDICATIONS FOR SPECIALIST REFERRAL

With adequate training, the vast majority of asthma may be successfully managed in the primary care setting.[76] However, specialist referral may be warranted in some cases, especially in patients with persistently uncontrolled or severe asthma, or in patients in whom the diagnosis of asthma is unclear. Involvement of specialist care, through either pulmonology or allergy, has been associated with improved outcomes.[76,77] **Box 1** lists common indications for referral.

REFERENCES

1. Villarroel MA, Blackwell DL. Percentage of adults aged 18-64 years with current asthma,* by State-National Health Interview Survey,(Dagger) 2014-2016. Atlanta (GA): Centers Disease Control 1600 Clifton Rd; 2018. 30333 USA.
2. CDC - Asthma - Most recent asthma data. 2018. Available at: https://www.cdc.gov/asthma/most_recent_data.htm. Accessed September 14, 2018.
3. Mazurek JM. Prevalence of asthma, asthma attacks, and Emergency Department visits for asthma among working adults — national health interview survey, 2011–2016. MMWR Morb Mortal Wkly Rep 2018;67. https://doi.org/10.15585/mmwr.mm6713a1.
4. Winer RA, Qin X, Harrington T, et al. Asthma incidence among children and adults: findings from the behavioral risk factor surveillance system asthma callback survey—United States, 2006–2008. J Asthma 2012;49(1):16–22.
5. Huovinen E, Kaprio J, Koskenvuo M. Factors associated to lifestyle and risk of adult onset asthma. Respir Med 2003;97(3):273–80.
6. Guerra S, Sherrill DL, Martinez FD, et al. Rhinitis as an independent risk factor for adult-onset asthma. J Allergy Clin Immunol 2002;109(3):419–25.
7. Jamrozik E, Knuiman MW, James A, et al. Risk factors for adult-onset asthma: a 14-year longitudinal study. Respirology 2009;14(6):814–21.
8. Shen H, Hua W, Wang P, et al. A new phenotype of asthma: chest tightness as the sole presenting manifestation. Ann Allergy Asthma Immunol 2013;111(3):226–7.
9. Dixon AE. Rhinosinusitis and asthma: the missing link. Curr Opin Pulm Med 2009;15(1):19–24.
10. Vernon MK, Wiklund I, Bell JA, et al. What do we know about asthma triggers? a review of the literature. J Asthma 2012;49(10):991–8.
11. Henneberger PK, Redlich CA, Callahan DB, et al. An official American Thoracic Society statement: work-exacerbated asthma. Am J Respir Crit Care Med 2011;184(3):368–78.
12. Tarlo SM, Lemiere C. Occupational asthma. N Engl J Med 2014;370(7):640–9.
13. Work-related asthma: number of cases by classification and state, 2009–2012. Available at: https://wwwn.cdc.gov/eworld/Data/Work-related_asthma_Number_of_cases_by_classification_and_state_20092012/924. Accessed September 14, 2018.
14. Pellegrino R, Viegi G, Brusasco V, et al. Interpretative strategies for lung function tests. Eur Respir J 2005;26(5):948–68.
15. Bateman ED, Hurd SS, Barnes PJ, et al. Global strategy for asthma management and prevention: GINA executive summary (vol 31, pg 143, 2008). Eur Respir J 2018;51(2):143–78.
16. Busse WW, Boushey HA, Camargo CA, et al. Expert panel report 3: guidelines for the diagnosis and management of asthma. Washington (DC): US Department of Health and Human Services, National Heart Lung and Blood Institute; 2007. p. 1–417.

17. Borak J, Lefkowitz RY. Bronchial hyperresponsiveness. Occup Med (Lond) 2016; 66(2):95–105.
18. Cockcroft DW. Direct challenge tests: airway hyperresponsiveness in asthma: its measurement and clinical significance. Chest 2010;138(2, Supplement): 18S–24S.
19. Cockcroft DW, Murdock KY, Berscheid BA, et al. Sensitivity and specificity of histamine PC20 determination in a random selection of young college students. J Allergy Clin Immunol 1992;89(1, Part 1):23–30.
20. Aaron SD, Vandemheen KL, FitzGerald JM, et al. Reevaluation of diagnosis in adults with physician-diagnosed asthma. JAMA 2017;317(3):269–79.
21. Desai D, Brightling C. Cough due to asthma, cough-variant asthma and non-asthmatic eosinophilic bronchitis. Otolaryngol Clin North Am 2010;43(1):123–30.
22. Corrao W, Braman S, Irwin R. Chronic cough as the sole presenting manifestation of bronchial asthma. N Engl J Med 1979;300:633–7.
23. Niimi A. Cough and asthma. Curr Respir Med Rev 2011;7(1):47–54.
24. McFadden ER, Gilbert IA. Exercise-induced asthma. N Engl J Med 1994;330(19): 1362–7.
25. Rajan JP, Wineinger NE, Stevenson DD, et al. Prevalence of aspirin-exacerbated respiratory disease among asthmatic patients: a meta-analysis of the literature. J Allergy Clin Immunol 2015;135(3):676–81.e1.
26. Kenn K, Balkissoon R. Vocal cord dysfunction: what do we know? Eur Respir J 2011;37(1):194–200.
27. Schatz M, Sorkness CA, Li JT, et al. Asthma control test: reliability, validity, and responsiveness in patients not previously followed by asthma specialists. J Allergy Clin Immunol 2006;117(3):549–56.
28. Juniper EF, O'Byrne PM, Guyatt GH, et al. Development and validation of a questionnaire to measure asthma control. Eur Respir J 1999;14(4):902–7.
29. Cockcroft DW, Swystun VA. Asthma control versus asthma severity. J Allergy Clin Immunol 1996;98(6):1016–8.
30. Kitch BT, Paltiel AD, Kuntz KM, et al. A single measure of FEV1 is associated with risk of asthma attacks in long-term follow-up. Chest 2004;126(6):1875–82.
31. Osborne ML, Pedula KL, O'Hollaren M, et al. Assessing future need for acute care in adult asthmatics: the Profile of Asthma Risk Study: a prospective health maintenance organization-based study. Chest 2007;132(4):1151–61.
32. Petsky HL, Cates CJ, Kew KM, et al. Tailoring asthma treatment on eosinophilic markers (exhaled nitric oxide or sputum eosinophils): a systematic review and meta-analysis. Thorax 2018. https://doi.org/10.1136/thoraxjnl-2018-211540.
33. Gautier C, Charpin D. Environmental triggers and avoidance in the management of asthma. J Asthma Allergy 2017;10:47–56.
34. Gøtzsche PC, Johansen HK. House dust mite control measures for asthma. Cochrane Database Syst Rev 2008;(2). https://doi.org/10.1002/14651858. CD001187.pub3.
35. Platts-Mills TAE. Allergen avoidance in the treatment of asthma and rhinitis. N Engl J Med 2003;349(3):207–8.
36. Gibson PG, Henry R, Coughlan JJ. Gastro-oesophageal reflux treatment for asthma in adults and children. Cochrane Database Syst Rev 2003;(1). https://doi.org/10.1002/14651858.CD001496.
37. Taramarcaz P, Gibson PG. Intranasal corticosteroids for asthma control in people with coexisting asthma and rhinitis. Cochrane Database Syst Rev 2003;(3). https://doi.org/10.1002/14651858.CD003570.

38. Kim DK, Riley LE, Hunter P. Recommended immunization schedule for adults aged 19 years or older, United States, 2018. Ann Intern Med 2018;168(3):210–20.
39. Juel CT-B, Ali Z, Nilas L, et al. Asthma and obesity: does weight loss improve asthma control? a systematic review. J Asthma Allergy 2012;5:21–6.
40. Halm EA, Mora P, Leventhal H. No symptoms, no asthma: the acute episodic disease belief is associated with poor self-management among inner-city adults with persistent asthma. Chest 2006;129(3):573–80.
41. Chauhan BF, Ducharme FM. Addition to inhaled corticosteroids of long-acting beta2-agonists versus anti-leukotrienes for chronic asthma. Cochrane Database Syst Rev 2014;(1). https://doi.org/10.1002/14651858.CD003137.pub5.
42. Ducharme F, Ni Chroinin M, Greenstone I, et al. The addition of long-acting beta2-agonists to inhaled steroids compared to higher doses of inhaled steroids alone as maintenance treatment for chronic asthma. Cochrane Database Syst Rev 2010;(4). https://doi.org/10.1002/14651858.CD005533.pub2.
43. Kew K, Dahri K. Long-acting muscarinic antagonists (LAMA) added to combination long-acting beta2-agonists and inhaled corticosteroids (LABA/ICS) versus LABA/ICS for adults with asthma. Cochrane Database Syst Rev 2016;(1). https://doi.org/10.1002/14651858.CD011721.pub2.
44. Sobieraj DM, Baker WL, Nguyen E, et al. Association of inhaled corticosteroids and long-acting muscarinic antagonists with asthma control in patients with uncontrolled, persistent asthma: a systematic review and meta-analysis. JAMA 2018;319(14):1473–84.
45. Newman KB, Milne S, Hamilton C, et al. A comparison of albuterol administered by metered-dose inhaler and spacer with albuterol by nebulizer in adults presenting to an urban emergency department with acute asthma. Chest 2002;121(4):1036–41.
46. Newman SP. Spacer devices for metered dose inhalers. Clin Pharmacokinet 2004;43(6):349–60.
47. Sanchis J, Gich I, Pedersen S. Systematic review of errors in inhaler use: has patient technique improved over time? Chest 2016;150(2):394–406.
48. Price D, Bosnic-Anticevich S, Briggs A, et al. Inhaler competence in asthma: common errors, barriers to use and recommended solutions. Respir Med 2013;107(1):37–46.
49. CDC - Asthma - Using an asthma inhaler videos. 2018. Available at: https://www.cdc.gov/asthma/inhaler_video/default.htm. Accessed September 15, 2018.
50. Asthma patient resources and videos. Available at: http://www.lung.org/lung-health-and-diseases/lung-disease-lookup/asthma/patient-resources-and-videos/. Accessed September 15, 2018.
51. Bårnes CB, Ulrik CS. Asthma and adherence to inhaled corticosteroids: current status and future perspectives. Respir Care 2015. https://doi.org/10.4187/respcare.03200.
52. Dima AL, Hernandez G, Cunillera O, et al. Asthma inhaler adherence determinants in adults: systematic review of observational data. Eur Respir J 2015;45(4):994–1018.
53. Gamble J, Stevenson M, Heaney LG. A study of a multi-level intervention to improve non-adherence in difficult to control asthma. Respir Med 2011;105(9):1308–15.
54. Miller MR, Dickinson SA, Hitchings DJ. The accuracy of portable peak flow meters. Thorax 1992;47(11):904–9.
55. McKeever T, Mortimer K, Wilson A, et al. Quadrupling inhaled glucocorticoid dose to abort asthma exacerbations. N Engl J Med 2018;378:902–10.

56. Gibson PG, Powell H, Wilson A, et al. Self-management education and regular practitioner review for adults with asthma. Cochrane Database Syst Rev 2002;(3). https://doi.org/10.1002/14651858.CD001117.
57. Powell H, Gibson PG. Options for self-management education for adults with asthma. Cochrane Database Syst Rev 2002;(3). https://doi.org/10.1002/14651858.CD004107.
58. Asthma Action Plan | National Heart, Lung, and Blood Institute (NHLBI). Available at: https://www.nhlbi.nih.gov/health-topics/all-publications-and-resources/asthma-action-plan. Accessed September 17, 2018.
59. CDC - Asthma - tools for asthma control. 2018. Available at: https://www.cdc.gov/asthma/tools_for_control.htm. Accessed September 17, 2018.
60. Create an asthma action plan | American Lung Association. Available at: https://www.lung.org/lung-health-and-diseases/lung-disease-lookup/asthma/living-with-asthma/managing-asthma/create-an-asthma-action-plan.html. Accessed September 17, 2018.
61. Chung KF, Wenzel SE, Brozek JL, et al. International ERS/ATS guidelines on definition, evaluation and treatment of severe asthma. Eur Respir J 2014;43(2): 343–73.
62. Thomson NC, Chaudhuri R. Omalizumab: clinical use for the management of asthma. Clin Med Insights Circ Respir Pulm Med 2012;6:27–40.
63. Ortega HG, Liu MC, Pavord ID, et al. Mepolizumab treatment in patients with severe eosinophilic asthma. N Engl J Med 2014;371(13):1198–207.
64. Castro M, Zangrilli J, Wechsler ME, et al. Reslizumab for inadequately controlled asthma with elevated blood eosinophil counts: results from two multicentre, parallel, double-blind, randomised, placebo-controlled, phase 3 trials. Lancet Respir Med 2015;3(5):355–66.
65. FitzGerald JM, Bleecker ER, Nair P, et al. Benralizumab, an anti-interleukin-5 receptor α monoclonal antibody, as add-on treatment for patients with severe, uncontrolled, eosinophilic asthma (CALIMA): a randomised, double-blind, placebo-controlled phase 3 trial. Lancet 2016;388(10056):2128–41.
66. Lin SY, Azar A, Suarez-Cuervo C, et al. The role of immunotherapy in the treatment of asthma. Rockville (MD): Agency for Healthcare Research and Quality (US); 2018. Available at: http://www.ncbi.nlm.nih.gov/books/NBK513535/. Accessed September 16, 2018.
67. Dombret M-C, Alagha K, Boulet LP, et al. Bronchial thermoplasty: a new therapeutic option for the treatment of severe, uncontrolled asthma in adults. Eur Respir Rev 2014;23(134):510–8.
68. Chupp G, Laviolette M, Cohn L, et al. Long-term outcomes of bronchial thermoplasty in subjects with severe asthma: a comparison of 3-year follow-up results from two prospective multicentre studies. Eur Respir J 2017;50(2). https://doi.org/10.1183/13993003.00017-2017.
69. Dougherty RH, Fahy JV. Acute exacerbations of asthma: epidemiology, biology and the exacerbation-prone phenotype. Clin Exp Allergy 2009;39(2):193–202.
70. Cates CJ, Bara A, Crilly JA, et al. Holding chambers versus nebulisers for beta-agonist treatment of acute asthma. Cochrane Database Syst Rev 2003;(2). https://doi.org/10.1002/14651858.CD000052.
71. Strauss L, Hejal R, Galan G, et al. Observations on the effects of aerosolized albuterol in acute asthma. Am J Respir Crit Care Med 1997;155(2):454–8.
72. McFadden ER, Elsanadi N, Dixon L, et al. Protocol therapy for acute asthma: therapeutic benefits and cost savings. Am J Med 1995;99(6):651–61.

73. Krishnan JA, Davis SQ, Naureckas ET, et al. An umbrella review: corticosteroid therapy for adults with acute asthma. Am J Med 2009;122(11):977–91.
74. O'Byrne P, Pedersen S, Lamm CJ, et al. Severe Exacerbations and decline in lung function in asthma | American Journal of Respiratory and Critical Care Medicine. Am J Respir Crit Care Med 2008;179:19–24.
75. Bai TR, Vonk JM, Postma DS, et al. Severe exacerbations predict excess lung function decline in asthma. Eur Respir J 2007;30(3):452–6.
76. Wu AW, Young Y, Skinner EA, et al. Quality of care and outcomes of adults with asthma treated by specialists and generalists in managed care. Arch Intern Med 2001;161(21):2554–60.
77. Laforest L, Ganse EV, Devouassoux G, et al. Management of asthma in patients supervised by primary care physicians or by specialists. Eur Respir J 2006;27(1): 42–50.

Chronic Obstructive Pulmonary Disease
Evaluation and Management

Sean P. Duffy, MD*, Gerard J. Criner, MD

KEYWORDS

- COPD • Emphysema • Chronic bronchitis • Acute exacerbation

KEY POINTS

- COPD is a common, preventable disease of fixed airflow limitation that accounts for the third most deaths of any disease process in the United States.
- Cigarette smoking is by far the most important risk factor in the development of COPD and smoking cessation is the intervention with the greatest impact on the natural history of the disease.
- Pharmacologic therapy with inhaled corticosteroids and long-acting bronchodilators has proven to reduce exacerbations and improve symptoms.
- Advanced treatments, such as lung volume reduction surgery and bronchoscopic lung volume reduction, have been shown to improve symptoms in patients with significant hyperinflation and gas trapping.

BURDEN OF DISEASE

As the third leading cause of death in the United States in 2014, chronic obstructive pulmonary disease (COPD) presents a significant challenge to the health care provider.[1] Worldwide, it is the fourth leading cause of death.[2] It is estimated that up to 40% of these deaths are attributed to smoking.[3] Additionally, the financial burden of COPD is significant accounting for nearly $50 billion in US government spending in 2010.[3] As a result, a great deal of emphasis has been placed on combatting the morbidity and mortality associated with COPD. The Global Initiative for Chronic Obstructive Lung Disease (GOLD) 2017 defines COPD as a common, preventable disease characterized by airflow limitation and frequent respiratory symptoms.[4]

Disclosure Statement: S.P. Duffy, none. G.J. Criner reports grants from Boehringer Ingelheim, Novartis, AstraZeneca, Respironics, MedImmune, Actelion, Forest, Pearl, Ikaria, Aeris, PneumRx, and Pulmonx; other from HGE Health Care Solutions, Inc, Amirall, Boehringer-Ingelheim, and Holaira outside the submitted work.
Department of Thoracic Medicine and Surgery, Lewis Katz School of Medicine at Temple University, 3401 North Broad Street, 7th Floor Parkinson Pavilion, Philadelphia, PA 19140, USA
* Corresponding author.
E-mail address: Sean.duffy2@tuhs.temple.edu

OVERVIEW OF PATHOPHYSIOLOGY

The chronic airflow obstruction characteristic of COPD is a result of chronic lung inflammation and occurs as a result of two distinct, but often overlapping processes[5]:

- Small airways disease: this refers to obstructive bronchiolitis, airway remodeling, and narrowing and loss of the peripheral airways
- Emphysema: this refers to parenchymal destruction that causes loss of alveolar units and the characteristic gas trapping and hyperinflation that is found in patients with COPD

Lung inflammation that causes COPD is most commonly caused by cigarette smoke but can also be induced by other harmful particles, such as smoke from biomass fuels. In patients with COPD the normal inflammatory response of the lung is amplified because of factors that are genetically determined but not fully understood at present. Accelerated lung inflammation is mediated by multiple types of inflammatory cells including macrophages, neutrophils, and T and B lymphocytes that populate the airway lumen in COPD.[6] A minority of patients with COPD have been found to have eosinophil-mediated inflammation, an important distinction because this cohort may respond more favorably to corticosteroids.[7] Additionally, systemic inflammation is increased in COPD, especially in severe disease and during exacerbation as evidenced by increased levels of inflammatory biomarkers. Persistent systemic inflammation is associated with the development of comorbid cardiac disease and poorer clinical outcomes.[8] Further study is warranted in this field because the identification of therapeutic phenotypes could improve personalization of therapy and clinical response.

RISK FACTORS

Cigarette smoking is the most well-established risk factor for the development of COPD. However, lifelong nonsmokers can develop COPD and less than half of heavy smokers go on to develop COPD.[9] Despite reaching normal peak lung function in early adulthood, some patients develop COPD because of accelerated lung function decline presumably caused by inhalation of noxious particles. Another mechanism of development of chronic airflow limitation is related to poor lung growth and development with subsequent normal lung function decline with aging. This may be a contributory mechanism in nonsmokers.[10] Additional risk factors for the development of chronic airflow limitation include

- Occupational exposures: 10% to 20% of COPD cases[11]
  - Dust
  - Chemical agents
  - Fumes
- Indoor air pollution
  - Biomass fuel
  - Wood burning stove
- Asthma and airway hyperresponsiveness
  - Second leading risk factor to cigarette smoking when studied in a group of young adults aged 20 to 44[12]

Genetic risk factors also contribute to the development of airflow limitation. Most notably, hereditary α_1-antitrypsin deficiency contributes to chronic airflow obstruction and emphysema.[13] Additional genes have been studied and implicated in the development of airflow obstruction, but a causal relationship has not been established.[4]

CLINICAL PRESENTATION

The clinical presentation can vary widely in COPD, although most patients are at least 40 years of age and have a significant cigarette smoking or exposure history. According to a large European study of patients with COPD, the most commonly reported symptoms are as follows[14]:

- Dyspnea
  - Reported by more than 70%
  - Typically, worse with exertion
- Chronic cough
  - Reported by nearly 60% of patients
  - Often dismissed as "smoker's cough" by patients
- Mucous production
  - Reported by 63% of patients
  - May be indicative of chronic bronchitis if occurring for more than 3 months in two consecutive years[15]

The patients reported that symptoms were most problematic on awakening but also reported significant day-to-day and week-to-week variability.[14] Wheezing and chest tightness have also been noted as highly variable yet commons symptoms.[14] Physical examination is not likely to be helpful in establishing the diagnosis of mild or moderate COPD. Wheezing may be present but is subject to significant variability. Often physical examination signs, such as poor air movement, accessory muscle use, and muscle wasting, are not apparent until the patient has entered the advanced stage of disease.[16]

DIAGNOSIS AND TESTING

Spirometry is necessary for the diagnosis of COPD and should be the initial test of choice. Values are reported as raw measures of flow and as percentage of predicted after correction for height, age, and sex. The diagnosis is established by finding the forced expiratory volume in 1 second (FEV_1) to forced vital capacity (FVC) ratio (FEV_1/FVC) is less than 70%. Severity of airflow obstruction is then established by the FEV_1 as (GOLD)[4]:

- GOLD 1: mild obstructive defect, $FEV_1 \geq 80\%$ predicted
- GOLD 2: moderate obstructive defect, $50\% \leq FEV_1$ less than 80%
- GOLD 3: severe obstructive defect, $30\% \leq FEV_1$ less than 50%
- GOLD 4: very severe obstructive defect, $FEV_1 < 30\%$

Symptomatic patients with risk factors for COPD should certainly be sent for spirometry. Screening the general population is not recommended because this endeavor has not proven to benefit asymptomatic patients regarding management of symptoms or clinical outcomes.[17] Complete lung function testing with lung volumes and diffusion capacity is not necessary for diagnosis but is performed to assess for hyperinflation, gas trapping, and gas exchange abnormalities. Symptoms should be assessed at each office visit because FEV_1 does not provide a strong correlation with symptoms on an individual level.[18] The most commonly used and validated scales are the modified British Medical Research Council (mMRC) questionnaire and the COPD Assessment Test (CAT). The mMRC provides a simple assessment of breathlessness with a 0 to 5 score ranging from "breathless only with strenuous exercise" to "too breathless to leave the house."[19] The CAT is an eight-item assessment score with a maximum possible score of 40. The assessment accounts for a wider range of symptoms, such as cough, phlegm, chest tightness, sleep quality, and energy level.[20] A score of 10 or greater on the CAT is consistent with significant symptoms.[21]

Patients should also be assessed for exacerbation history. The 2017 GOLD update has categorized COPD patients into four (ABCD) groups based on symptoms and exacerbation history. The ABCD groups are listed next (GOLD):

- Group A: low symptom score, low exacerbation risk
  - mMRC 0 or 1, CAT <10
  - 0 to 1 exacerbation in past year, no hospitalizations
- Group B: high symptom score, low exacerbation risk
  - mMRC $\geq$2, CAT $\geq$10
  - 0 to 1 exacerbation in past year, no hospitalizations
- Group C: low symptom score, high exacerbation risk
  - mMRC 0 or 1, CAT <10
  - $\geq$2 exacerbations in past year or one or more hospitalizations
- Group D: high symptom score, high exacerbation risk
  - mMRC $\geq$2, CAT $\geq$10
  - $\geq$2 exacerbations in past year or one or more hospitalizations

These groups should be used in combination with spirometry to classify patients with COPD. For instance, a patient with an FEV_1 of 56% predicted, CAT score of 12, and one mild exacerbation the past year is categorized as GOLD grade 2, group B.

MANAGEMENT OF CHRONIC OBSTRUCTIVE PULMONARY DISEASE

The therapeutic intervention with the greatest impact on COPD is smoking cessation. Smoking cessation has been shown to improve lung function in the year after quitting and reduce the rate of decline by half over the long term when compared with continuing smokers.[22] Additionally, smoking cessation has been shown to improve mortality when compared with continued smoking in patients with COPD.[23]

The goal of pharmacologic treatment in stable COPD is to prevent acute exacerbations of COPD (AECOPD), to reduce symptoms, and to minimize the rate of lung function decline. Inhaled corticosteroids (ICS) and long-acting bronchodilators, long-acting β-agonists (LABA), and long-acting muscarinic antagonists (LAMA) are the mainstays of therapy. Symptomatic patients often require some combination of inhaled therapy. Therapy should be tailored to the individual patient with respect to insurance coverage, device preference, and the side effect profile of the medications (GOLD).[4] Current data suggest that the best initial therapy in most stable mild-to-moderate patients with COPD (GOLD group A) is combination inhaled LAMA/LABA. The combination has proven to be more effective at reducing exacerbations than either bronchodilator alone[24] and ICS/LABA combination inhaler in patients with a prior low burden of exacerbations.[25] Triple inhaler therapy (ICS/LABA/LAMA) has been shown to be superior compared with ICS/LABA and LAMA/LABA in reducing the risk of moderate or severe COPD exacerbations in a population of symptomatic patients with moderate or severe airflow limitation and a prior history of frequent or severe exacerbations.[26] There is a slight increase in the risk of pneumonia in the study cohort receiving ICS; ICS therapy should be carefully considered in patients with a significant history of pneumonia.[26] **Table 1** provides a guideline for the initiation of therapy by GOLD grade. The treatment options, risks, adverse effects, and potential benefits should be discussed with the patient and treatment decisions should be tailored to the individual.

Table 1
Initial treatment options by GOLD grade for COPD

COPD Severity	SABD (Rescue)	LAMA	LAMA or LABA	LAMA + LABA	LABA + ICS	LAMA + LABA + ICS
Group A	√		√			
Group B	√		√			
Group C	√	√				
Group D	√			√	√ (asthma features)	√

Abbreviation: SABD, short-acting bronchodilator.

Data from Global Strategy for the Diagnosis, Management and Prevention of COPD, Global Initiative for Chronic Obstructive Lung Disease (GOLD) 2017. Available at: http://goldcopd.org/gold-2017-global-strategy-diagnosis-management-prevention-copd/. Accessed September 5, 2018.

Patients with more severe obstruction, frequent exacerbations (>1 per year), or persistent symptoms despite first-line inhaler therapy may require adjunctive therapies. For instance, patients with chronic bronchitis tend to have increased rates of exacerbation when compared with the general COPD population.[27] In this population roflumilast, a phosphodiesterase-4 inhibitor designed to reduce inflammation,[28] has been shown to reduce the rate of moderate and severe exacerbations, especially in those with prior repeated hospitalizations.[29,30] Daily azithromycin, a macrolide antibiotic, has also been studied and shown to reduce the exacerbation rate in an at-risk COPD population by up to 30%, especially in those that are not current smokers.[31] Pulmonary rehabilitation incorporates exercise training, education, and behavioral disease management strategies and has been shown to improve dyspnea and exercise tolerance especially in patients with moderate-to-severe disease.[32]

ACUTE EXACERBATION OF CHRONIC OBSTRUCTIVE PULMONARY DISEASE

AECOPD confers a substantial negative impact on patients' health status and quality of life.[33] AECOPD is defined as an acute increase in respiratory symptoms requiring therapy. They are classified by severity as follows[4]:

- Mild: treated as an outpatient with increased frequency of short-acting bronchodilators
- Moderate: treated as an outpatient with short-acting bronchodilators plus antibiotics and/or oral corticosteroids
- Severe: requires hospitalization or emergency room care

The most common trigger for an AECOPD is an upper respiratory infection and the most commonly isolated organism is rhinovirus.[34] Short-acting bronchodilators and oral corticosteroids are the mainstay of therapy in exacerbation. A 5-day course of 40 mg of oral prednisone has been shown to be as efficacious as a 14-day course of glucocorticoid in preventing recurrent exacerbation within 6 months.[35] Historically, antibiotics have been a controversial topic in treatment of AECOPD, but recent guidelines endorse the use of a 5- to 7-day course of antibiotics if patients have increased purulence of sputum along with dyspnea or increased volume of sputum.[4] Adjunctive therapies, such as noninvasive ventilation and high-flow nasal cannula, may prevent intubation[36] and reintubation[37] in patients with respiratory failure (**Fig. 1**).

ADVANCED THERAPIES FOR SEVERE CHRONIC OBSTRUCTIVE PULMONARY DISEASE

Advanced therapies, such as lung volume reduction surgery and bronchoscopic lung volume reduction, are treatments that aim to reduce hyperinflation by decreasing the volume of emphysematous lung tissue in patients with severe COPD with significant hyperinflation and gas trapping. Lung volume reduction surgery has been shown to improve mortality in patients with COPD with severe, predominantly upper lobe emphysema who have low exercise tolerance.[38] Despite the evidence, lung volume reduction surgery remains an uncommonly performed procedure because of the surgical morbidity, specialized nature of the surgery, and difficulty identifying suitable candidates in the community.[39] Bronchoscopic lung volume reduction has since been developed as a less-invasive means of achieving lung volume reduction. Endobronchial valves placed into the airways of emphysematous lung tissue have proven to effectively reduce the target lobe volume of emphysematous lung.[40] This has proven to be an effective means of symptom relief and quality of life improvement in patients with severe heterogenous[40] and homogenous emphysema.[41] Finally, lung transplant

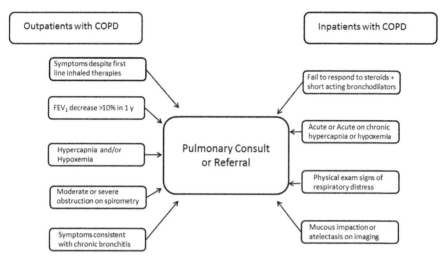

Fig. 1. Indications for a pulmonary consultation or referral.

evaluation remains an option in patients with severe COPD, typically FEV_1 less than 25%, hypercapnia, and/or frequent COPD-related hospitalizations.[42] These advanced therapeutic options should be undertaken in a specialized center after thorough evaluation by a multidisciplinary team.

SUMMARY

COPD is a highly prevalent and heterogeneous disease with high morbidity and mortality that imparts a significant burden on health care providers worldwide. It is a chronic progressive illness that accounts for a large and increasing percentage of deaths worldwide. Pharmacologic and nonpharmacologic treatment options abound although rarely do these therapies confer a mortality benefit to the patient. Smoking cessation remains the most impactful therapeutic and preventative intervention in the care of these patients. Thus, smoking cessation and abstinence should be a key focus of any physician-patient interaction that involves a current or former smoker. Otherwise, COPD may continue to rise in the ranks of worldwide causes of death.

REFERENCES

1. National Center for Health Statistics. Health, United States 2015 with special feature on racial and ethnic health disparities. Hyattsville (MD): US Dept Health and Human Services; 2016.
2. Lozano R, Naghavi M, Foreman K, et al. Global and regional mortality from 235 causes of death for 20 age groups in 1990 and 2010: a systematic analysis for the Global Burden of Disease Study 2010. Lancet 2012;380:2095–128.
3. Adeloye D, Chua S, Lee C, et al, Global Health Epidemiology Reference Group. Global and regional estimates of COPD prevalence: systematic review and meta-analysis. J Glob Health 2015;5:020415.
4. GOLD 2017. Global Strategy for the Diagnosis, Management and Prevention of COPD. Available at: http://goldcopd.org/gold-2017-global-strategy-diagnosis-management- prevention-copd/. Accessed September 5, 2018.

5. Barnes PJ. Inflammatory mechanisms in patients with chronic obstructive pulmonary disease. J Allergy Clin Immunol 2016;138:16–27.
6. Hogg JC, Chu F, Utokaparch S, et al. The nature of small-airway obstruction in chronic obstructive pulmonary disease. N Engl J Med 2004;350:2645–53.
7. Postma DS, Rabe KF. The asthma-COPD overlap syndrome. N Engl J Med 2015; 373:1241–9.
8. Thomsen M, Dahl M, Lange P, et al. Inflammatory biomarkers and comorbidities in chronic obstructive pulmonary disease. Am J Respir Crit Care Med 2012;186:982–8.
9. Rennard SI, Vestbo J. COPD: the dangerous underestimate of 15%. Lancet 2006; 367(9518):1216–9.
10. Lange P, Celli B, Agusti A, et al. Lung-function trajectories leading to chronic obstructive pulmonary disease. N Engl J Med 2015;373:111–22.
11. Eisner MD, Anthonisen N, Coultas D, et al. An Official American Thoracic Society Public Policy Statement: novel risk factors and the global burden of chronic obstructive pulmonary disease. Am J Respir Crit Care Med 2010;182:693–718.
12. De Marco R, Accordini S, Macron A, et al. Risk factors for chronic obstructive pulmonary disease in a European cohort of young adults. Am J Respir Crit Care Med 2011;183(7):891–7.
13. Stoller JK, Abbousouan LS. Alpha 1-antitrypsin deficiency. Lancet 2005; 365(9478):2225–36.
14. Kessler R, Partridge MR, Miravitlles M, et al. Symptom variability in patients with severe COPD: a pan-European cross-sectional study. Eur Respir J 2011;37(2):264–72.
15. Medical Research Council Committee on the Aetiology of Chronic bronchitis. Definition and classification of chronic bronchitis for clinical and epidemiological purposes. A report to the Medical Research Council by their Committee on the aetiology of chronic bronchitis. Lancet 1965;1(7389):775–9.
16. Holleman DR Jr, Simel DL. Does the clinical examination predict airflow limitation? JAMA 1995;273(4):313–9.
17. Siu AL, Bibbins-Domingo K, Grossman DC, et al. Screening for chronic obstructive pulmonary disease: US preventive services task force recommendation statement. JAMA 2016;315(13):1372–7.
18. Han MK, Muellerova H, Curran-Everett D, et al. GOLD 2011 disease severity classification in COPDGene: a perspective cohort study. Lancet Respir Med 2013; 1(1):43–50.
19. Fletcher CM. Standardised questionnaire on respiratory symptoms: a statement prepared and approved by the MRC Committee on the Aetiology of Chronic Bronchitis (MRC breathlessness score). BMJ 1960;2:1662.
20. Jones PW, Harding G, Berry P, et al. Development and first validation of the COPD assessment test. Eur Respir J 2009;34(3):648–54.
21. Jones PW, Tabberer M, Chen WH. Creating scenarios of the impact of COPD and their relationship to COPD Assessment Test (CAT) scores. BMC Pulm Med 2011; 11:42.
22. Scanlon PD, Connett JE, Waller L, et al. Smoking cessation and lung function in mild-to-moderate chronic obstructive pulmonary disease: the lung health study. Am J Respir Crit Care Med 2000;161(2):381–90.
23. Godtfredsen NS, Lam TH, Hansel TT, et al. COPD-related morbidity and mortality after smoking cessation: status of the evidence. Eur Respir J 2008;32:844–53.
24. Wedzicha JA, Decramer M, Ficker JH, et al. Analysis of chronic obstructive pulmonary disease exacerbations with the dual bronchodilator QVA149 compared with glycopyrronium and tiotropium (SPARK): a randomized, double-blind, parallel group study. Lancet Respir Med 2013;1(3):199–209.

25. Wedzicha JA, Banerji D, Chapman KR, et al. Indacaterol-glycopyrronium versus salmeterol-fluitcasone for COPD. N Engl J Med 2016;374(23):2222–34.
26. Lipson DA, Barnhart F, Brealey N, et al. Once-daily single-inhaler triple versus dual therapy in patients with COPD. N Engl J Med 2018;378:1671–80.
27. Kim V, Han MK, Vance GB, et al. The chronic bronchitic phenotype of COPD: an analysis of the COPDGene Study. Chest 2011;140(3):626–33.
28. Rabe KF. Update on roflumilast, a phosphodiesterase 4 inhibitor for the treatment of chronic obstructive pulmonary disease. Br J Pharmacol 2011;163(1):53–67.
29. Calverley PM, Rabe KF, Goehring UM, et al. Roflumilast in symptomatic chronic obstructive pulmonary disease: two randomized clinical trials. Lancet 2009; 374(9691):685–94.
30. Fabbri LM, Calverley PM, Izquierdo-Alonso JL, et al. Roflumilast in moderate to severe chronic obstructive pulmonary disease treated with long acting broncho-dilators: two randomized clinical trials. Lancet 2009;374(9691):695–703.
31. Albert RK, Connett J, Bailey WC, et al. Azithromycin for the prevention of exacerbations of COPD. N Engl J Med 2011;365(8):689–98.
32. McCarthy B, Casey D, Devane D, et al. Pulmonary rehabilitation for chronic obstructive pulmonary disease. Cochrane Database Syst Rev 2015;(2):CD003793.
33. Seemungal TA, Donaldson GC, Paul EA, et al. Effect of exacerbation on quality of life in patients with chronic obstructive pulmonary disease. Am J Respir Crit Care Med 1998;157(5):1418–22.
34. White AJ, Gompertz S, Stockley RA. Chronic obstructive pulmonary disease. 6: The aetiology of exacerbations of chronic obstructive pulmonary disease. Thorax 2003;58(1):73–80.
35. Leuppi JD, Scheutz P, Bingisser R, et al. Short-term vs. conventional glucocorti-coid therapy in acute exacerbations of chronic obstructive pulmonary disease: the REDUCE randomized clinical trial. JAMA 2013;309(21):2223–31.
36. Lightowler JV, Wedzicha JA, Elliott MW, et al. Non-invasive positive pressure ventilation to treat respiratory failure resulting from exacerbations of chronic obstructive pulmonary disease: Cochrane systematic review and meta-analysis. BMJ 2003;326(7382):185.
37. Hernandez G, Vaquero C, Colinas L, et al. Effect of postextubation high-flow nasal cannula vs. noninvasive ventilation on reintubation and postextubation res-piratory failure in high risk patients: a randomized clinical trial. JAMA 2016; 316(15):1565–74.
38. Fishman A, Martinez F, Naunheim K, the National Emphysema Treatment Trial Research Group. A randomized trial comparing lung-volume-reduction surgery with medical therapy for severe emphysema. N Engl J Med 2003;348:2059–73.
39. Criner GJ, Cordova F, Sternberg A, et al. The National Emphysema Treatment Trial (NETT). Part II: Lessons learned about lung volume reduction surgery. Am J Respir Crit Care Med 2011;184:881–93.
40. Criner GJ, Sue R, Wright S, et al. A multicenter RCT of Zephyr endobronchial valve treatment in heterogeneous emphysema (LIBERATE). Am J Respir Crit Care Med 2018. https://doi.org/10.1164/rccm.201803-0590OC.
41. Valipour A, Slebos D, Herth F, et al. Endobronchial valve therapy in patients with homogeneous emphysema. Results from the IMPACT study. Am J Respir Crit Care Med 2016;194(9):1073–82.
42. Weill D, Benden C, Corris PA, et al. A consensus document for the selection of lung transplant candidates: 2014—an update from the Pulmonary Transplantation Council of the International Society for Heart and Lung Transplantation. J Heart Lung Transplant 2015;34(1):1–15.

Lung Cancer

Faria Nasim, MD, Bruce F. Sabath, MD, George A. Eapen, MD*

KEYWORDS

- Lung cancer • Smoking • Screening • Staging • Chemotherapy

KEY POINTS

- Lung cancer is the leading cancer killer in the world.
- Smoking is the predominant risk factor, but other risk factors exist.
- Low-dose computed tomography for lung cancer screening improves mortality.
- Various modalities exist for diagnosis and staging of lung cancer.
- Treatment depends on several factors and is best guided by a multidisciplinary team to determine the best approach for a given patient.

INTRODUCTION

Lung cancer is the world's leading cause of cancer death.[1] This is largely because it is initially asymptomatic and typically discovered at advanced stages. Screening for lung cancer by low-dose computed tomography (LDCT) has recently been shown to have a mortality benefit, and implementation of this practice is growing. Once suspected, lung cancer must be diagnosed and staged, and there are recent guidelines to aid in this process. Treatment is determined by subtype and stage of cancer and there are several personalized therapies that did not exist just a few years ago. This review provides a broad outline of this disease, helping clinicians identify such patients and familiarizing them with lung cancer care so they are better equipped to guide their patients along this challenging journey.

EPIDEMIOLOGY

Worldwide, lung cancer continues to be the most common cause of cancer death.[1] Approximately 1.8 million new people were diagnosed in 2012, with 1.6 million fatalities. It is estimated that, in 2018, the United States alone will have had more than 230,000 new cases, and that lung cancer will lead to more deaths than breast,

Disclosure Statement: The authors have no commercial or financial conflicts of interest nor any relevant funding sources.
Department of Pulmonary Medicine, The University of Texas MD Anderson Cancer Center, Unit 1462, 1515 Holcombe Boulevard, Houston, TX 77030, USA
* Corresponding author.
E-mail address: geapen@mdanderson.org

Med Clin N Am 103 (2019) 463–473
https://doi.org/10.1016/j.mcna.2018.12.006
0025-7125/19/© 2019 Elsevier Inc. All rights reserved.

prostate, and colon cancers combined.[2] Lung cancer is relatively rare before the fifth decade of life; risk increases with age thereafter.[2] Men are more affected than women. Interestingly, although smoking is the exposure most closely tied to lung cancer (an estimated 80%–90% of cases are caused by this), only approximately 15% of smokers develop lung cancer, suggesting a genetic susceptibility.[3] Smoking intensity (eg, how many cigarettes per day) and lifetime duration affect risk proportionately.[4] As a corollary, smoking cessation reduces lung cancer risk. For patients who cannot quit completely, even reducing the number of cigarettes smoked daily has a demonstrated benefit.[5] Generally speaking, any form of smoking exposure increases lung cancer risk, including secondhand smoke and cigar and pipe smoking.[6] The association of marijuana is less clear due to conflicting results, and that of electronic cigarettes is also uncertain, in part due to confounding from prior or concurrent cigarette use, and the lack of long-term data.[7] Asbestos exposure acts synergistically with tobacco use, being associated with higher rates of lung malignancy than either risk factor alone. Other risk factors include radon exposure and some forms of interstitial lung disease. The presence of chronic obstructive lung disease and a family history are also associated with lung cancer, even after adjustment for tobacco exposure.[6]

SCREENING

Until recently, no effective method of lung cancer screening was available. Several studies have investigated the role of LDCT, the largest of which is the National Lung Screening Trial (NLST), which included more than 50,000 patients and had longer follow-up compared with other randomized controlled trials.[8] Researchers demonstrated a 20% reduction in lung cancer mortality by annual LDCT compared with chest radiograph (CXR) with a decrease in overall mortality by 6.7%. A concern raised with screening by LDCT is the high rate of benign nodules detected (more than 90% in most studies). In the NLST, for example, approximately one-quarter of the scans revealed nodules, with 96.4% of these being benign; a similarly high false-positive rate was found in the CXR arm. Another concern with repeated LDCT screening tests is accumulating radiation exposure. It is estimated that a single LDCT will expose a patient to 1.5 mSv of radiation. The average total exposure for each NLST participant over 3 years was approximately 8 mSv. By way of comparison, the average annual dose provided by background radiation (in the United States) is 3 to 4 mSv.[9] Even with the high false-positive rates and radiation risks, available evidence indicates that the reductions in cancer death brought about by screening outweigh the possible risks. Based on these findings, the US Preventive Services Task Force recommends lung cancer screening with LDCT in adults of age 55 to 80 years who have a 30 pack-year smoking history and are currently smoking or have quit within the past 15 years.[10] Approximately 8 million Americans are eligible to receive annual screening with LDCT using these criteria.[11] The current National Comprehensive Cancer Network (NCCN) Clinical Practice Guidelines in Oncology for Lung Cancer Screening also considers it reasonable to use a statistical risk prediction model (https://brocku.ca/lung-cancer-risk-calculator) to quantify lung cancer risk for individuals who do not meet the NLST criteria but may be at similar risk to the NLST cohort.[12] Because the benefits of screening decrease at lower-risk thresholds, but the harms of screening remain constant, it is challenging to determine the ideal balance of benefit and harm, particularly as the impact of the benefit and harms can vary markedly with patient preferences.[13] The American Thoracic Society/American College of Chest Physicians policy statement on lung cancer screening provides guidelines for implementation of a successful screening program that include structured reporting and a smoking cessation program. Screening should be discontinued once an individual has not smoked for 15 years or develops a health problem that substantially limits life expectancy or the ability or willingness to have curative treatment.[14]

INCIDENTAL VERSUS SCREEN-DETECTED PULMONARY NODULE MANAGEMENT

There are important distinctions between nodules found incidentally and those found on screening LDCT. The Fleischner Society guidelines are typically used for management of incidental detected pulmonary nodules on computed tomography (CT). The more recent guidelines revised in 2017 recommend longer intervals between scans even for high-risk individuals with nodules >6 mm. To estimate high risk, the American College of Chest Physicians intermediate-risk (5%–65% risk) and high-risk (>65% risk) categories are combined into one category. High-risk factors include older age, heavy smoking, larger nodule size, irregular or spiculated margins, and upper lobe location. The NCCN clinical practice guidelines in oncology provide management recommendations for screen-detected nodules. In 2018, the NCCN cutoff thresholds for lung nodules were revised to reflect the Lung Imaging Reporting and Data System (Lung-RADS) cutoffs. Lung-RADS is a structured decision-oriented reporting system published in 2014 that aimed to reduce the false-positive result rate and suggest management recommendations based on estimated lung cancer risk.[15] **Table 1** summarizes the current recommendations based on these guidelines.

CLINICAL MANIFESTATIONS

Occurring in approximately half of patients with lung cancer, a new cough in a smoker or former smoker should raise concern for lung cancer. Recurrent pneumonia in the same anatomic location or frequent exacerbations of chronic obstructive pulmonary disease also should trigger concern for neoplasm as a root cause.[18] Dyspnea is present in approximately one-third to one-half of patients with lung cancer, and could be

Table 1
Guidelines for pulmonary nodule management

Nodule type	Size, mm	Fleischner 2017[16]	NCCN 2018[12]	Lung-RADS 2014[17]
		Recommended Follow-up, mo		
Applicable population	All	Incidental	LDCT screening	LDCT Screening
Solid	<6	None for low risk, 12 mo optional for high risk	AS	AS
	6–8	6–12 mo, 18–24 mo	6 mo	6 mo, AS
	>8	3 mo, PET, or tissue sampling	3 mo, PET, tissue sampling for high risk	3 mo, AS
Part solid	<6	None	AS	AS
	≥6	3–6 mo, every 12 mo × 5 y	Based on size of solid component	Based on size of solid component
Ground glass	<6	None	AS	AS
	≥6	6–12 mo, every 24 mo until 5 y	AS	AS up to 20 mm

Abbreviations: AS, annual screening; LDCT, low-dose computed tomography; Lung-RADS, lung imaging reporting and data system; NCCN, national comprehensive cancer network.

due to direct malignant airway, or parenchymal or pleural involvement. Patients also are at risk of developing pulmonary emboli, pneumothoraces, pleural effusions, and/ or pericardial effusions. Other less common symptoms include chest pain from regional tumor invasion and hoarseness from involvement of the recurrent laryngeal nerve. Hemoptysis is the presenting symptom in approximately one-quarter of patients with lung cancer and is rarely massive.[19] Other manifestations of intrathoracic spread are the superior vena cava syndrome, dysphagia, or arm/shoulder pain; these are all due to mass effect on various structures. Patients also can present with symptoms from extrathoracic metastases. Often these are nonspecific, such as weight loss, anorexia, and fatigue.[18] Bone metastases are frequently painful; brain metastases can be asymptomatic, although neurologic sequelae do manifest based on size and location. Finally, paraneoplastic syndromes can occur, including the syndrome of inappropriate antidiuretic hormone, neurologic syndromes, such as Lambert-Eaton myasthenic syndrome and cerebellar ataxia, or hypercalcemia from bone metastases or secretion of parathyroid hormone–related protein.[20]

Box 1 reviews when a pulmonary consultation should be considered.

DIAGNOSIS AND STAGING

All patients with known or suspected non–small-cell lung cancer (NSCLC) should have a thorough clinical evaluation and a CT chest with contrast.[21] If both clinical evaluation and CT scan are without extrathoracic abnormalities, a PET scan is recommended to evaluate for metastases.[9] Notably, a PET scan may not be required if the primary lung lesion is a ground glass opacity or a peripheral nodule 3 cm or smaller, as these have a low likelihood of metastasis, assuming negative intrathoracic nodal involvement on CT.[21] Such patients may proceed directly to curative-intent treatment immediately after tissue confirmation. For patients who do not clearly have very early or advanced NSCLC, staging of intrathoracic lymph nodes is recommended. However, if the mediastinum is extensively infiltrated, invasive staging may not be necessary.[21] When sampling is needed, endobronchial ultrasound (EBUS)-guided bronchoscopic sampling is recommended over surgical staging by mediastinoscopy. Direct comparison trials have shown EBUS-guided sampling of thoracic lymph nodes to perform as well as or better than surgical sampling while also being less invasive and having fewer complications.[22] However, if suspicion of nodal involvement remains after a negative result by bronchoscopy, surgical confirmation should be performed.[21] Given the previously described complexities, it is advisable that any patient with suspected lung cancer be referred to a pulmonologist, and multidisciplinary care is recommended.

Various methods for diagnosis and staging (bronchoscopic, surgical, and transthoracic) exist, and a pulmonologist can provide guidance for further steps as needed.

Box 1
Recommendations on when to call a pulmonary consultation

To determine a patient's candidacy for lung cancer screening

To decide how to approach the diagnosis of a lung nodule (or if a diagnosis is necessary)

History of pneumonia that does not resolve completely (either symptomatically or radiographically)

The presence of any pleural effusion, particularly if exudative without a clear etiology

Any patient with lung cancer with shortness of breath

Hemoptysis

Table 2 summarizes the various diagnostic modalities along with their diagnostic yield. Minimizing invasive procedures is desirable, such as attempting to diagnose and stage with a single procedure if possible. For example, if a patient with a lung mass has any sign of metastasis (eg, enlarged mediastinal lymph nodes, pleural effusion, and adrenal mass), the highest-stage location should be sampled first, if feasible and technically safe to do so.[23] The reason is that the finding of lung cancer at a metastatic site would adequately provide both diagnostic and staging information. Finally, the aforementioned diagnostic approaches apply largely to NSCLC rather than small-cell lung cancer (SCLC). Current guidelines suggest that if SCLC is suspected (based on certain characteristics, such as massive adenopathy, direct mediastinal invasion, or the presence of a paraneoplastic syndrome, for example), then diagnosis should be sought via the least-invasive method.[23]

BRIEF UPDATE ON THE EIGHTH EDITION TUMOR-NODE-METASTASIS CLASSIFICATION OF LUNG CANCER

The eighth edition of the tumor-node-metastasis (TNM) classification for lung cancer has some clinically important updates. There are 24 T descriptors and the "p" or "c" T-stage designators correspond to the pathologic versus the clinical stage, respectively. Size measurement in part-solid nodules uses the size of solid component for clinical size, and size of invasive component for pathologic size. Tumor size itself is a descriptor in all T categories and every centimeter increment in size affects prognosis.[28] To ensure accurate radiographic assessment of T stage, the International Association for the Study of Lung Cancer recommends that tumor size be measured in the lung window. The new T categories are Tis, denoting carcinoma in situ (squamous or adenocarcinoma), and T1a (mi), for minimally invasive adenocarcinoma. T2 and T3 endobronchial tumors have similar prognosis, even with total atelectasis and pneumonitis. T3 with involvement of the diaphragm has been reclassified as a T4 tumor.[29]

For the N component, it is important to quantify nodal disease both clinically and pathologically. Apart from keeping the seventh edition N descriptors as they are, new subclass descriptors have been added for prospective testing and validation. pN1a will denote involvement of single pN1 nodal station, whereas pN1b will be assigned to involvement of multiple pN1 nodal stations. pN2a1 will be designated for involvement of single pN2 nodal station without pN1 (skip pN2), and pN2a2 will

Table 2
Diagnostic modalities for tissue diagnosis of lung cancer and their yield

Diagnostic Modality	Yield, %
Convex probe endobronchial ultrasound transbronchial needle aspiration[24]	94.5
Peripheral bronchoscopy with radial probe[25]	53–84
Electromagnetic navigation bronchoscopy[26]	38–71
Computed tomography–guided transthoracic needle aspiration[27]	90
Image-guided closed pleural biopsy[23]	75–88
Pleuroscopy with pleural biopsy[23]	95–97
Thoracentesis[23]	72
Conventional bronchoscopy with endobronchial biopsy, brushings, and washings[23]	88

be involvement of single pN2 nodal station with pN1. Last, pN2b will be involvement of multiple pN2 nodal stations.

Finally, for the M component, number of metastases is more important than their location. Cancers with multiple lesions are defined by disease pattern. For multiple primary tumors, 1 TNM is assigned for each tumor. These changes in the eighth edition of the TNM classification of lung cancer aim to facilitate more homogeneous tumor classification and collection of prospective data to improve tumor stratification for future research trials.[30]

TREATMENT

For early-stage lung cancer, surgical resection is the preferred treatment.[31] The extent of resection depends on the size and location of the tumor as well as the patient's preoperative pulmonary reserve. Adjuvant chemotherapy is recommended for completely resected stage II NSCLC but not usually stage I. Postoperative radiation is not recommended except for incomplete resection. For those with early-stage NSCLC who are not surgical candidates, stereotactic ablative body radiotherapy (SABR), can be considered.[32] Comparative studies are under way as to whether this is equivalent to surgery in terms of long-term outcomes.[33,34] An alternative to SABR is percutaneous ablation for select peripheral tumors, but there is scant evidence of efficacy and a substantial pneumothorax rate.[35] Transbronchial ablation may have certain advantages and is currently in investigational stages.[36]

Stage III NSCLC encompasses a heterogeneous group of patients. Patients with limited nodal (N1) involvement may be candidates for surgical resection upfront followed by chemotherapy and/or radiation.[37] Those with more advanced nodal (N2) involvement may still be candidates for surgery, although usually only after induction therapy because data have consistently shown better outcomes with this approach.[38] Nevertheless, whether there is greater benefit from tri-modality therapy (surgery, chemotherapy, radiation) versus chemo-radiation alone is still unclear, and further studies of subgroups of patients with N2 disease are needed.[38] Patients with most advanced nodal (N3) involvement are not generally considered to be surgical candidates.

For patients with stage IV NSCLC, chemotherapy with platinum-based (eg, cisplatin, carboplatin) 2-drug, regimens is standard, but the past several years have seen the significant additional therapies directed at specific driver mutations.[39] As such, efforts should be made to not only determine the histologic subtype but also to obtain sufficient tissue for molecular analysis. Each institution has its own approach to molecular testing, but typically, testing tumor tissue for epidermal growth factor receptor gene mutations, anaplastic lymphoma kinase gene rearrangements, reactive oxygen species proto-oncogene-1 gene rearrangements, B-raf proto-oncogene point mutations and KRAS proto-oncogene (KRAS) point mutations is recommended.[37] The presence of such genetic alterations can guide the choice of targeted therapies, as they can predict responsiveness (or lack thereof) to certain agents. In addition, testing for programmed death ligand-1 expression levels can be used to guide treatment with certain immunotherapies. Indeed, the armamentarium against stage IV disease is greater than it has ever been. This will all be managed by a medical oncologist, but it is useful for the referring clinician to be familiar with the options. **Table 3** summarizes the commonly used molecular targeted therapies and immunotherapies currently approved by the Food and Drug Administration.

Aside from systemic therapy, local treatment is sometimes needed in stage IV disease if a given metastatic focus is causing localized symptoms.[37,40] Airway

Table 3
Molecularly targeted therapies and immunotherapeutics currently approved by the Food and Drug Administration

Lung Cancer	Target	Drug	Type of Therapy
NSCLC	The anti-programmed death-1 (PD-1)/PD-ligand 1 pathway[44]	Nivolumab, pembrolizumab, atezolizumab, durvalumab, avelumab	Immunotherapy
	Anti-cytotoxic T-lymphocyte-associated antigen 4 (CTLA-4) pathway[44]	Ipilimumab, tremelimumab	
	Epidermal growth factor receptor (EGFR)+[45]	Tyrosine kinase inhibitors: erlotinib, gefitinib, afatinib, osimertinib	Molecular targeted therapy
	Anaplastic lymphoma kinase (ALK)+ [46]	Tyrosine kinase inhibitors: crizotinib, ceritinib, alectinib, brigatinib	
	B-raf proto-oncogene [47]	Dabrafenib and trametinib combination	
	Vascular endothelial growth factor (VEGF) receptor[45]	Ramucirumab	
SCLC	Mammalian target of rapamycin (mTOR)[48]	Everolimus	
	PD-1 pathway[49]	Nivolumab	

Abbreviations: NSCLC, non–small-cell lung cancer; SCLC, small-cell lung cancer.

obstruction by tumor may cause dyspnea, postobstructive pneumonia, or hemoptysis, for example, An interventional pulmonologist may be able to alleviate these symptoms and possibly improve performance status, thereby improving candidacy for systemic therapy.[41] Bone or brain metastases may undergo radiation therapy or even surgical treatment in specific circumstances.[40] Recurrent, symptomatic malignant pleural effusions are usually best treated with tunneled pleural catheters or chemical pleurodesis, but repeated thoracentesis is an alternative if a patient's life expectancy is very short.

SCLC is treated with a more simplified approach compared with NSCLC; all patients receive systemic therapy.[42] Those with confirmed limited stage disease also receive radiation. Patients with extensive disease initially receive systemic therapy alone, although palliative radiation can be given at sites in which tumor burden is causing clinically significant symptoms. Surgical resection is reserved for fewer than 5% of all SCLC where stage I disease is found and confirmed with invasive nodal staging and PET scan.[42] Even in these cases, adjuvant postoperative chemotherapy is given. Prophylactic cranial irradiation is usually offered to all patients who have had some response to therapy, regardless of initial stage, as this confers a survival benefit.[43]

PROGNOSIS

In the United States, from 2007 to 2013, the overall 5-year relative survival rate was 23.6% for NSCLC and only 7% for SCLC.[50] Given these statistics, guidelines recommend that physicians begin discussions about a patient's prognosis and goals of care at the time of lung cancer diagnosis, and that they continue such conversations throughout treatment.[51] Particularly for advanced disease, initiation of palliative care is recommended to be done as early as possible. In fact, there are data to suggest that the addition of palliation to usual care may prolong survival compared with usual care alone in addition to improving quality of life.[40,52]

SUMMARY

Lung cancer remains a highly lethal disease. The implementation of widespread lung cancer screening holds promise for the future. Given the nonspecific clinical presentation, clinicians should consider the diagnosis in any former or current smoker who presents with worrisome symptoms. If lung cancer is suspected, referral to a pulmonologist is strongly recommended. There are various minimally invasive diagnostic and staging modalities currently available and there has been tremendous advancement in our understanding of lung cancer biology leading to various new treatment options.

REFERENCES

1. World Health Organization. Lung cancer. Available at: http://globocan.iarc.fr/Pages/fact_sheets_cancer.aspx. Accessed August 11, 2018.
2. Siegel RL, Miller KD, Jemal A. Cancer statistics, 2018. CA Cancer J Clin 2018; 68(1):7–30.
3. Spitz MR, Wei Q, Dong Q, et al. Genetic susceptibility to lung cancer: the role of DNA damage and repair. Cancer Epidemiol Biomarkers Prev 2003;12(8):689–98.
4. Mattson ME, Pollack ES, Cullen JW. What are the odds that smoking will kill you? Am J Public Health 1987;77(4):425–31.
5. Godtfredsen NS, Prescott E, Osler M. Effect of smoking reduction on lung cancer risk. JAMA 2005;294(12):1505–10.
6. Alberg AJ, Brock MV, Ford JG, et al. Epidemiology of lung cancer: diagnosis and management of lung cancer, 3rd ed: American College of Chest Physicians evidence-based clinical practice guidelines. Chest 2013;143(5 Suppl):e1S–29S.
7. de Groot PM, Wu CC, Carter BW, et al. The epidemiology of lung cancer. Transl Lung Cancer Res 2018;7(3):220–33.
8. Aberle DR, Adams AM, Berg CD, et al. Reduced lung-cancer mortality with low-dose computed tomographic screening. N Engl J Med 2011;365(5):395–409.
9. Detterbeck FC, Mazzone PJ, Naidich DP, et al. Screening for lung cancer: diagnosis and management of lung cancer, 3rd ed: American College of Chest Physicians evidence-based clinical practice guidelines. Chest 2013;143(5 Suppl): e78S–92S.
10. Moyer VA, U.S. Preventive Services Task Force. Screening for lung cancer: U.S. preventive services task force recommendation statement. Ann Intern Med 2014; 160(5):330–8.
11. Cheung LC, Katki HA, Chaturvedi AK, et al. Preventing lung cancer mortality by computed tomography screening: the effect of risk-based versus U.S. Preventive Services Task Force eligibility criteria, 2005-2015. Ann Intern Med 2018;168(3): 229–32.
12. Wood DE, Kazerooni EA, Baum SL, et al. Lung cancer screening, version 3.2018, NCCN clinical practice guidelines in oncology. J Natl Compr Canc Netw 2018; 16(4):412–41.
13. Kanodra NM, Pope C, Halbert CH, et al. Primary care provider and patient perspectives on lung cancer screening. A qualitative study. Ann Am Thorac Soc 2016;13(11):1977–82.
14. Wiener RS, Gould MK, Arenberg DA, et al. An official American Thoracic Society/American College of Chest Physicians policy statement: implementation of

low-dose computed tomography lung cancer screening programs in clinical practice. Am J Respir Crit Care Med 2015;192(7):881–91.

15. Pinsky PF, Gierada DS, Black W, et al. Performance of lung-RADS in the National Lung Screening Trial: a retrospective assessment. Ann Intern Med 2015;162(7): 485–91.

16. MacMahon H, Naidich DP, Goo JM, et al. Guidelines for management of incidental pulmonary nodules detected on CT images: from the Fleischner Society 2017. Radiology 2017;284(1):228–43.

17. Lung-RADS Assessment Categories, Version 1.0. American College of Radiology. Lung CT Screening Reporting and Data System (Lung-RADS™). Available at: http://www.acr.org/Quality-Safety/Resources/LungRADS. Release date April 28, 2014. Accessed March 10, 2019.

18. Ost DE, Jim Yeung SC, Tanoue LT, et al. Clinical and organizational factors in the initial evaluation of patients with lung cancer: diagnosis and management of lung cancer, 3rd ed: American College of Chest Physicians evidence-based clinical practice guidelines. Chest 2013;143(5 Suppl):e121S–41S.

19. Kocher F, Hilbe W, Seeber A, et al. Longitudinal analysis of 2293 NSCLC patients: a comprehensive study from the TYROL registry. Lung Cancer 2015;87(2): 193–200.

20. Kanaji N, Watanabe N, Kita N, et al. Paraneoplastic syndromes associated with lung cancer. World J Clin Oncol 2014;5(3):197–223.

21. Silvestri GA, Gonzalez AV, Jantz MA, et al. Methods for staging non-small cell lung cancer: diagnosis and management of lung cancer, 3rd ed: American College of Chest Physicians evidence-based clinical practice guidelines. Chest 2013;143(5 Suppl):e211S–50S.

22. Um SW, Kim HK, Jung SH, et al. Endobronchial ultrasound versus mediastinoscopy for mediastinal nodal staging of non-small-cell lung cancer. J Thorac Oncol 2015;10(2):331–7.

23. Rivera MP, Mehta AC, Wahidi MM. Establishing the diagnosis of lung cancer: diagnosis and management of lung cancer, 3rd ed: American College of Chest Physicians evidence-based clinical practice guidelines. Chest 2013;143(5 Suppl):e142S–65S.

24. Labarca G, Folch E, Jantz M, et al. Adequacy of samples obtained by EBUS-TBNA for molecular analysis in patients with non-small cell lung cancer: systematic review and meta-analysis. Ann Am Thorac Soc 2018;15(10):1205–16.

25. Kokkonouzis I, Strimpakos AS, Lampaditis I, et al. The role of endobronchial ultrasound in lung cancer diagnosis and staging: a comprehensive review. Clin Lung Cancer 2012;13(6):408–15.

26. Patrucco F, Gavelli F, Daverio M, et al. Electromagnetic navigation bronchoscopy: where are we now? five years of a single-center experience. Lung 2018;196(6): 721–7.

27. Deng CJ, Dai FQ, Qian K, et al. Clinical updates of approaches for biopsy of pulmonary lesions based on systematic review. BMC Pulm Med 2018;18(1):146.

28. Goldstraw P, Chansky K, Crowley J, et al. The IASLC lung cancer staging project: proposals for revision of the TNM stage groupings in the forthcoming (eighth) edition of the TNM classification for lung cancer. J Thorac Oncol 2016;11(1):39–51.

29. Detterbeck FC, Boffa DJ, Kim AW, et al. The eighth edition lung cancer stage classification. Chest 2017;151(1):193–203.

30. Detterbeck FC, Chansky K, Groome P, et al. The IASLC lung cancer staging project: methodology and validation used in the development of proposals for

revision of the stage classification of NSCLC in the forthcoming (eighth) edition of the TNM classification of lung cancer. J Thorac Oncol 2016;11(9):1433–46.

31. Howington JA, Blum MG, Chang AC, et al. Treatment of stage I and II non-small cell lung cancer: diagnosis and management of lung cancer, 3rd ed: American College of Chest Physicians evidence-based clinical practice guidelines. Chest 2013;143(5 Suppl):e278S–313S.

32. Stokes WA, Rusthoven CG. Surgery vs. SBRT in retrospective analyses: confounding by operability is the elephant in the room. J Thorac Dis 2018; 10(Suppl 17):S2007–10.

33. Detterbeck FC. The eighth edition TNM stage classification for lung cancer: what does it mean on main street? J Thorac Cardiovasc Surg 2018;155(1):356–9.

34. Bryant AK, Mundt RC, Sandhu AP, et al. Stereotactic body radiation therapy versus surgery for early lung cancer among US veterans. Ann Thorac Surg 2018;105(2):425–31.

35. Ye X, Fan W, Wang H, et al. Expert consensus workshop report: guidelines for thermal ablation of primary and metastatic lung tumors (2018 edition). J Cancer Res Ther 2018;14(4):730–44.

36. Casal RF, Walsh G, McArthur M, et al. Bronchoscopic laser interstitial thermal therapy: an experimental study in normal porcine lung parenchyma. J Bronchology Interv Pulmonol 2018;25(4):322–9.

37. National Comprehensive Cancer Network. Non-small cell lung cancer (Version 6.2018). Available at. https://www.nccn.org/professionals/physician_gls/pdf/nscl.pdf. Accessed September 21, 2018.

38. Ramnath N, Dilling TJ, Harris LJ, et al. Treatment of stage III non-small cell lung cancer: diagnosis and management of lung cancer, 3rd ed: American College of Chest Physicians evidence-based clinical practice guidelines. Chest 2013;143(5 Suppl):e314S–40S.

39. Socinski MA, Evans T, Gettinger S, et al. Treatment of stage IV non-small cell lung cancer: diagnosis and management of lung cancer, 3rd ed: American College of Chest Physicians evidence-based clinical practice guidelines. Chest 2013;143(5 Suppl):e341S–68S.

40. Simoff MJ, Lally B, Slade MG, et al. Symptom management in patients with lung cancer: diagnosis and management of lung cancer, 3rd ed: American College of Chest Physicians evidence-based clinical practice guidelines. Chest 2013;143(5 Suppl):e455S–97S.

41. Sabath BF, Ost DE. Update on airway stents. Curr Opin Pulm Med 2018;24(4): 343–9.

42. National Comprehensive Cancer Network. Small cell lung cancer (Version 2.2018). Available at: https://www.nccn.org/professionals/physician_gls/pdf/sclc.pdf. Accessed September 21, 2018.

43. Jett JR, Schild SE, Kesler KA, et al. Treatment of small cell lung cancer: diagnosis and management of lung cancer, 3rd ed: American College of Chest Physicians evidence-based clinical practice guidelines. Chest 2013;143(5 Suppl): e400S–19S.

44. Qin H, Wang F, Liu H, et al. New advances in immunotherapy for non-small cell lung cancer. Am J Transl Res 2018;10(8):2234–45.

45. Gridelli C, Ascierto PA, Grossi F, et al. Second-line treatment of advanced non-small cell lung cancer non-oncogene addicted: new treatment algorithm in the era of novel immunotherapy. Curr Clin Pharmacol 2018;13(2):76–84.

46. Sullivan I, Planchard D. ALK inhibitors in non-small cell lung cancer: the latest evidence and developments. Ther Adv Med Oncol 2016;8(1):32–47.

47. Mayekar MK, Bivona TG. Current landscape of targeted therapy in lung cancer. Clin Pharmacol Ther 2017;102(5):757–64.

48. Pavel ME, Singh S, Strosberg JR, et al. Health-related quality of life for everolimus versus placebo in patients with advanced, non-functional, well-differentiated gastrointestinal or lung neuroendocrine tumours (RADIANT-4): a multicentre, randomised, double-blind, placebo-controlled, phase 3 trial. Lancet Oncol 2017;18(10):1411–22.

49. Antonia SJ, Lopez-Martin JA, Bendell J, et al. Nivolumab alone and nivolumab plus ipilimumab in recurrent small-cell lung cancer (CheckMate 032): a multicentre, open-label, phase 1/2 trial. Lancet Oncol 2016;17(7):883–95.

50. Howlader N, Noone AM, Krapcho M, et al. SEER Cancer Statistics Review, 1975-2014, National Cancer Institute. Bethesda, MD. Available at: https://seer.cancer.gov/csr/1975_2014/, based on November 2016 SEER data submission, posted to the SEER web site, April 2017. Accessed September 21, 2018.

51. Ford DW, Koch KA, Ray DE, et al. Palliative and end-of-life care in lung cancer: diagnosis and management of lung cancer, 3rd ed: American College of Chest Physicians evidence-based clinical practice guidelines. Chest 2013;143(5 Suppl):e498S–512S.

52. Temel JS, Greer JA, Muzikansky A, et al. Early palliative care for patients with metastatic non-small-cell lung cancer. N Engl J Med 2010;363(8):733–42.

Update in the Management of Pleural Effusions

Matthew Aboudara, MD, Fabien Maldonado, MD*

KEYWORDS

- Pleural effusion • Malignant pleural effusion • Empyema • Pleuroscopy
- Indwelling pleural catheters

KEY POINTS

- Thoracic ultrasound always should be performed in the evaluation of a pleural effusion. It can help characterize the complexity of the effusion and identify a safe access point for thoracentesis.
- Pleural fluid studies should be ordered with the intent of ruling out an exudative effusion by Light's criteria. An exudative effusion of unknown cause should prompt a pulmonologist consultation.
- Medical pleuroscopy is a safe and minimally invasive technique performed by expert pulmonologists in the evaluation of unexplained exudative effusions with high diagnostic yield for malignancy.
- Indwelling pleural catheters are useful in the palliation of malignant pleural effusions. They are effective in symptom control and appear to be cost-effective with long-term use.
- Complex parapneumonic effusions require prompt diagnosis and treatment with antibiotics, chest tube drainage, intrapleural fibrinolytic therapy when indicated, and surgical intervention.

INTRODUCTION

Primary care physicians are frequently asked to manage pleural effusions. Approximately 1.5 million pleural effusions are diagnosed annually in the United States alone, among which 500,000 are attributed to congestive heart failure (CHF) and 150,000 to malignancy.[1] Of the 1 million individuals diagnosed with pneumonia every year in the United States, approximately 32,000 will develop an empyema.[2] **Table 1** lists the most common causes of pleural effusions.

Disclosure Statement: F. Maldonado received an unrestricted research grant from Centurion Medical (digital manometer).
Division of Allergy, Pulmonary and Critical Care Medicine, Vanderbilt University Medical Center, The Vanderbilt Clinic, 1301 Medical Center Drive, B-817 The Vanderbilt Clinic, Nashville, TN 37232-5735, USA
* Corresponding author.
E-mail address: Fabien.maldonado@vumc.org

Med Clin N Am 103 (2019) 475–485
https://doi.org/10.1016/j.mcna.2018.12.007
0025-7125/19/© 2018 Elsevier Inc. All rights reserved.

Table 1 Common etiologies of pleural effusions	
Transudates	**Exudates**
Congestive heart failure	Pneumonia
Cirrhosis with ascites	Malignancy
Pulmonary embolism	Post coronary artery bypass surgery
Nephrotic syndrome	Viral pneumonia
Hypoalbuminemia	Pulmonary embolism
Trapped lung	Collagen vascular disease

Data from Light RW. Pleural Diseases, 6th edition. Philadelphia(PA): Lippincott Williams & Wilkins; 2013.

The pleural space is a reservoir for approximately 15 mL of fluid per hemothorax, constantly turned over, purported to serve as a lubricant to optimize the mechanical coupling of lung and chest wall.[3] Although the obliteration of the pleural space (ie, pleurodesis) does not appear to cause major issues, pathologic expansion of the pleural space from fluid can cause significant breathlessness and impair quality of life, both of which can be improved with fluid removal.

A considerable body of evidence has emerged in the past decade and has led to a paradigm shift in the management of pleural diseases, specifically with regard to pleural effusions. The goal of this review was to update the primary care physician on recent advances in the diagnosis, imaging evaluation, and treatment of pleural effusions. This review addresses 6 key questions of practical relevance to primary care physicians (**Box 1**).

SHOULD I ALWAYS USE POINT OF CARE ULTRASOUND TO ASSESS A PLEURAL EFFUSION?

Pathologic accumulation of pleural fluid occurs when fluid production outpaces absorption, absorption is impaired, or, more commonly, as a combination of both.[4] A comprehensive history and detailed physical examination are of utmost importance, as 75% of effusions can be attributed to CHF, pneumonia, or malignancy,[1] diagnoses that can often be entertained before pleural fluid analysis.

Initial radiographic imaging typically consists of a chest radiograph, obtained to elucidate the cause of breathlessness, the most common symptom experienced by patients with pleural effusion and understood to result from restricted diaphragmatic

---

Box 1
Six key clinical questions in pleural effusion management

- Should I always use point-of-care ultrasound to assess for a pleural effusion?
- When should I pursue a diagnostic thoracentesis?
- What test should I order on the fluid?
- What is the role for medical pleuroscopy and when should I refer?
- What is the role for indwelling pleural catheters?
- When do I chose between chest tube with intrapleural therapy versus surgery for an empyema or complicated parapneumonic effusion not responding to antibiotics and chest tube drainage alone?

excursion. When the chest radiograph suggests an effusion, a thoracic ultrasound (TUS) examination should be performed next, as it can confirm the presence of and quantify pleural fluid, reveal septations and loculations, and identify a flattened or inverted diaphragm predictive of symptomatic improvement after thoracentesis.[5] A computed tomography (CT) scan of the chest with contrast is generally recommended if the pleural fluid has complex ultrasonographic features (such as septations and loculations), which may suggest parapneumonic effusion or malignancy (**Figs. 1** and **2**).

The use of TUS for the initial evaluation of pleural effusions has become the standard of care, and procedures performed without are medicolegally indefensible.[6] In a systematic review of more than 6000 thoracenteses, the use of TUS was the strongest predictor of a reduction in the rate of pneumothorax (4.0% vs 9.5%).[7] Thoracic ultrasound allows identification of the liver, spleen, diaphragm, and underlying lung, thereby allowing the operator to readily identify the safest point of entry (**Fig. 3**). Although real-time ultrasound during the procedure is ideal, most clinicians use the "mark-and-go" method, although the patient should not move between identification of the entry site and needle entry. Thoracic ultrasound at the end of the procedure can confirm complete fluid evacuation and exclude an iatrogenic pneumothorax. The use of TUS for the management of pleural diseases has been reviewed elsewhere.[5]

WHEN SHOULD I PURSUE A DIAGNOSTIC THORACENTESIS?

Traditional teaching recommends performing a thoracentesis if the thickness of the pleural effusion exceeds 10 mm on a lateral decubitus radiograph or 2 cm on CT scan or ultrasound, and the effusion is not thought to be secondary to CHF. It is important to act promptly in patients with possible parapneumonic effusions, as these effusions can progress quickly from simple, free-flowing effusions to complex, septated effusions or empyema within 12 to 24 hours.[8]

When addressing a pleural effusion, one must consider whether performing the thoracentesis is intended to be therapeutic, diagnostic, or both, as this may impact the amount of fluid removed. In general, the clinician should attempt to remove the largest amount of fluid possible to provide relief and delay the need for subsequent procedures. The maximal amount of fluid that may be safely drained in one setting is unclear. Complications related to large-volume thoracentesis, such as reexpansion

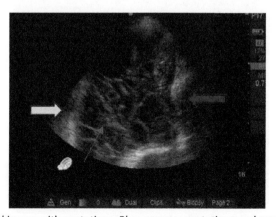

Fig. 1. Ultrasound image with septations. Blue arrow = septations; red arrow = diaphragm; yellow arrow = compressed lung.

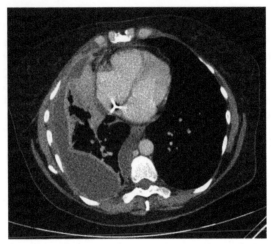

Fig. 2. CT of the chest demonstrating loculated lung consistent with empyema.

pulmonary edema (REPE), pneumothorax ex vacuo, and chest discomfort, are thought to be secondary to the development of excessively negative pleural pressures, rather than to the absolute volume drained. REPE is a rare entity (0.5%)[9] of unclear pathogenesis but carries a mortality rate of 20%.[10] Accordingly, some advocate the routine use of manometry to detect the development of dangerously low pleural pressures (defined as <20 cm H_2O).[11] As negative pressures correlate with chest discomfort, most prefer discontinuing the procedure when patients start reporting pain. As we await the result of a clinical trial addressing this question (ClinicalTrials.gov Identifier: NCT02677883), it seems prudent to recommend limiting thoracentesis to 1000 mL.

WHAT TEST SHOULD I ORDER ON THE FLUID?

An algorithmic approach to pleural fluid evaluation and when to consult a pulmonologist is outlined in **Fig. 4**. Pleural fluid analysis should be based on the Light criteria,

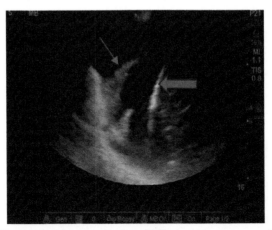

Fig. 3. Ultrasound image showing simple pleural effusion. Blue arrow = diaphragm; orange arrow = compressed lung by surrounding fluid (*black*).

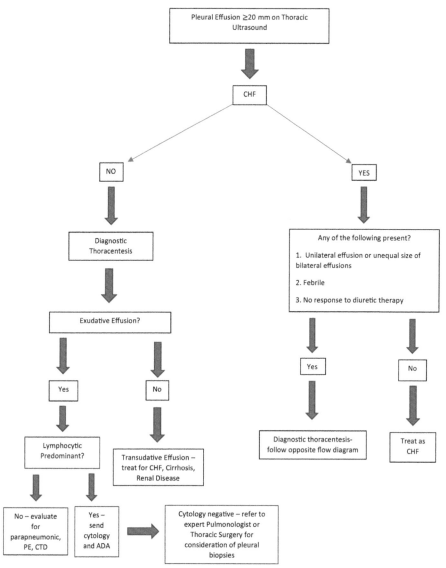

Fig. 4. Diagnostic approach to pleural effusions. ADA, adenosine deaminase; PE, pleural effusion; CTD, connective tissue disease. (*Modified from* Light RW. Clinical practice. Pleural effusion. N Engl J Med 2002;346(25):1973.)

which have a high sensitivity for exudative effusions. An effusion is considered exudative when any one of the following three criteria are met: pleural/serum total protein ratio > 0.5, pleural/serum lactate dehydrogenase (LDH) > 0.6, or pleural LDH > two-thirds the upper limit of normal.[12] As approximately 25% of pleural effusions due to CHF may be misclassified as an exudate, a serum to pleural albumin gradient should be calculated. If >1.2 g/L, the effusion may be a so-called pseudo-exudate and be due to a diuretic effect. If albumin is unavailable, a protein gradient greater than 3.1 g/L may have the same diagnostic value. Some have recommended a pleural fluid

N-terminal pro b-type natriuretic peptide, as a level greater than 1500 pg per mL has a sensitivity and specificity of 91% and 93%, respectively, for a transudate.[13] There does not appear to be much difference between elevated pleural and serum levels, however, so that serum values are typically preferred.

Pleural fluid cultures should be obtained if infection is suspected. Aerobic and anaerobic blood culture bottles should be inoculated at the bedside, as this increases the yield from 40% to 60%.[14] A neutrophilic effusion in a context of recent respiratory infection, fever, or chills is suggestive of parapneumonic effusion. Parapneumonic effusions with low pH (<7.2), low glucose (<40 mg/dL), or empyema (identified by the presence of pus or positive cultures) require chest tube drainage in addition to aerobic and anaerobic antibiotic coverage, and a multidisciplinary management including expert consultation with pulmonology and thoracic surgery is recommended.

Pleural fluid cytology should be sent whenever malignant pleural effusion (MPE) is possible or if the patient has a lymphocytic exudative effusion. The sensitivity of cytology is 60% with 1 sample, and 75% with 2. A third pleural fluid cytology does not increase the diagnostic yield and may delay diagnosis and treatment.[14] Recent data suggest that diagnostic yield of cytology depends on the type of malignancy: higher with adenocarcinomas, and lower with squamous cell carcinomas and sarcomas.[15] Repeating thoracenteses unnecessarily may increase pleural space septations, making future diagnostic and therapeutic interventions difficult. As such, patients with unexplained exudative pleural effusions after a maximum of 2 thoracenteses should be referred for pleuroscopy with pleural biopsies or image-guided pleural biopsies.

A lymphocytic exudative effusion also should prompt consideration for mycobacterium tuberculosis (TB) when risk factors are present. Acid-fast cultures have a low yield for pleural TB and biopsies are generally needed. A pleural fluid adenosine deaminase has good test characteristics (sensitivity of 92%, specificity 90%[16]) and may be helpful in ruling out TB in patients with low pretest probability, but should not be used to establish the diagnosis, as treatment should be based on cultures and sensitivities.

WHAT IS THE ROLE OF PLEUROSCOPY AND WHEN SHOULD I REFER PATIENTS?

Pleuroscopy is a minimally invasive procedure performed by expertly trained pulmonologists in which a semirigid or rigid videoscope is introduced through a single port into the pleural space under moderate sedation in a spontaneously breathing patient (http://medical.olympusamerica.com/procedure/pleuroscopy). Compared with surgery, pleuroscopy obviates the need for general anesthesia, single lung ventilation, and operating room time and expense. Although no head-to-head comparison exists, the diagnostic yield of pleuroscopy approaches that of video-assisted thoracoscopic surgery, estimated at approximately 90% to 95%. The indications for pleuroscopy are listed in **Table 2**. The yield for malignancy is 92.6% and 93.0% for TB pleuritis in low-prevalence regions.[17] The high yield is attributed to direct visualization and biopsy of pleural abnormalities (**Figs. 5** and **6**).

It is a low-risk procedure, with complications reported in 1.8% of cases, and a mortality rate of 0.34%,[14] although mortality in strictly diagnostic procedures has not been reported. An important consideration with pleuroscopy is the diagnosis of nonspecific pleuritis, an entity with unclear clinical implications diagnosed in approximately 25% of cases in large series. Several series have suggested that 5% to 10% of patients diagnosed with nonspecific pleuritis via pleuroscopy or

Table 2	
Indications for medical pleuroscopy	
Diagnostic	**Therapeutic**
Cytologic negative lymphocytic exudative effusion	Talc poudrage to achieve pleurodesis
Staging	Drainage of pleural fluid/space
Additional tissue for molecular analysis	Complex parapneumonic effusion

Data from Rahman NM, Ali NJ, Brown G, et al. Local anaesthetic thoracoscopy: British Thoracic Society Pleural Disease guideline 2010. Thorax 2010;65(Suppl 2):ii54–60.

surgery ultimately develop MPE, usually in the form of malignant pleural mesothelioma. Accordingly, radiologic follow-up with chest CT for at least 2 years is recommended in this situation.

WHAT IS THE ROLE FOR INDWELLING PLEURAL CATHETERS?

MPEs typically portend a poor prognosis with median survival of 3 to 12 months.[1] Accordingly, the primary goal of management is symptom palliation. Current guidelines recommend a definitive intervention for symptom relief from an MPE if:

1. The effusion recurs quickly after thoracentesis (generally no more than 2 or 3),
2. Symptoms are relieved after therapeutic thoracentesis, and
3. The patient has a life expectancy of more than 30 days.[18]

Definitive treatment can be achieved with either a tunneled indwelling pleural catheter (IPC), talc pleurodesis (achieved by chest tube or thoracoscopy), or combination

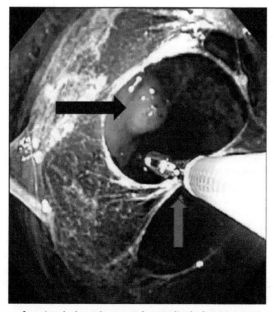

Fig. 5. Visualization of parietal pleural tumors by medical pleuroscopy in a patient with malignant mesothelioma. Tumor on parietal pleura/chest wall (*black arrow*); flexible forceps were used to remove simple adhesions (*blue arrow*).

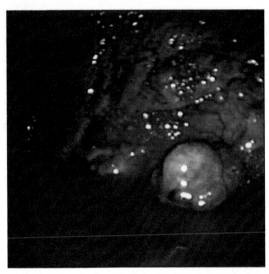

Fig. 6. Medical pleuroscopy image of metastatic thyroid cancer on chest wall.

thereof. Although both procedures are equivalent in symptom relief and achieving pleurodesis,[19] IPCs have become the procedure of choice in the United States, as they have been demonstrated to have a more favorable profile in reducing hospital length of stay as compared with talc pleurodesis,[20] and are not associated with rare but potentially deadly complications from talc pleurodesis (acute respiratory distress syndrome). Furthermore, an estimated 25% of patients with MPE have unexpandable lung, and are therefore not suitable candidates for pleurodesis, which requires apposition of the visceral and parietal pleura. IPCs are, however, associated with a 5% risk of pleural space infection, which usually respond well to antibiotics alone.

Interestingly, IPCs appear to be cost-effective from a third-party payer perspective compared with alternative strategies when the patient's life expectancy exceeds 6 months. A validated clinical prediction score, the LENT score, may facilitate the decision-making process in this situation.[21] Ultimately, the decision should be tailored to the patient's unique situation and preferences.

WHEN DO I CHOSE BETWEEN CHEST TUBE WITH INTRAPLEURAL THERAPY VERSUS SURGERY FOR AN EMPYEMA OR COMPLICATED PARAPNEUMONIC EFFUSION NOT RESPONDING TO ANTIBIOTICS AND CHEST TUBE DRAINAGE ALONE?

Of the 1 million people hospitalized in the United States annually with pneumonia, up to 40% will have a parapneumonic effusion and close to 10% will progress to empyema. Mortality approaches 20%, and up to 30% in patients with comorbidities,.[20] The prevalence of empyema is increasing, which may be attributed to a replacement phenomenon as a result of community pneumococcal vaccination programs, allowing the emergence of more virulent serotypes.[22] A clinical risk stratification tool has been developed that may predict those who are at increased risk for morbidity and mortality and may benefit from an early and more aggressive intervention.[23]

Prompt antibiotic administration and drainage of the pleural space are the cornerstones of therapy. For community-acquired infections, antibiotics should target the most commonly identified organisms (streptococcal species 52% and anaerobes 20%) whereas *Staphylococcus* and gram-negative organisms are more common in the hospital setting.[22] The duration of antibiotics varies from 2 to 6 weeks depending on the response to drainage. Follow-up CT scan of the chest is generally recommended 4 to 6 weeks after adequate therapy to ensure resolution of the infection and to assess for any underlying predisposing processes.

The indications for tube thoracostomy, intrapleural therapy, and surgery are listed in **Table 3**. Simple parapneumonic effusions can be managed with thoracentesis alone with the goal of complete evacuation of the pleural space, if feasible. In contrast, complicated parapneumonic effusions have radiographic, bacteriologic, or pleural chemistry features predictive of a poor outcome (eg, sepsis, entrapped lung, respiratory failure, death) and require intervention with a chest tube or surgery. Generally speaking, this includes patients with frank pus, septations and/or loculations, lactate dehydrogenase greater than 1000, positive Gram stain or culture, pH <7.15, or glucose less than 40 mg/dL[3].

A complicated parapneumonic effusion requires a multidisciplinary approach with pulmonology and thoracic surgery experts. The decision to proceed with up-front surgery versus intrapleural therapy is guided by current guidelines as we await the results of ongoing trials.[2,24] Regardless of the approach taken, source control with drainage via a small-bore chest tube is recommended based on data suggesting no difference in failure rates between small-bore and large-bore tubes, but with the advantage of less pain with small-bore tubes.[25]

In the presence of a complicated parapneumonic effusion or empyema, a thoracic surgeon should be consulted for consideration of surgery.[2,24] If the patient is not a surgical candidate, then intrapleural instillation of tissue plasminogen activator and deoxyribonuclease for 3 days should be considered based on results from the MIST 2 study, which showed a reduction in size of the pleural effusion on chest radiograph

Table 3
Interventions for parapneumonic effusions

Effusion Type	Pleural Fluid Characteristics	Thoracentesis	Small-Bore Chest Tube (8.5–14F)	tPA and DNAse	VATS
Simple parapneumonic effusion	>10 mm fluid, pH >7.20, negative Gram stain and culture	Yes	No	No	No
Complex parapneumonic effusion	Large free-flowing effusion, loculated lung; pH <7.15, glucose <40 mg/dL	No	Yes	±Yes[b]	Yes[c]
Empyema	Pus or positive Gram stain/culture	No	Yes[a]	No	Yes

Abbreviations: DNAse, deoxyribonuclease; tPA, tissue plasminogen activator; VATS, video-assisted thoracoscopic surgery

[a] Chest tube is placed for source control pending definitive surgical intervention.
[b] If patient is not a surgical candidate, tPA plus DNAse is recommended.
[c] Preferred intervention in this category.

Data from Shen KR, Bribriesco A, Crabtree T, et al. The American Association for Thoracic Surgery consensus guidelines for the management of empyema. J Thorac Cardiovasc Surg 2017;153:e129–46 and Scarci M, Abah U, Solli P, et al. EACTS expert consensus statement for surgical management of pleural empyema. Eur J Cardiothorac Surg 2015;48:642–53.

and a reduction in surgical interventions.[26] It should be emphasized that the clinically relevant endpoints in the MIST 2 were secondary endpoints, and its encouraging results will need to be further validated.

SUMMARY

Pleural effusions are a common clinical entity for the primary care physician. Prompt evaluation with TUS and a diagnostic thoracentesis are essential. Pleural fluid studies should focus on ruling out an exudative effusion and unexplained exudates should be referred for further evaluation, particularly if there remains a clinical concern for malignancy. Pleuroscopy is a minimally invasive procedure performed by expertly trained pulmonologists with a high yield in MPE. Indwelling pleural catheters are an effective therapeutic option for some patients in the palliation of MPE. Finally, complex parapneumonic effusions require prompt initiation of antibiotics, intrapleural therapy when indicated, and surgical consultation.

REFERENCES

1. Light RW. Pleural disease. 6th edition. Philadelphia: Lippincott Williams & Wilkins; 2013.
2. Shen KR, Bribriesco A, Crabtree T, et al. The American Association for Thoracic Surgery consensus guidelines for the management of empyema. J Thorac Cardiovasc Surg 2017;153:e129–46.
3. Feller-Kopman D, Light R. Pleural disease. N Engl J Med 2018;378:1754.
4. Feller-Kopman D, Parker MJ, Schwartzstein RM. Assessment of pleural pressure in the evaluation of pleural effusions. Chest 2009;135:201–9.
5. Thomas R, Jenkins S, Eastwood PR, et al. Physiology of breathlessness associated with pleural effusions. Curr Opin Pulm Med 2015;21:338–45.
6. Corcoran JP, Tazi-Mezalek R, Maldonado F, et al. State of the art thoracic ultrasound: intervention and therapeutics. Thorax 2017;72:840–9.
7. Gordon CE, Feller-Kopman D, Balk EM, et al. Pneumothorax following thoracentesis: a systematic review and meta-analysis. Arch Intern Med 2010;170:332–9.
8. Sahn SA, Light RW. The sun should never set on a parapneumonic effusion. Chest 1989;95:945–7.
9. Feller-Kopman D, Berkowitz D, Boiselle P, et al. Large-volume thoracentesis and the risk of reexpansion pulmonary edema. Ann Thorac Surg 2007;84:1656–61.
10. Mahfood S, Hix WR, Aaron BL, et al. Reexpansion pulmonary edema. Ann Thorac Surg 1988;45:340–5.
11. Feller-Kopman D. Point: should pleural manometry be performed routinely during thoracentesis? Yes. Chest 2012;141:844–5.
12. Light RW. Clinical practice. Pleural effusion. N Engl J Med 2002;346:1971–7.
13. Porcel JM, Martinez-Alonso M, Cao G, et al. Biomarkers of heart failure in pleural fluid. Chest 2009;136:671–7.
14. Menzies SM, Rahman NM, Wrightson JM, et al. Blood culture bottle culture of pleural fluid in pleural infection. Thorax 2011;66:658–62.
15. Grosu HB, Kazzaz F, Vakil E, et al. Sensitivity of initial thoracentesis for malignant pleural effusion stratified by tumor type in patients with strong evidence of metastatic disease. Respiration 2018;96(4):363–9.
16. Liang QL, Shi HZ, Wang K, et al. Diagnostic accuracy of adenosine deaminase in tuberculous pleurisy: a meta-analysis. Respir Med 2008;102:744–54.

17. Rahman NM, Ali NJ, Brown G, et al. Local anaesthetic thoracoscopy: British Thoracic Society Pleural Disease guideline 2010. Thorax 2010;65(Suppl 2): ii54–60.

18. Simoff MJ, Lally B, Slade MG, et al. Symptom management in patients with lung cancer: diagnosis and management of lung cancer, 3rd ed: American College of Chest Physicians evidence-based clinical practice guidelines. Chest 2013;143: e455S–97S.

19. Davies HE, Mishra EK, Kahan BC, et al. Effect of an indwelling pleural catheter vs chest tube and talc pleurodesis for relieving dyspnea in patients with malignant pleural effusion: the TIME2 randomized controlled trial. JAMA 2012;307:2383–9.

20. Shafiq M, Frick KD, Lee H, et al. Management of malignant pleural effusion: a cost-utility analysis. J Bronchology Interv Pulmonol 2015;22:215–25.

21. Clive AO, Kahan BC, Hooper CE, et al. Predicting survival in malignant pleural effusion: development and validation of the LENT prognostic score. Thorax 2014;69:1098–104.

22. Corcoran JP, Wrightson JM, Belcher E, et al. Pleural infection: past, present, and future directions. Lancet Respir Med 2015;3:563–77.

23. Rahman NM, Kahan BC, Miller RF, et al. A clinical score (RAPID) to identify those at risk for poor outcome at presentation in patients with pleural infection. Chest 2014;145:848–55.

24. Scarci M, Abah U, Solli P, et al. EACTS expert consensus statement for surgical management of pleural empyema. Eur J Cardiothorac Surg 2015;48:642–53.

25. Rahman NM, Maskell NA, Davies CW, et al. The relationship between chest tube size and clinical outcome in pleural infection. Chest 2010;137:536–43.

26. Rahman NM, Maskell NA, West A, et al. Intrapleural use of tissue plasminogen activator and DNase in pleural infection. N Engl J Med 2011;365:518–26.

Community-acquired Pneumonia and Hospital-acquired Pneumonia

Charles W. Lanks, MD[a],*, Ali I. Musani, MD[b], David W. Hsia, MD[a]

KEYWORDS

- Community-acquired pneumonia • Hospital-acquired pneumonia • Pneumonia
- CAP • HAP

KEY POINTS

- Pneumonia is a common disease that requires a deep understanding of pathophysiology, epidemiology, and pharmacology to properly manage.
- Diagnostic strategies for pneumonia range from simple to highly complex depending on disease severity and likelihood of altering the empiric antibiotic regimen.
- Pneumonia management plans are tailored to each individual patient encounter and incorporate knowledge of health care setting, pathogen type, and risk factors for antibiotic resistance.
- Complications from pneumonia are common and should prompt consultation with a pulmonary specialist when necessary.

INTRODUCTION

Pneumonia is consistently among the leading causes of morbidity and mortality worldwide.[1] Defined as acute infection of the lung parenchyma, it is caused by a wide variety of microorganisms, including bacteria, viruses, and fungi.[2] Common categories of pneumonia include:

- Community-acquired pneumonia (CAP): infection acquired outside of the hospital setting.
- Hospital-acquired pneumonia (HAP): infection acquired after at least 48 hours of hospitalization.[3]

Disclosure: The authors have no financial conflicts of interest.
[a] Division of Respiratory and Critical Care Physiology and Medicine, Harbor-UCLA Medical Center, 1000 West Carson Street, Box 402, Torrance, CA 90509, USA; [b] Division of Pulmonary Sciences and Critical Care Medicine, University of Colorado Hospital, 12631 East 17th Street, Office #8102, Aurora, CO 80045, USA
* Corresponding author.
E-mail address: clanks@dhs.lacounty.gov

Med Clin N Am 103 (2019) 487–501
https://doi.org/10.1016/j.mcna.2018.12.008
0025-7125/19/© 2019 Elsevier Inc. All rights reserved.

- Ventilator-associated pneumonia (VAP): subcategory of HAP that occurs in patients receiving mechanical ventilation. Because of major differences in pathophysiology, microbiology, and therapy in VAP compared with non-VAP HAP, it is outside the scope of this review.
- Health care–associated pneumonia (HCAP): infection acquired in lower-acuity health care settings such as nursing homes and dialysis centers.[3] It is now recognized that patients acquiring pneumonia in lower-acuity health care settings are not at increased risk for multidrug-resistant (MDR) pathogens[4]; therefore, HCAP was not included in the most recent treatment guidelines for CAP or HAP.[2,5]

PATHOPHYSIOLOGY

Pathogens such as *Streptococcus pneumoniae*, *Haemophilus influenzae*, and gram-negative bacilli typically enter the lower respiratory tract through aspiration of oropharyngeal secretions. Microaspiration can occur on a regular basis, even in healthy individuals and particularly during sleep, but progression to pneumonia is rare. Progression largely depends on the inoculum of pathogenic bacteria, volume of aspirate, frequency of aspiration, and virulence of aspirated bacteria relative to the host immune system.[6] Colonization of the oropharynx with virulent organisms is affected by comorbidities such as chronic malnutrition, alcoholism, and diabetes. These comorbidities lead to defects in the host immune response, such as deficiencies in local immunoglobulins, complement, and salivary fibronectins, which prevent bacterial surface binding.

Intracellular bacteria (*Mycoplasma pneumoniae*, *Chlamydia pneumoniae*, *Legionella* spp) and viruses tend to enter the lower respiratory tract via the inhalational route. Progression to infection again depends on the inoculum of pathogenic organisms. However, the microparticles in which that inoculum is suspended must also be small enough (typically <5 μm) to facilitate transit into the lower airways while continuing to evade local host defenses.

EPIDEMIOLOGY

Pneumonia remains a leading cause of hospitalization and death worldwide. In 2015, pneumonia was the eighth leading cause of death in the United States,[1] the fourth leading cause of death worldwide, and leading cause of death in low-income countries.[7] However, the true incidence of CAP is likely underestimated. Patients with mild infections are less likely to seek medical attention and diagnosis may therefore go unrecognized.

Microbiology

Among patients who seek medical attention, *S pneumoniae* is by far the most commonly isolated bacterial pathogen, accounting for more than 25% of cases of CAP worldwide.[8] The likelihood of disease being caused by a specific organism varies with disease severity (**Table 1**). Milder presentations are more likely to be caused by *M pneumonia*, *C pneumoniae*, and viruses, although *S pneumoniae* still predominates.[9] More severe presentations commonly involve *Staphylococcus aureus*, *Legionella*, and *H influenzae* (see **Table 1**). This rough association between causative organism and disease severity lays the groundwork for empiric antimicrobial therapy.[2]

The spectrum of causative organisms in HAP also includes gram-positive cocci such as *S aureus* and *S pneumoniae*[10] but is more likely to involve gram-negative bacilli such as *Pseudomonas aeruginosa*, *Klebsiella pneumoniae*, *Enterococcus coli*,

Table 1 Causative organisms and suggested diagnostics by pneumonia type and severity		
	Common Causative Organisms	**Suggested Diagnostics**
CAP: outpatient	*M pneumoniae, S pneumoniae, Chlamydophila pneumoniae*, respiratory viruses[a]	• None routinely
CAP: non-ICU, low severity	*S pneumoniae, M pneumoniae, C pneumoniae*, respiratory viruses[a]	• Sputum bacterial culture • Respiratory viral PCR
CAP: non-ICU, moderate severity	*S pneumoniae, Staphylococcus aureus, H influenzae, Legionella* species, respiratory viruses[a]	• Sputum bacterial culture • Blood bacterial culture • Respiratory viral PCR • Pneumococcal urinary Ag • *Legionella* urinary Ag
CAP: ICU, high severity	*S pneumoniae*, enteric gram-negative bacilli,[b] *S aureus, H influenzae, Legionella* species, respiratory viruses[a], *Pseudomonas aeruginosa*	• Sputum bacterial culture • Blood bacterial culture • Respiratory viral PCR • Pneumococcal urinary Ag • *Legionella* urinary Ag • Consider bronchoscopy
HAP (non-VAP)	*S pneumoniae*, enteric gram-negative bacilli, *S aureus, P aeruginosa*	• Sputum bacterial culture • Blood bacterial culture • Respiratory viral PCR • Pneumococcal urinary Ag

Abbreviations: Ag, antigen; ICU, intensive care unit; PCR, polymerase chain reaction.
[a] Such as influenza, parainfluenza, and respiratory syncytial virus.
[b] Such as *Klebsiella pneumoniae, Enterococcus coli*, and *Enterobacter* spp.

and *Enterobacter* spp.[11] The presence of multidrug resistance is affected by a combination of patient-specific and hospital-specific risk factors such as recent antibiotic use, length of current hospitalization, presence of structural lung disease, and local hospital resistance patterns. Commonly encountered MDR pathogens include methicillin-resistant *S aureus* (MRSA), *Pseudomonas*, and extended-spectrum β-lactamase (ESBL)–producing gram-negative enteric bacteria.[12,13]

Viruses, including influenza, are common causative organisms depending on seasonal variations.[14] In addition, viruses have been found to play an increasingly recognized role in HAP.[15] However, it should be noted that the mere detection of a viral pathogen does not guarantee causality because there is a strong association between viral infection and secondary bacterial coinfection.[16]

Less commonly encountered organisms include *Mycobacterium tuberculosis*, nontuberculous mycobacteria, *Chlamydophila* spp, *Coxiella*, and fungi such as *Coccidioides, Blastomyces, Histoplasma, Cryptococcus*, and *Aspergillus*. Suspicion for these should depend on individual patient risk factors, including immunosuppression and travel history.

Risk Factors and Genetics

The risk of acquiring pneumonia increases with patient age and the presence of comorbidities.[17] These comorbidities include chronic respiratory diseases, such as chronic obstructive pulmonary disease and bronchiectasis, as well as nonrespiratory problems such as cardiovascular and renal diseases. Comorbidities such as epilepsy, dementia, and stroke increase pneumonia risk as well, possibly via increased risk of aspiration. Lifestyle-related factors such as tobacco use, alcohol use, chronic malnutrition, and poor dental hygiene also confer increased risk.[18] The presence of structural lung disease, recent antibiotic use, and corticosteroid use are risk factors for gram-negative infection.[19]

More recently, several genetic risk factors for CAP have also been identified.[20] Variants in the proto-oncogene tyrosine-protein kinase FER gene, which regulates cell adhesion, migration, and chemotaxis, have been associated with reduced risk of death from pneumonia.[21]

CLINICAL PRESENTATION

The classic or typical presentation of pneumonia is characterized by the acute onset of infectious lower respiratory tract symptoms in conjunction with consistent radiographic findings. Fever, cough, pleurisy, dyspnea, and increased sputum production are common symptoms of pneumonia. In many patients, the presentation of pneumonia can be atypical and characterized predominantly by nonrespiratory symptoms such as malaise, myalgia, confusion, and diarrhea. In elderly individuals, this type of presentation may occur with increased frequency,[22,23] leading to delays in therapy and increased mortality.[24]

The grouping of clinical presentations into typical and atypical categories was previously thought to be useful in predicting type of causative organism and, therefore, guiding choice of empiric antibiotic therapy. Typical presentations were thought to more likely be caused by the so-called typical pathogens (ie, S pneumoniae, H influenzae, S aureus, and Moraxella catarrhalis) and atypical presentations by so-called atypical pathogens (ie, Legionella, M pneumoniae, and C pneumoniae). It has since been shown that the breakdown of presentation types into typical and atypical categories has little value in predicting type of causative organism.[25] Despite this, the typical versus atypical naming system is still widely used, but physicians should understand its limitations.

DIAGNOSTICS
Imaging

Radiographic evidence of parenchymal lung involvement is needed to establish the diagnosis of pneumonia. The radiographic appearance of pneumonia can be highly variable (Fig. 1). Although computed tomography (CT) is the gold standard for detection of pulmonary infiltrates, plain chest radiographs are more frequently obtained, especially in the outpatient setting. Although CT imaging can elucidate more specific findings than plain chest radiography (see Figs. 1D–F), it also exposes patients to significantly more radiation, cannot be performed at the bedside, and cannot be interpreted in real time by most clinicians.

The sensitivity of plain chest radiographs for detecting infiltrates is low, ranging from 38% to 75%.[26,27] In critically ill patients, the suboptimal anteroposterior view is most often used. Quality is further degraded by poor inspiratory effort, obese body habitus, and suboptimal patient positioning.

Point-of-care ultrasonography has more recently emerged as a viable alternative to plain chest radiographs for the detection of lung consolidations (Fig. 2A). Advantages include the ability to perform and interpret images at the bedside in real time, no radiation exposure, and improved sensitivity compared with plain chest radiographs. Distinguishing between lung consolidation and pleural effusion is also more easily done with ultrasonography (Fig. 2B). However, sensitivities exceeding 95% reported in the literature[26,27] require time-intensive evaluations of the lungs from multiple angles by experienced practitioners.

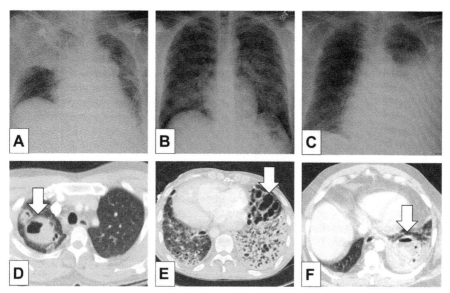

Fig. 1. Variations in radiographic appearance of pneumonia. (*A*) Lobar consolidation of the right upper lobe. (*B*) Bilateral interstitial infiltrates. (*C*) Large left parapneumonic pleural effusion. (*D*) Right upper lobe cavitary lesions (*white arrow*). (*E*) Diffuse bronchiectasis involving primarily the anterior left lower lobe (*white arrow*). (*F*) Pulmonary abscess with air fluid level in the posterior left lower lobe (*white arrow*).

Laboratory

In patients with suspected pneumonia, routine laboratory testing is typically indicated, particularly when hospitalization is required. Complete blood cell count may reveal a leukocytosis or bandemia suggestive of acute infection.[28] Serum chemistry can provide insight into associated organ involvement, such as hepatic or renal dysfunction, and provides useful data for pneumonia severity stratification.

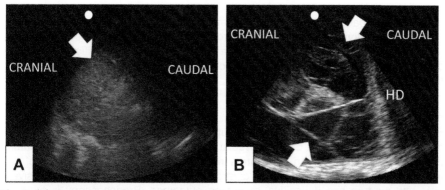

Fig. 2. (*A*) Tissue sign indicating lobar consolidation in pneumonia as imaged by point-of-care ultrasonography (*white arrow*). (*B*) Septations in pleural space (*white arrows*) suggestive of complicated parapneumonic effusion as imaged with point-of-care ultrasonography. HD, hemidiaphragm.

Procalcitonin (PCT) is a serum protein that is released in response to bacterial infection. In viral infections, PCT release is downregulated via the release of the inhibitory cytokine interferon gamma. This quality makes PCT a useful biomarker for discriminating between viral and bacterial causes of CAP.[29] In studies of both outpatient and inpatient populations, using a lower threshold value of PCT to discourage antibiotic initiation resulted in decreased antibiotic usage without a negative impact on mortality.[30] However, given the high morbidity and mortality associated with delaying or withholding necessary antibiotics in pneumonia, there is not widespread agreement as to how PCT should be used routinely in this context and its use was not included in the most recent treatment guidelines.[2,5]

Microbiologic

Isolating a causative organism can be of tremendous value when it leads to a change in management. Diagnostic strategies vary depending on disease severity and suspected pathogen (see **Table 1**). Most clinicians agree that, in the outpatient setting, microbiologic tests are likely to be low yield and add little to the choice and duration of antibiotics.[31] In hospitalized patients, particularly those with severe sepsis or septic shock, determining a causative organism can significantly improve mortality.[32] All hospitalized patients with purulent sputum should have it sent for Gram stain and culture.[2] In patients without purulent sputum or who are unable to provide lower respiratory tract samples, culture results can be inaccurate and commonly represent upper airway or oropharyngeal colonizers rather than true pathogens. Blood cultures are positive in only 20% of cases and should only be performed in cases of moderate to high severity, including all patients admitted to the intensive care unit (ICU). Every effort should be made to collect cultures before initiation of antibiotics in order to increase their diagnostic yield.[33]

Urinary antigen testing is a useful tool for the identification of S pneumoniae and Legionella pneumophila serogroup 1 in patients hospitalized with pneumonia. Although these tests should not be used in lieu of conventional cultures because of their lack of resistance data, they do hold several advantages. The sensitivity and specificity of both tests for their respective pathogens is high: approximately 74% for S pneumoniae and 97% for Legionella.[34,35] In addition, these tests are less affected by being on antibiotics than conventional cultures[36] and turnaround time is fairly rapid.

Polymerase chain reaction (PCR) testing is now a widely available technique for detecting respiratory pathogens in sputum. It can simultaneously test for a variety of viruses and bacteria, including C pneumoniae and M pneumoniae. Studies using PCR in conjunction with conventional microbiologic studies have achieved detection rates of 65%.[15] However, although PCR is a highly sensitive and specific test, it cannot discriminate between lower respiratory tract pathogens and colonizers, which potentially leads to false-positive tests.

Bronchoscopy

Flexible bronchoscopy does not have a routine role in the initial diagnosis or management of CAP and HAP. A bronchoalveolar lavage can be performed when sputum collection fails to provide an adequate sample. Although this occurs in 40% of patients, in the absence of randomized controlled trials, it is unclear whether invasively obtaining sputum has a positive impact on outcomes. Bronchoscopy is typically reserved for immunosuppressed patients or those failing initial therapy and unable to produce sputum. In these cases, an organism can be identified in a large percentage of patients.[37]

THERAPEUTIC APPROACH
Severity Scores

Severity scoring indices seek to standardize the decision to treat patients with CAP in the outpatient versus inpatient settings by predicting mortality. Determination of disease severity is often the first branch point in the management algorithm for CAP (**Fig. 3**). The PSI (Pneumonia Severity Index) and CURB-65 (confusion, urea nitrogen,

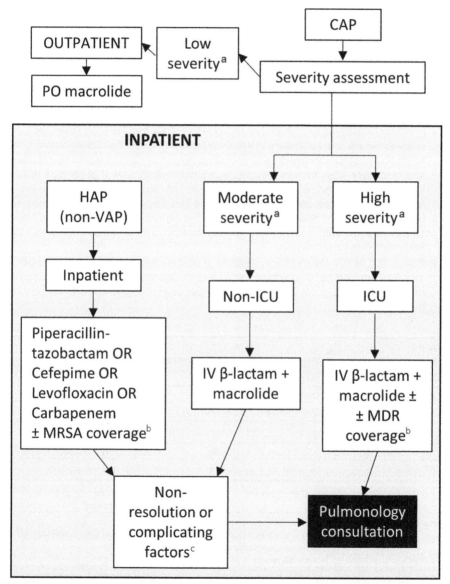

Fig. 3. Management algorithm for CAP and HAP. [a] Based on clinical judgment and severity score such as Pneumonia Severity Index or CURB-65 (confusion, urea nitrogen, respiratory rate, blood pressure, age ≥65 years). [b] Dependent on patient-specific and unit-specific risk factors for drug resistance. [c] See **Box 1**. IV, intravenous; PO, by mouth.

respiratory rate, blood pressure, age $\geq$ 65 years) scoring systems are the most widely used of these tools. The PSI includes 20 different variables and may be cumbersome to apply. CURB-65, by comparison, only includes 5 variables but is less accurate in predicting mortality.[38] No severity scoring system has been well validated in patients with HAP. The Clinical Pulmonary Infection Score consists of 6 variables and has been applied to patients with VAP but not non-VAP HAP.[39]

Choice of Antibiotics

Once the diagnosis of pneumonia is established, antibiotic treatment should be initiated without delay. Rushing diagnostic processes in order to initiate antibiotics as early as possible may provoke errors in medical decision making.[40] Key points from pneumonia treatment guidelines include (**Table 2**):

- In otherwise healthy patients with CAP treated in the outpatient setting, monotherapy with either a macrolide or doxycycline is recommended if local rates of S pneumoniae macrolide resistance are less than 25%.[2]
- In immunosuppressed individuals, those with risk factors for drug resistance, or in areas where rates of macrolide resistance are greater than 25%, outpatients should be treated with a respiratory fluoroquinolone or combination of a β-lactam and macrolide. Risk factors for drug resistance include use of antibiotics within the previous 90 days; chronic heart, lung, liver, or renal disease; diabetes; alcoholism; malignancies; or exposure to a child in a day care center.[2]
- In patients who are hospitalized with CAP but do not require ICU level of care, empiric therapy with a respiratory fluoroquinolone or combination of a β-lactam and macrolide is appropriate.
- If admitted to ICU level of care, patients should be treated with either a respiratory fluoroquinolone or combination of a β-lactam and macrolide, but assessment of risk factors for infection with MRSA or P aeruginosa infection should be performed.[2]

Table 2
Recommended empiric antibiotics by pneumonia type and severity

Pneumonia Type	Preferred Regimen	Alternative Regimen
CAP: outpatient	Oral macrolide	Oral doxycycline
CAP: outpatient with risk factors for macrolide resistance[a]	Oral β-lactam + macrolide	Oral respiratory fluoroquinolone
CAP: inpatient, non-ICU	IV β-lactam + macrolide	IV respiratory fluoroquinolone
CAP: inpatient, ICU	IV β-lactam + macrolide, ± antipseudomonal, MRSA, ESBL coverage[b]	IV β-lactam + respiratory fluoroquinolone, ±antipseudomonal, MRSA, ESBL coverage[b]
HAP (non-VAP)	Piperacillin-tazobactam or cefepime or respiratory fluoroquinolone or carbapenem ± MRSA coverage[b]	Aztreonam or aminoglycoside ± MRSA coverage[b]

Abbreviation: IV, intravenous.
[a] Including immunosuppression, recent antibiotic use, local rates of macrolide resistance greater than 25%.
[b] Dependent on patient-specific and unit-specific risk factors for drug resistance.

- In patients with HAP, empiric therapy is guided primarily by individual risk factors for antibiotic resistance rather than disease severity (see **Fig. 3**). Empiric antibiotics should cover *S aureus*, *Pseudomonas*, and other nosocomial gram-negative bacilli. The agent chosen to cover *S aureus* depends on risk factors for methicillin resistance, including antibiotic use within 90 days and unit MRSA prevalence greater than 20%. If MRSA is suspected, an antibiotic regimen containing either vancomycin or linezolid is recommended.[2]
- In patients with risk factors for fungal, mycobacterial, and viral infections, empiric bacterial coverage should still be administered but targeted diagnostic studies and empiric coverage for fungal, viral, or mycobacterial infection should be considered early. Delays in therapy may be linked to increased morbidity and mortality in these patients.[41,42]

Duration

Antibiotics for CAP should be administered for at least 5 days.[2] Some studies support shorter treatment duration, but these strategies have not entered into common practice. For example, macrolides have been administered in courses as short as 3 days.[43] However, because of the long half-lives of this class of antibiotics, results should not be widely extrapolated. Compared with longer antibiotic courses (>7 days), 5 days has been shown to have equal efficacy in prospective trials.[44] However, in patients who fail to improve clinically or who experience complications, longer courses are warranted.

For HAP, antibiotics should be administered for 7 days or less. This recommendation is extrapolated from data on VAP because no high-quality studies exist for non-VAP HAP. In VAP, shorter antibiotic courses did not significantly affect mortality and had lower rates of recurrence with MDR organisms.[5]

De-escalation

Antibiotic regimens should routinely be reassessed and narrowed as new microbiologic data become available. Antibiotic stewardship leads to decreased antibiotic use and antibiotic resistance, and curbs the negative side effects of unnecessary antibiotic administration.[45]

There is substantial evidence supporting the use of PCT in the de-escalation and discontinuation of antibiotics. In patients who have improved clinically, a decline in PCT by greater than 80% to a level less than 0.25 ng/mL is consistent with a positive response to antibiotics and could prompt their discontinuation. This strategy has been shown to decrease total antibiotic use with no significant effect on mortality.[46]

Adjunctive Therapies

Noninvasive positive pressure ventilation (NIPPV) has been evaluated in patients with pneumonia and acute respiratory failure. NIPPV has been shown to decrease mortality and intubation rates in ICU patients[47,48] but should only be considered in patients who are alert and able to manage their secretions.

Oxygen delivered through high-flow nasal cannula (HFNC) has also been studied in patients with acute respiratory failure. It has been shown to decrease intubation rates and reduce mortality[49] but has not specifically been studied in CAP or HAP. HFNC may be more effective than NIPPV at preventing intubation.[50]

Corticosteroids may decrease mortality in patients with severe CAP.[51] Steroids should be avoided in patients with suspected viral, fungal, or mycobacterial pneumonia because risk versus benefit has not been well defined in these patients and they might cause harm.[52,53]

COMPLICATIONS

Complications of pneumonia frequently occur. Although not all cases of pneumonia require pulmonary consultation, when complicating factors are evident at the time of initial presentation or arise during treatment, consultation with a pulmonary specialist should be considered (**Box 1**).

Parapneumonic effusions frequently complicate pneumonia. Most of these are sterile inflammatory exudates and do not require a change in management. However, when microorganisms transit into the pleural space, a more complicated fluid collection can develop, which occasionally progresses to empyema. In these cases, prompt drainage should be performed to both hasten clinical recovery and prevent residual functional limitations of the lungs.[54]

Lung abscesses can result from aspiration of oral anaerobes or necrotizing lung infections. Percutaneous drainage is generally not recommended because seeding of the previously uninvolved pleural space may occur. Endobronchial drainage has been described but is not routinely performed.[55] Surgical intervention may require lobectomy or pneumonectomy and is typically reserved for very large abscesses exerting mass effect on nearby structures.

Cardiovascular events occur with increased frequency in patients hospitalized with pneumonia. These events include myocardial infarction and arrhythmia, particularly atrial fibrillation, and are associated with increased mortality.[56]

PREVENTION

For pneumonia prevention, behavioral risk factors such as smoking and alcoholism should be addressed. Vaccines for influenza and S pneumoniae are routinely used in select patient populations. Annual influenza vaccination is recommended in all individuals more than 6 months of age with priority given to older adults, immunocompromised patients, those with medical comorbidities, and health care workers.[57]

Conjugate (PCV13) and polysaccharide (PPSV23) vaccines against S pneumonia are available. Disease caused by S pneumoniae has decreased following the introduction of conjugate vaccines in children and adults.[58,59] PCV13 confers a more robust and longer-lasting immune response compared with PPSV23. The Advisory Committee on Immunization Practices recommends vaccination with both PCV13 and PPSV23 for all adults more than 65 years of age. For adults younger than 65 years,

---

Box 1
Common reasons for pulmonology consultation

- Failed outpatient antibiotics
- Lack of improvement after 48 to 72 hours
- Unusual radiographic appearance (eg, cavitation, bronchiectasis)
- Suspected airway obstruction with mass or foreign body
- Multiple recurrent episodes in same or different lobe
- Suspected noninfectious cause (eg, organizing pneumonia, eosinophilic pneumonia)
- Concomitant severe obstructive/restrictive lung disease
- Immunosuppression (eg, human immunodeficiency virus, neutropenia)
- Complications from pneumonia (eg, complicated parapneumonic effusion, empyema, lung abscess, significant hemoptysis)

recommendations depend on patient-specific risk factors for pneumococcal disease. Individuals at intermediate risk for pneumococcal disease should receive PPSV23 and those at high risk should receive PCV13 in addition to PPSV23.[60]

OUTCOMES

Mortality from CAP in the ambulatory, inpatient, and ICU settings is approximately 5%, 15%, and 36%, respectively.[61] Overall mortality is approximately 10%, with half of the deaths occurring after hospital discharge.[62] Gram-negative organisms and *S aureus* have the highest mortalities.[61] Thirty-day readmission rates are between 7% and 18% and result from both recurrent pneumonia as well as exacerbations of preexisting comorbidities.[63–65] Patients who survive beyond 30 days have substantially higher mortalities at 1 year.[66]

SUMMARY

Although pneumonia is a commonly encountered problem in clinical practice, variability in presentation, causative organism, and severity make appropriate diagnosis and treatment extremely challenging. There have been many recent advances in diagnostic techniques such as PCR testing and point-of-care ultrasonography, but recommendations for antimicrobial treatment are largely unchanged in the last decade. Particular attention should be paid to multidrug resistance and development of complications, both of which may affect morbidity and mortality if unrecognized.

REFERENCES

1. Heron M. Deaths: leading causes for 2015. Natl Vital Stat Rep 2017;66(5):1–76.
2. Mandell LA, Wunderink RG, Anzueto A, et al. Infectious Diseases Society of America/American Thoracic Society consensus guidelines on the management of community-acquired pneumonia in adults. Clin Infect Dis 2007;44(Suppl 2): S27–72.
3. Kalil AC, Syed A, Rupp ME, et al. Is bacteremic sepsis associated with higher mortality in transplant recipients than in nontransplant patients? A matched case-control propensity-adjusted study. Clin Infect Dis 2015;60(2):216–22.
4. Chalmers JD, Taylor JK, Singanayagam A, et al. Epidemiology, antibiotic therapy, and clinical outcomes in health care-associated pneumonia: a UK cohort study. Clin Infect Dis 2011;53(2):107–13.
5. Kalil AC, Metersky ML, Klompas M, et al. Executive summary: management of adults with hospital-acquired and ventilator-associated pneumonia: 2016 clinical practice guidelines by the Infectious Diseases Society of America and the American Thoracic Society. Clin Infect Dis 2016;63(5):575–82.
6. Scheld WM. Developments in the pathogenesis, diagnosis and treatment of nosocomial pneumonia. Surg Gynecol Obstet 1991;172(Suppl):42–53.
7. Available at: http://www.who.int/news-room/fact-sheets/detail/the-top-10-causes-of-death. World Health Organization. Accessed September 5, 2018.
8. Said MA, Johnson HL, Nonyane BA, et al. Estimating the burden of pneumococcal pneumonia among adults: a systematic review and meta-analysis of diagnostic techniques. PLoS One 2013;8(4):e60273.
9. Beović B, Bonac B, Kese D, et al. Aetiology and clinical presentation of mild community-acquired bacterial pneumonia. Eur J Clin Microbiol Infect Dis 2003; 22(10):584–91.

10. Weber DJ, Sickbert-Bennett EE, Brown V, et al. Comparison of hospitalwide surveillance and targeted intensive care unit surveillance of healthcare-associated infections. Infect Control Hosp Epidemiol 2007;28(12):1361–6.
11. Arancibia F, Bauer TT, Ewig S, et al. Community-acquired pneumonia due to gram-negative bacteria and *Pseudomonas aeruginosa*: incidence, risk, and prognosis. Arch Intern Med 2002;162(16):1849–58.
12. Webb BJ, Dascomb K, Stenehjem E, et al. Predicting risk of drug-resistant organisms in pneumonia: moving beyond the HCAP model. Respir Med 2015;109(1): 1–10.
13. Prina E, Ranzani OT, Polverino E, et al. Risk factors associated with potentially antibiotic-resistant pathogens in community-acquired pneumonia. Ann Am Thorac Soc 2015;12(2):153–60.
14. Johnstone J, Majumdar SR, Fox JD, et al. Viral infection in adults hospitalized with community-acquired pneumonia: prevalence, pathogens, and presentation. Chest 2008;134(6):1141–8.
15. Luchsinger V, Ruiz M, Zunino E, et al. Community-acquired pneumonia in Chile: the clinical relevance in the detection of viruses and atypical bacteria. Thorax 2013;68(11):1000–6.
16. Centers for Disease Control and Prevention (CDC). Bacterial coinfections in lung tissue specimens from fatal cases of 2009 pandemic influenza A (H1N1) - United States, May-August 2009. MMWR Morb Mortal Wkly Rep 2009;58(38):1071–4.
17. Cillóniz C, Polverino E, Ewig S, et al. Impact of age and comorbidity on cause and outcome in community-acquired pneumonia. Chest 2013;144(3):999–1007.
18. Torres A, Peetermans WE, Viegi G, et al. Risk factors for community-acquired pneumonia in adults in Europe: a literature review. Thorax 2013;68(11):1057–65.
19. Falguera M, Carratalà J, Ruiz-Gonzalez A, et al. Risk factors and outcome of community-acquired pneumonia due to Gram-negative bacilli. Respirology 2009;14(1):105–11.
20. Wunderink RG. Slow response times: is it the pneumonia or the physician? Crit Care Med 2005;33(6):1429–30.
21. Rautanen A, Mills TC, Gordon AC, et al. Genome-wide association study of survival from sepsis due to pneumonia: an observational cohort study. Lancet Respir Med 2015;3(1):53–60.
22. Zalacain R, Torres A, Celis R, et al. Community-acquired pneumonia in the elderly: Spanish multicentre study. Eur Respir J 2003;21(2):294–302.
23. Marrie TJ, Lau CY, Wheeler SL, et al. Predictors of symptom resolution in patients with community-acquired pneumonia. Clin Infect Dis 2000;31(6):1362–7.
24. Waterer GW, Kessler LA, Wunderink RG. Delayed administration of antibiotics and atypical presentation in community-acquired pneumonia. Chest 2006; 130(1):11–5.
25. Bochud PY, Moser F, Erard P, et al. Community-acquired pneumonia. A prospective outpatient study. Medicine (Baltimore) 2001;80(2):75–87.
26. Parlamento S, Copetti R, Di Bartolomeo S. Evaluation of lung ultrasound for the diagnosis of pneumonia in the ED. Am J Emerg Med 2009;27(4):379–84.
27. Xirouchaki N, Magkanas E, Vaporidi K, et al. Lung ultrasound in critically ill patients: comparison with bedside chest radiography. Intensive Care Med 2011; 37(9):1488–93.
28. Wanahita A, Goldsmith EA, Musher DM. Conditions associated with leukocytosis in a tertiary care hospital, with particular attention to the role of infection caused by *Clostridium difficile*. Clin Infect Dis 2002;34(12):1585–92.

29. Self WH, Balk RA, Grijalva CG, et al. Procalcitonin as a marker of etiology in adults hospitalized with community-acquired pneumonia. Clin Infect Dis 2017;65(2): 183–90.

30. Christ-Crain M, Stolz D, Bingisser R, et al. Procalcitonin guidance of antibiotic therapy in community-acquired pneumonia: a randomized trial. Am J Respir Crit Care Med 2006;174(1):84–93.

31. van der Eerden MM, Vlaspolder F, de Graaff CS, et al. Value of intensive diagnostic microbiological investigation in low- and high-risk patients with community-acquired pneumonia. Eur J Clin Microbiol Infect Dis 2005;24(4):241–9.

32. Uematsu H, Hashimoto H, Iwamoto T, et al. Impact of guideline-concordant microbiological testing on outcomes of pneumonia. Int J Qual Health Care 2014;26(1):100–7.

33. Musher DM, Montoya R, Wanahita A. Diagnostic value of microscopic examination of Gram-stained sputum and sputum cultures in patients with bacteremic pneumococcal pneumonia. Clin Infect Dis 2004;39(2):165–9.

34. Sinclair A, Xie X, Teltscher M, et al. Systematic review and meta-analysis of a urine-based pneumococcal antigen test for diagnosis of community-acquired pneumonia caused by Streptococcus pneumoniae. J Clin Microbiol 2013;51(7): 2303–10.

35. Shimada T, Noguchi Y, Jackson JL, et al. Systematic review and metaanalysis: urinary antigen tests for legionellosis. Chest 2009;136(6):1576–85.

36. Harris AM, Bramley AM, Jain S, et al. Influence of antibiotics on the detection of bacteria by culture-based and culture-independent diagnostic tests in patients hospitalized with community-acquired pneumonia. Open Forum Infect Dis 2017;4(1):ofx014.

37. Ortqvist A, Kalin M, Lejdeborn L, et al. Diagnostic fiberoptic bronchoscopy and protected brush culture in patients with community-acquired pneumonia. Chest 1990;97(3):576–82.

38. Abers MS, Musher DM. Clinical prediction rules in community-acquired pneumonia: lies, damn lies and statistics. QJM 2014;107(7):595–6.

39. Fartoukh M, Maitre B, Honoré S, et al. Diagnosing pneumonia during mechanical ventilation: the clinical pulmonary infection score revisited. Am J Respir Crit Care Med 2003;168(2):173–9.

40. Welker JA, Huston M, McCue JD. Antibiotic timing and errors in diagnosing pneumonia. Arch Intern Med 2008;168(4):351–6.

41. Garey KW, Rege M, Pai MP, et al. Time to initiation of fluconazole therapy impacts mortality in patients with candidemia: a multi-institutional study. Clin Infect Dis 2006;43(1):25–31.

42. Kethireddy S, Light RB, Mirzanejad Y, et al. Mycobacterium tuberculosis septic shock. Chest 2013;144(2):474–82.

43. Rizzato G, Montemurro L, Fraioli P, et al. Efficacy of a three day course of azithromycin in moderately severe community-acquired pneumonia. Eur Respir J 1995; 8(3):398–402.

44. Dunbar LM, Wunderink RG, Habib MP, et al. High-dose, short-course levofloxacin for community-acquired pneumonia: a new treatment paradigm. Clin Infect Dis 2003;37(6):752–60.

45. Barlam TF, Cosgrove SE, Abbo LM, et al. Executive summary: implementing an antibiotic stewardship program: guidelines by the Infectious Diseases Society of America and the Society for Healthcare Epidemiology of America. Clin Infect Dis 2016;62(10):1197–202.

46. Schuetz P, Müller B, Christ-Crain M, et al. Procalcitonin to initiate or discontinue antibiotics in acute respiratory tract infections. Cochrane Database Syst Rev 2012;(9):CD007498.

47. Hilbert G, Gruson D, Vargas F, et al. Noninvasive ventilation in immunosuppressed patients with pulmonary infiltrates, fever, and acute respiratory failure. N Engl J Med 2001;344(7):481–7.

48. Confalonieri M, Potena A, Carbone G, et al. Acute respiratory failure in patients with severe community-acquired pneumonia. A prospective randomized evaluation of noninvasive ventilation. Am J Respir Crit Care Med 1999;160(5 Pt 1): 1585–91.

49. Ou X, Hua Y, Liu J, et al. Effect of high-flow nasal cannula oxygen therapy in adults with acute hypoxemic respiratory failure: a meta-analysis of randomized controlled trials. CMAJ 2017;189(7):E260–7.

50. Ni YN, Luo J, Yu H, et al. Can high-flow nasal cannula reduce the rate of endotracheal intubation in adult patients with acute respiratory failure compared with conventional oxygen therapy and noninvasive positive pressure ventilation?: A systematic review and meta-analysis. Chest 2017;151(4):764–75.

51. Stern A, Skalsky K, Avni T, et al. Corticosteroids for pneumonia. Cochrane Database Syst Rev 2017;(12):CD007720.

52. Rodrigo C, Leonardi-Bee J, Nguyen-Van-Tam J, et al. Corticosteroids as adjunctive therapy in the treatment of influenza. Cochrane Database Syst Rev 2016;(3):CD010406.

53. Parody R, Rabella N, Martino R, et al. Upper and lower respiratory tract infections by human enterovirus and rhinovirus in adult patients with hematological malignancies. Am J Hematol 2007;82(9):807–11.

54. Colice GL, Curtis A, Deslauriers J, et al. Medical and surgical treatment of parapneumonic effusions: an evidence-based guideline. Chest 2000;118(4):1158–71.

55. Herth F, Ernst A, Becker HD. Endoscopic drainage of lung abscesses: technique and outcome. Chest 2005;127(4):1378–81.

56. Corrales-Medina VF, Alvarez KN, Weissfeld LA, et al. Association between hospitalization for pneumonia and subsequent risk of cardiovascular disease. JAMA 2015;313(3):264–74.

57. Grohskopf LA, Sokolow LZ, Broder KR, et al. Prevention and control of seasonal influenza with vaccines: recommendations of the Advisory Committee on Immunization Practices—United States, 2018–19 influenza season. MMWR Recomm Rep 2018;67(3):1–20.

58. Weil-Olivier C, van der Linden M, de Schutter I, et al. Prevention of pneumococcal diseases in the post-seven valent vaccine era: a European perspective. BMC Infect Dis 2012;12:207.

59. Moberley S, Holden J, Tatham DP, et al. Vaccines for preventing pneumococcal infection in adults. Cochrane Database Syst Rev 2013;(1):CD000422.

60. Tomczyk S, Bennett NM, Stoecker C, et al. Use of 13-valent pneumococcal conjugate vaccine and 23-valent pneumococcal polysaccharide vaccine among adults aged ≥65 years: recommendations of the Advisory Committee on Immunization Practices (ACIP). MMWR Morb Mortal Wkly Rep 2014;63(37):822–5.

61. Fine MJ, Smith MA, Carson CA, et al. Prognosis and outcomes of patients with community-acquired pneumonia. A meta-analysis. JAMA 1996;275(2):134–41.

62. Metersky ML, Waterer G, Nsa W, et al. Predictors of in-hospital vs postdischarge mortality in pneumonia. Chest 2012;142(2):476–81.

63. Bruns AH, Oosterheert JJ, El Moussaoui R, et al. Pneumonia recovery: discrepancies in perspectives of the radiologist, physician and patient. J Gen Intern Med 2010;25(3):203–6.
64. Capelastegui A, España Yandiola PP, Quintana JM, et al. Predictors of short-term rehospitalization following discharge of patients hospitalized with community-acquired pneumonia. Chest 2009;136(4):1079–85.
65. Jasti H, Mortensen EM, Obrosky DS, et al. Causes and risk factors for rehospitalization of patients hospitalized with community-acquired pneumonia. Clin Infect Dis 2008;46(4):550–6.
66. Bruns AH, Oosterheert JJ, Cucciolillo MC, et al. Cause-specific long-term mortality rates in patients recovered from community-acquired pneumonia as compared with the general Dutch population. Clin Microbiol Infect 2011;17(5): 763–8.

Orphan Lung Diseases

Muhammad Sajawal Ali, MD, MS[a],*, Uzair Khan Ghori, MD[a],
Ali I. Musani, MD[b]

KEYWORDS

- Orphan lung diseases • Rare lung diseases • Pleuroparenchymal fibroelastosis
- Pulmonary alveolar proteinosis • Lymphangioleiomyomatosis • Yellow nail syndrome
- Mounier–Kuhn syndrome

KEY POINTS

- Orphan lung diseases include pulmonary disorders that have received little attention from the scientific community; therefore, there is a dearth of understanding about their pathogenesis and treatment options.
- Most of the orphan lung disease are also rare (prevalence of <1 in 2000).
- Pleuroparenchymal fibroelastosis, pulmonary alveolar proteinosis, lymphangioleiomyomatosis, yellow nail syndrome, and Mounier–Kuhn syndrome, are rare lung disease that are discussed in detail in this article.

Orphan lung diseases refer to pulmonary disorders that have only attracted limited scientific investigation and, therefore, are poorly understood. Typically, there are limited therapeutic interventions available for orphan diseases, which adds to the plight of the patients. Although orphan diseases can be very prevalent, most of these are rare diseases. A disease is defined as being rare if its prevalence is less than 1 in 2000. For the purpose of this article, we will focus on some of the rare orphan lung diseases.

There are hundreds of rare orphan lung diseases and discussing all of them is beyond the scope of this article. We highlight five rare orphan lung diseases herein, one from each of the five major categories of pulmonary disorders:

- Pleuroparenchymal fibroelastosis (PPFE; a rare diffuse parenchymal lung disease),
- Pulmonary alveolar proteinosis (PAP; a rare autoimmune and diffuse parenchymal lung disease),

Disclosure Statement: The authors have no conflicts of interest to disclose with regards to this publication.
[a] Division of Pulmonary & Critical Care Medicine, Medical College of Wisconsin, HUB for Collaborative Medicine, 8701 West Watertown Plank Road, Milwaukee, WI 53226, USA;
[b] Division of Pulmonary Sciences & Critical Care Medicine, University of Colorado, Denver, Academic Office 1, 12631 East 17th Avenue, M/S C323, Office # 8102, Aurora, CO 80045, USA
* Corresponding author.
E-mail address: muali@mcw.edu

Med Clin N Am 103 (2019) 503–515
https://doi.org/10.1016/j.mcna.2018.12.009
0025-7125/19/© 2018 Elsevier Inc. All rights reserved.

- Lymphangioleiomyomatosis (LAM; a rare cystic lung disease),
- Yellow nail syndrome (YNS; a rare pleural disease), and
- Mounier–Kuhn syndrome (MKS; a rare airway disorder).

PLEUROPARENCHYMAL FIBROELASTOSIS

The term pleuroparenchymal fibroelastosis (PPFE) was introduced in 2004 by Frankel and colleagues[1] to describe a rare upper lobe predominant interstitial lung disease. Since then, there have been close to a hundred cases of PPFE described in literature and the disorder has now been included in the American Thoracic Society/European Respiratory Society consensus statement for the multidisciplinary diagnosis of interstitial lung diseases.[2,3]

Two distinct forms of PPFE are recognized. An idiopathic form, where a specific cause cannot be identified, and a secondary form. Bone marrow transplant, lung transplant, and exposure to certain chemotherapeutic agents have been reported as the most common causes of secondary PPFE.[4]

Presentation and Diagnosis

The patients with PPFE typically present with dyspnea, cough, chest pain, and weight loss. They often have bilateral lung crackles, and finger clubbing is typically absent.[5] PPFE is diagnosed based on its unique radiographic, histologic, and pulmonary function test (PFT) patterns. On imaging, PPFE is characterized by upper lobe predominant pleural thickening and subpleural fibrosis. The middle and lower lobes tend to be relatively preserved[6] (Fig. 1). Pathologic examination reveals intense fibrosis of the pleural and subpleural parenchyma, along with elastosis of the alveolar septa.[2] Few inflammatory infiltrates and fibroblastic foci are seen, and there is a sharp demarcation between diseased and healthy lung.[1] PFTs reveal a restrictive pattern with low total lung capacity and vital capacity; however, the residual volume is preserved. As a result, the patients with PPFE characteristically have a high residual volume/total lung capacity ratio.[7]

Treatment

Unfortunately, no good medical treatments have been validated for PPFE. Investigators have extrapolated the idiopathic pulmonary fibrosis (IPF) data and there have been case reports of some response to pirfenidone and nintedanib.[8,9] However, these agents have not consistently been shown to be beneficial.[10] Steroids, cyclosporin, and cyclophosphamide have also been tried, but with little success.[10] Early lung transplant evaluation is warranted because, for select advanced cases, lung transplant might be the only option.[10]

Prognosis

Prognosis is variable, with some patients having a rapid progression, and others experiencing a gradual decline. In one case series, survival of the patients with PPFE ranged from 1.8 to 14.8 years after the onset of symptoms.[11] Data on the long-term outcomes of the lung transplant recipients is limited, but some reports suggest patients with PPFE have been doing well up to 2 to 3 years after transplantation.

PULMONARY ALVEOLAR PROTEINOSIS

Pulmonary alveolar proteinosis (PAP) was first described by Rosen and colleagues[12] in 1958 in a series of 27 patients who had presented with progressive respiratory symptoms and were found to have alveoli filled with periodic acid-Schiff–positive, lipid-rich

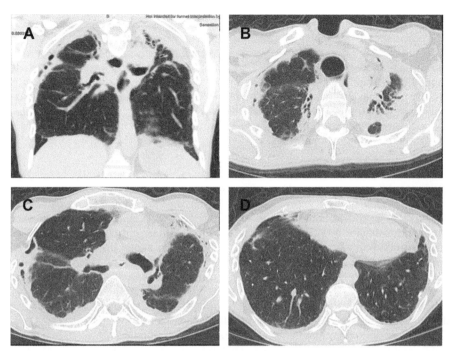

Fig. 1. Computed tomography (CT) images of a patient with biopsy-proven pleuroparenchymal fibroelastosis. (*A*) Coronal and (*B–D*) axial cuts are seen. Marked pleural thickening and upper lobe predominant fibrosis with relatively preserved lower lobes can be appreciated. These changes are hallmarks of pleuroparenchymal fibroelastosis .

proteinaceous material. Based on human and animal studies, great strides have been made in our understanding of the disease and three distinct types of PAP are now recognized, namely, acquired, secondary, and congenital.[13]

The acquired form of PAP is considered an autoimmune process where antibodies against granulocyte–macrophage colony–stimulating factor (GM–CSF) are found. GM–CSF is an essential mediator for macrophage maturation, surfactant homeostasis and lung immunity.[13] Disruption of GM–CSF and its downstream regulation of macrophages leads to unchecked accumulation of surfactant in the alveoli.[14] The acquired or the autoimmune form account for 90% of all PAP cases.[15] The secondary form of PAP is caused by deranged surfactant metabolism, which in turn is a consequence of another disease process, such as a hematologic malignancy, dust inhalation (eg, silica, aluminum), and pharmacologic immunosuppression.[13] The congenital form of PAP can be caused by a number of mutations effecting surfactant either directly or via impaired GM–CSF.[16–18] The consequence of all of these pathogenic mechanisms is the unchecked accumulation of surfactant in the alveoli and distal airways. This process leads to a loss of effective surface area for gas exchange, respiratory symptoms, and an increased risk of opportunistic infections.

The incidence of PAP is 0.5 per million population, and its prevalence is 6.2 to 6.9 per million population.[15,19] A large Japanese series reported a 2.1:1.0 (male to female ratio); however, in other studies both genders were equally affected.[15,20] There does not seem to be an ethnic predilection and large series have been reported from Iran, Israel, Japan, and the United States.

Presentation

The most common presenting symptom is dyspnea, which is seen in 54.3% to 79.0% of the patients.[15,21] Cough, hemoptysis, and chest pain are present in 79%, 17%, and 13% of the patients, respectively. Other commonly reported symptoms include sputum production, fatigue, weight loss, and fever. The disease onset is insidious with symptoms evolving over weeks to months. Crackles are often appreciated on examination; however, this is not always the case, especially if the distal airways are flooded with surfactant to the point where air movement is impaired. Cyanosis and clubbing are also uncommonly seen.

Diagnosis

Like most diffuse parenchymal lung diseases, the diagnosis is established based on the constellation of history, physical examination, and radiographic and pathologic findings. Chest radiographs reveal bilateral diffuse air space opacities; however, a computed tomography (CT) scan will reveal diffuse areas of ground glass opacities that are superimposed on a background of interlobular septal thickening[22] (**Fig. 2**). These changes are present in a "geographic" distribution, resembling irregularly laid out cobblestones on a pavement. Hence, this pattern has been referred to as the crazy paving pattern.[23]

Bronchoscopy reveals normal airways, however, bronchoalveolar lavage (BAL) produces a milky, viscous effluent that gives a thick sediment if allowed to stand.[24] Cytologic evaluation reveals that this effluent is positive for periodic acid-Schiff and is rich in eosinophils. It is essentially composed of surfactant and sloughed off mucosal cells. If transbronchial biopsies are performed, pathologic examination shows well-

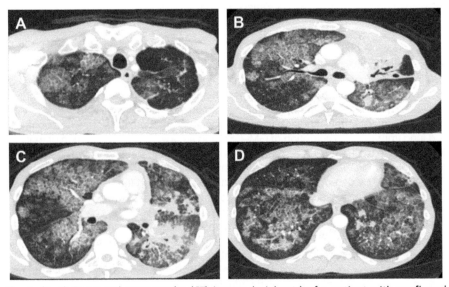

Fig. 2. (A–D) Computed tomography (CT) images (axial cuts) of a patient with confirmed pulmonary alveolar proteinosis. Bilateral patches of ground glass opacities on a background of septal thickening can be seen. This pattern has been described as "crazy paving" and is often seen in pulmonary alveolar proteinosis. In (B, C) the cavitary and consolidative changes in the left upper and lower lobes were attributed to superimposed nocardia infection in this patient, and as such are not typical for pulmonary alveolar proteinosis.

preserved pulmonary architecture, but alveoli are inundated with a periodic acid-Schiff–positive, lipoproteinaceous substance.[25,26] Of note, there is a lack of inflammation. BAL and transbronchial biopsies can help make the diagnosis in a majority of the patients; however, in some of the prior studies a significant number of the patients underwent surgical lung biopsies.[21] BAL evaluation also allows to rule out superimposed infections.

If available, assays for checking anti–GM–CSF antibodies in serum are an excellent noninvasive tool for diagnosing acquired PAP. Their reported sensitivity and specificity are 100% and 98%, respectively.[27]

Treatment

Active intervention is not always needed; in a significant number of the patients, symptoms are low grade and resolve spontaneously. However, when moderate to severe symptoms are present or the patients demonstrate marked hypoxia and PFT abnormalities, whole lung lavage (WLL) remains the gold standard treatment.[28] WLL is performed under general anesthesia and only one lung is treated at a time. The other lung is treated after a gap of about two weeks.[24] In one study, 70% of the patients remained symptom-free after WLL at 7 years follow-up.[28]

If the patients with acquired PAP do not respond adequately to WLL or if it is not available, they can be treated with recombinant GM–CSF. A recent meta-analysis revealed excellent response and low recurrence rates.[29] Of note corticosteroids have no role in the treatment of PAP.[30]

Prognosis

In one study, the 5-year survival with PAP was 85% without treatment and 94% with WLL.[24] 72% of the deaths were due to progressive respiratory failure, and 18% of deaths were attributed to superimposed infections. The relapse rate for PAP has been reported to be around 24.4%.[20]

LYMPHANGIOLEIOMYOMATOSIS

Lymphangioleiomyomatosis (LAM) is a rare, multisystem neoplastic disorder characterized by cystic lung disease, chylous fluid accumulations (pleural and ascitic), angiomyolipomas, and lymphangioleiomyomas.[31] LAM can either be associated with tuberous sclerosis complex (TSC) or can occur sporadically.[32,33]

Patients with both the sporadic and TSC-associated LAM have mutations in the TSC-1 and TSC-2 genes. These genes regulate the mechanistic target of rapamycin pathway. Loss of TSC-1 and TSC-2 genes, leads to unchecked activation of mechanistic target of rapamycin pathway, with activation of downstream kinases, leading to the proliferation of LAM cells.[34] Studies have shown LAM cells from the patients to be of monoclonal origin, therefore supporting the neoplastic nature of the disease. LAM cells are essentially smooth muscle–like cells that, in addition to smooth muscle markers, also demonstrate melanocytic markers such as gp 100.[35]

The disease primarily affects women of childbearing age. Its prevalence has been reported to be 3.4 to 7.8 per million women, and its incidence has been reported to be 0.23 to 0.31 per million women.[36] However, there have been a few reports of the disease occurring in male patients as well.[37]

Presentation

LAM typically presents in the third to fourth decade of life with an overwhelmingly greater proportion of female patients.[38] Presentation depends on whether the disease is sporadic or associated with TSC. In a large US series of patients with LAM, TSC-associated LAM was only present in 14.8% of the cases with the rest being sporadic.[39] In the same series, pulmonary complaints such as dyspnea and cough were the presenting symptoms in about two-thirds of the patients, whereas spontaneous pneumothorax was the sentinel event in one-third the patients. Pleural effusion was present in 21% of the patients at presentation. Very few patients presented with just extrapulmonary symptoms resulting from abdominal tumors (angiomyolipomas and lymphangioleiomyomas), in the absence of pulmonary complaints.[40] In addition, patients with TSC-associated LAM will also have additional neurocutaneous manifestations, such as shagreen patches, hypopigmented macules, seizures, and mental retardation.

There are no characteristic PFT findings. About one-third of the patients can have normal spirometry, whereas in others LAM may present as obstructive, restrictive, or mixed patterns. Diffusion capacity, however, is often abnormal. Findings on a chest radiograph are again too nonspecific to provide meaningful diagnostic clues. CT scans reveal multiple, bilateral, thin-walled, regular appearing cysts[41,42] (**Fig. 3**). There is no definite cutoff for the number of cysts that are needed for diagnosis; however, most experts agree that ten or more cysts should be considered significant.[43] Of note, the lung parenchyma between the cysts is normal and no lung nodules are seen; this feature helps in differentiating LAM from other cystic lung diseases, such as pulmonary Langerhans cell histiocytosis.

Diagnosis

Based on the American Thoracic Society/Japanese Respiratory Society consensus guidelines, patients can be diagnosed with LAM in the presence of typical cystic

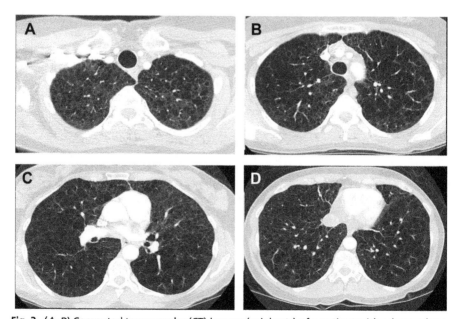

Fig. 3. (A–D) Computed tomography (CT) images (axial cuts) of a patient with advanced sporadic lymphangioleiomyomatosis (LAM). Most of the lung parenchyma is riddled with regular thin-walled cysts. Of note, no lung nodules or other lung parenchymal abnormalities are seen.

lung disease on the CT scan, if additional confirmatory clinical findings are present.[33] These additional findings include signs consistent with TSC, chylous fluid accumulations, or abdominal tumors (angiomyolipomas and lymphangioleiomyomas). If these confirmatory findings are not present lymphangiogenic vascular endothelial growth factor-D (VEGF-D) should be checked in serum. VEGF-D levels of 800 pg/mL or greater are associated with a sensitivity of 73% and a specificity of 100% for diagnosing LAM.[44] If suspicion for LAM remains despite a negative workup, the patients should preferably undergo surgical lung biopsy which will show abnormal smooth muscle–like cells that are also HMB-45 positive.

Treatment

If the symptoms are minimal and PFTs preserved (forced expiratory volume in 1 second [FEV_1] >70% of predicted, rate of FEV_1 decline <100 mL/y, and diffusion capacity of >80% of predicted), it is recommended to observe the patients with serial clinical examinations and PFTs. Otherwise, mechanistic target of rapamycin pathway inhibitor sirolimus is the first-line therapy.[33] For the patients who do not tolerate sirolimus or whose disease progresses while on sirolimus, everolimus can be tried. In the patients with advanced respiratory symptoms not responding to medical management, an evaluation for lung transplantation should be considered. However, because LAM is a neoplastic disorder, there is risk of disease recurrence in transplanted lungs.

Prognosis

Pulmonary disease in LAM is slowly progressive with a 10-year survival rate of 91%.[45] The annual rate of decline of FEV_1 and diffusion capacity is 2.4 ± 0.4% of predicted and 1.7 ± 0.4% of predicted, respectively.[46] At this rate, it takes about 9 to 10 years before dyspnea progresses to a level where the patients get dyspneic walking on a flat surface.[45]

YELLOW NAIL SYNDROME

Yellow nail syndrome (YNS) is a rare disorder with fewer than 400 cases reported in the medical literature. The first case of YNS was reported in 1927.[47] YNS is characterized by a triad of yellow thickened nails, respiratory manifestations, and lymphedema.[48]

The majority of the patients are 50 years or older at the time of presentation, with an equal gender distribution. No geographic predilection is seen with regard to its occurrence. Congenital cases of YNS have been reported in literature, but the bulk of the patients acquire the syndrome later in their lives. Familial clustering of YNS has been observed, but no specific attributable genetic mutation has so far been identified. YNS has been reported in patients suffering from cancer and autoimmune disorders, but no specific causative factor has been confirmed. Recent data suggests an association with titanium exposure, but more research is needed to determine if the association is causative.[49]

Presentation and Pathogenesis

During the initial presentation, all components of the triad might not be present, but appear subsequently. Maldonado and colleagues[50] and Pavlidakey and colleagues[51] in their case series reported the incidence of various clinical manifestation in YNS:

1. Yellow nails (85%–100%);
2. Lymphedema (63%–72%);
3. Chronic pulmonary manifestations (39%–56%); and
4. Complete triad (27%–60%).

The most frequent clinical manifestation is yellow discoloration of nails as evident by the name of the syndrome.[52] It is postulated that impaired lymphatic drainage results in lipid accumulation and oxidation, which manifests as yellow nail discoloration.[53] It has been observed that nail growth is impaired longitudinally, but nail thickness is doubled.

Bronchiectasis, chronic cough, pleural effusions, and sinusitis are the frequently encountered respiratory problems in YNS. **Fig. 4** shows the CT scan images of a patient with YNS with a large, right-sided pleural effusion. It is postulated that dysfunctional lymphatic drainage also hampers the clearance of pathogens, which results in the patients with YNS suffering from recurrent infections such as pneumonia and sinusitis. Recurrent pneumonias can lead to bronchiectasis. Pleural effusion occurs in less than one-half of the patients with YNS, and they are typically exudative in nature; lymphocytic predominant and serous or milky in appearance. PFTs can demonstrate a restrictive pattern if pleural effusions are significantly large.[54] Lower limb predominant lymphedema has been reported as one of the first manifestations of YNS in some cases. Impaired lymphatic drainage and fibrosis caused by lymph stasis are considered culprits for the development of lymphedema.

Treatment and Prognosis

In the patients with YNS, treatment is centered around addressing the specific symptoms. Yellow discoloration of the nails may have to be treated for aesthetic reasons. Vitamin E[53] has been shown to be promising in reversing nail color changes, although some experts also advocate the use of antifungal agents, even though studies have shown mixed results. In about one-third of the patients, the resolution of nail symptomology happens without any intervention.

Bronchiectasis exacerbations and sinus infections are treated with appropriate antibiotics. For recurrent exacerbations of bronchiectasis, prophylactic antibiotics such as azithromycin can be used. Airway clearance can be accomplished with postural drainage, flutter valve devices, and chest physiotherapy. Regular nasal saline irrigation

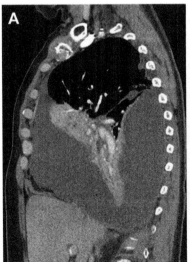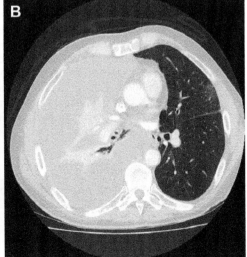

Fig. 4. Computed tomography images with (A) sagittal and (B) axial view showing a large right-sided effusion with lung collapse in a patient with yellow nail syndrome (YNS).

along with antibiotics can be tried for chronic sinusitis. Pneumococcal and annual flu vaccinations are also recommended[55] for the patients with YNS with bronchiectasis. Drainage of pleural effusion might be indicated in cases of empyema or large pleural effusions causing respiratory compromise. Extreme cases might necessitate surgical pleurodesis or in-dwelling pleural catheters. A review of the literature reveals octreotide being used in the management of YNS-related pleural effusions with promising results.[55]

Compressive bandages and other physical methods of improving lymphatic drainage are regularly used in the management of lymphedema. In cases of YNS associated with malignancy, symptoms might resolve with the treatment of underlying cancer. Clearly, more research is needed to better understand the pathogenic mechanisms behind this syndrome and assist with the development of novel therapeutic options.

MOUNIER–KUHN SYNDROME

Mounier-Kuhn syndrome (MKS) or tracheobronchomegaly is a rare disorder that is characterized by dilation of the trachea and central bronchi.[56] The disease course can be complicated by recurrent lower respiratory tract infections. Mounier–Kuhn described this clinical syndrome for the first time in 1932.[57]

It is a rare disease with just over 300 documented cases in medical literature. However, it is possible that many more patients have the disease but suffer from minimal or no symptoms. MKS is a male-predominant disease and commonly presents in third and fourth decades of life.[58] A genetic cause for MKS is yet to be identified, but it is associated with connective tissue diseases like Ehlers-Danlos syndrome, Marfan syndrome, and cutis laxa.[59] The exact etiology of MKS is unknown, but biopsy studies of the trachea and main bronchi have demonstrated atrophy of the elastic tissue and smooth muscles, which compromises the structural integrity, leading to tracheobronchomegaly.

Diagnosis and Presentation

MKS is diagnosed based on the radiographic features. CT imaging criteria for MKS include tracheal diameter of greater than 3 cm, a right main stem diameter of greater than 2 cm, and a left main stem bronchial diameter of greater than 1.8 cm.[60,61] Two of these three criteria need to be present in a patient for the diagnosis. Bronchoscopy can also aid in the diagnosis of tracheobronchomegaly by demonstrating dilated large airways and excessive dynamic airway collapse during expiration. **Fig. 5** shows the typical radiographic and bronchoscopic features of MKS.

MKS can be further divided into three subtypes. Type 1 is characterized by symmetric dilation of trachea and main bronchi, type 2 is characterized by diverticular dilation of trachea and main bronchi, and in type 3 dilated diverticulae and saccules extend to the distal bronchi.[62]

MKS can be diagnosed in asymptomatic patients when abnormalities are incidentally discovered during chest imaging performed for unrelated indications. Clinical manifestations, when present, are mostly due to ineffective mucociliary airway clearance. As a consequence of ineffective airway clearance, the patients may develop a chronic nonresolving cough, recurrent lower respiratory tract infections, and bronchiectasis. Bronchiectasis can in turn predispose these patients to hemoptysis. The PFTs typically demonstrate an obstructive pattern initially, but if recurrent infections lead to lung fibrosis, concomitant restriction might also be present. In asymptomatic patients, PFTs can be completely normal.

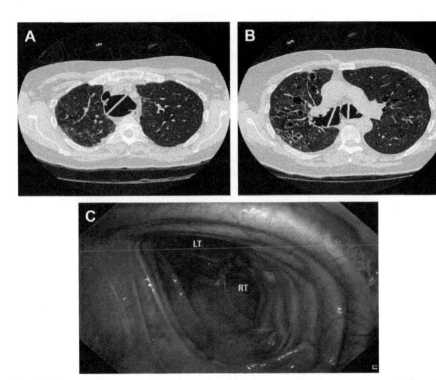

Fig. 5. Computed tomography (CT) images of (*A*) dilation of main trachea greater than 3 cm (*yellow line*) and (*B*) dilated right main bronchus (>2 cm) and left main bronchus (>1.8 cm). (*C*) Bronchoscopic view of the same patient from trachea with right (RT) and left (LT) main-stem bronchi also visible.

Treatment

In the patients with minimal or no symptoms, specific treatment is not indicated. Airway clearance can be promoted with the help of flutter valve devices, chest physiotherapy, and expectorants when the patients present with significant respiratory complaints.[63] Appropriate antibiotics can be used for recurrent lower respiratory tract infections and exacerbations of bronchiectasis.[59] The having respiratory symptoms owing to excessive dynamic airway collapse may benefit from positive airway pressure therapy. In cases of severe excessive dynamic airway collapse, airway stenting and/or tracheobronchoplasty may have to be considered.

REFERENCES

1. Frankel SK, Cool CD, Lynch DA, et al. Idiopathic pleuroparenchymal fibroelastosis: description of a novel clinicopathologic entity. Chest 2004;126: 2007–13.
2. Bonifazi M, Montero MA, Renzoni EA. Idiopathic pleuroparenchymal fibroelastosis. Curr Pulmonol Rep 2017;6:9–15.
3. Travis WD, Costabel U, Hansell DM, et al. An official American Thoracic Society/ European Respiratory Society statement: update of the international multidisciplinary classification of the idiopathic interstitial pneumonias. Am J Respir Crit Care Med 2013;188:733–48.

4. Beynat-Mouterde C, Beltramo G, Lezmi G, et al. Pleuroparenchymal fibroelastosis as a late complication of chemotherapy agents. Eur Respir J 2014;44:523–7.
5. Watanabe K. Pleuroparenchymal fibroelastosis: its clinical characteristics. Curr Respir Med Rev 2013;9. 299–237.
6. Reddy TL, Tominaga M, Hansell DM, et al. Pleuroparenchymal fibroelastosis: a spectrum of histopathological and imaging phenotypes. Eur Respir J 2012;40: 377–85.
7. Watanabe S, Waseda Y, Takato H, et al. Pleuroparenchymal fibroelastosis: distinct pulmonary physiological features in nine patients. Respir Investig 2015; 53:149–55.
8. Nasser M, Chebib N, Philit F, et al. Treatment with nintedanib in patients with pleuroparenchymal fibroelastosis. Eur Respir J 2017;50:PA4876.
9. Sato S, Hanibuchi M, Takahashi M, et al. A patient with idiopathic pleuroparenchymal fibroelastosis showing a sustained pulmonary function due to treatment with pirfenidone. Intern Med 2016;55:497–501.
10. Huang H, Feng R, Li S, et al. A CARE-compliant case report: lung transplantation for a Chinese young man with idiopathic pleuroparenchymal fibroelastosis. Medicine (Baltimore) 2017;96:e6900.
11. Yoshida Y, Nagata N, Tsuruta N, et al. Heterogeneous clinical features in patients with pulmonary fibrosis showing histology of pleuroparenchymal fibroelastosis. Respir Investig 2016;54:162–9.
12. Rosen SH, Castleman B, Liebow AA. Pulmonary alveolar proteinosis. N Engl J Med 1958;258:1123–42.
13. Trapnell BC, Whitsett JA, Nakata K. Pulmonary alveolar proteinosis. N Engl J Med 2003;349:2527–39.
14. Punatar AD, Kusne S, Blair JE, et al. Opportunistic infections in patients with pulmonary alveolar proteinosis. J Infect 2012;65:173–9.
15. Inoue Y, Trapnell BC, Tazawa R, et al. Characteristics of a large cohort of patients with autoimmune pulmonary alveolar proteinosis in Japan. Am J Respir Crit Care Med 2008;177:752–62.
16. Nogee LM, Dunbar AE, Wert SE, et al. A mutation in the surfactant protein C gene associated with familial interstitial lung disease. N Engl J Med 2001;344:573–9.
17. Nogee LM, Garnier G, Dietz HC, et al. A mutation in the surfactant protein B gene responsible for fatal neonatal respiratory disease in multiple kindreds. J Clin Invest 1994;93:1860–3.
18. Dirksen U, Nishinakamura R, Groneck P, et al. Human pulmonary alveolar proteinosis associated with a defect in GM-CSF/IL-3/IL-5 receptor common beta chain expression. J Clin Invest 1997;100:2211–7.
19. McCarthy C, Avetisyan R, Carey BC, et al. Prevalence and healthcare burden of pulmonary alveolar proteinosis. Orphanet J Rare Dis 2018;13:129.
20. Kiani A, Parsa T, Adimi Naghan P, et al. An eleven-year retrospective cross-sectional study on pulmonary alveolar proteinosis. Adv Respir Med 2018;86: 7–12.
21. Goldstein LS, Kavuru MS, Curtis-McCarthy P, et al. Pulmonary alveolar proteinosis: clinical features and outcomes. Chest 1998;114:1357–62.
22. Holbert JM, Costello P, Li W, et al. CT features of pulmonary alveolar proteinosis. AJR Am J Roentgenol 2001;176:1287–94.
23. Kunal S, Gera K, Pilaniya V, et al. "Crazy-paving" pattern: a characteristic presentation of pulmonary alveolar proteinosis and a review of the literature from India. Lung India 2016;33:335–42.

24. Suzuki T, Trapnell BC. Pulmonary alveolar proteinosis syndrome. Clin Chest Med 2016;37:431–40.
25. Wang BM, Stern EJ, Schmidt RA, et al. Diagnosing pulmonary alveolar proteinosis. A review and an update. Chest 1997;111:460–6.
26. Schoch OD, Schanz U, Koller M, et al. BAL findings in a patient with pulmonary alveolar proteinosis successfully treated with GM-CSF. Thorax 2002;57:277–80.
27. Kitamura T, Uchida K, Tanaka N, et al. Serological diagnosis of idiopathic pulmonary alveolar proteinosis. Am J Respir Crit Care Med 2000;162:658–62.
28. Beccaria M, Luisetti M, Rodi G, et al. Long-term durable benefit after whole lung lavage in pulmonary alveolar proteinosis. Eur Respir J 2004;23:526–31.
29. Sheng G, Chen P, Wei Y, et al. Better approach for autoimmune pulmonary alveolar proteinosis treatment: inhaled or subcutaneous granulocyte-macrophage colony-stimulating factor: a meta-analyses. Respir Res 2018;19:163.
30. Akasaka K, Tanaka T, Kitamura N, et al. Outcome of corticosteroid administration in autoimmune pulmonary alveolar proteinosis: a retrospective cohort study. BMC Pulm Med 2015;15:88.
31. Torre O, Elia D, Caminati A, et al. New insights in lymphangioleiomyomatosis and pulmonary Langerhans cell histiocytosis. Eur Respir Rev 2017;26. https://doi.org/10.1183/16000617.0042-2017.
32. Thway K, Fisher C. PEComa: morphology and genetics of a complex tumor family. Ann Diagn Pathol 2015;19:359–68.
33. McCormack FX, Gupta N, Finlay GR, et al. Official American Thoracic Society/Japanese Respiratory Society clinical practice guidelines: lymphangioleiomyomatosis diagnosis and management. Am J Respir Crit Care Med 2016;194:748–61.
34. Inoki K, Corradetti MN, Guan K-L. Dysregulation of the TSC-mTOR pathway in human disease. Nat Genet 2005;37:19–24.
35. Zhe X, Schuger L. Combined smooth muscle and melanocytic differentiation in lymphangioleiomyomatosis. J Histochem Cytochem 2004;52:1537–42.
36. Harknett EC, Chang WYC, Byrnes S, et al. Use of variability in national and regional data to estimate the prevalence of lymphangioleiomyomatosis. QJM 2011;104:971–9.
37. Wakida K, Watanabe Y, Kumasaka T, et al. Lymphangioleiomyomatosis in a male. Ann Thorac Surg 2015;100:1105–7.
38. Baldi BG, Freitas CSG, Araujo MS, et al. Clinical course and characterisation of lymphangioleiomyomatosis in a Brazilian reference centre. Sarcoidosis Vasc Diffuse Lung Dis 2014;31:129–35.
39. Ryu JH, Moss J, Beck GJ, et al. The NHLBI lymphangioleiomyomatosis registry: characteristics of 230 patients at enrollment. Am J Respir Crit Care Med 2006;173:105–11.
40. Kebria M, Black D, Borelli C, et al. Primary retroperitoneal lymphangioleiomyomatosis in a postmenopausal woman: a case report and review of the literature. Int J Gynecol Cancer 2007;17:528–32.
41. Lenoir S, Grenier P, Brauner MW, et al. Pulmonary lymphangiomyomatosis and tuberous sclerosis: comparison of radiographic and thin-section CT findings. Radiology 1990;175:329–34.
42. Müller NL, Chiles C, Kullnig P. Pulmonary lymphangiomyomatosis: correlation of CT with radiographic and functional findings. Radiology 1990;175:335–9.
43. Johnson SR, Cordier JF, Lazor R, et al. European Respiratory Society guidelines for the diagnosis and management of lymphangioleiomyomatosis. Eur Respir J 2010;35:14–26.

44. Young LR, Vandyke R, Gulleman PM, et al. Serum vascular endothelial growth factor-D prospectively distinguishes lymphangioleiomyomatosis from other diseases. Chest 2010;138:674–81.
45. Johnson SR, Whale CI, Hubbard RB, et al. Survival and disease progression in UK patients with lymphangioleiomyomatosis. Thorax 2004;59:800–3.
46. Taveira-DaSilva AM, Stylianou MP, Hedin CJ, et al. Decline in lung function in patients with lymphangioleiomyomatosis treated with or without progesterone. Chest 2004;126:1867–74.
47. Heller J. Die Krankheiten der Nagel, Handbuch der Haut-u. Geschlechtskrankeiten. Berlin: Julius Springer; 1926. p. 13.
48. Emerson PA. Yellow nails, lymphoedema, and pleural effusions. Thorax 1966;21: 247–53.
49. Decker A, Daly D, Scher RK. Role of titanium in the development of yellow nail syndrome. Skin Appendage Disord 2015;1:28–30.
50. Maldonado F, Tazelaar HD, Wang C-W, et al. Yellow nail syndrome: analysis of 41 consecutive patients. Chest 2008;134:375–81.
51. Pavlidakey GP, Hashimoto K, Blum D. Yellow nail syndrome. J Am Acad Dermatol 1984;11:509–12.
52. Samman PD, White WF. The "yellow nail" syndrome. Br J Dermatol 1964;76: 153–7.
53. Norton L. Further observations on the yellow nail syndrome with therapeutic effects of oral alpha-tocopherol. Cutis 1985;36:457.
54. Valdés L, Huggins JT, Gude F, et al. Characteristics of patients with yellow nail syndrome and pleural effusion. Respirology 2014;19:985–92.
55. Brooks KG, Echevarria C, Cooper D, et al. Case-based discussion from North Tyneside General Hospital: somatostatin analogues in yellow nail syndrome associated with recurrent pleural effusions. Thorax 2014;69(10):967–8.
56. Mohammed A, Ghori U, Siddiqui N, et al. Mounier-Kuhn syndrome masquerading as obstructive lung disease. Chest 2018;154:720A.
57. Kachhawa S, Meena M, Jindal G, et al. Case report: Mounier-Kuhn syndrome. Indian J Radiol Imaging 2008;18:316–8.
58. Menon B, Aggarwal B, Iqbal A. Mounier-Kuhn syndrome: report of 8 cases of tracheobronchomegaly with associated complications. South Med J 2008;101:83–7.
59. Noori F, Abduljawad S, Suffin DM, et al. Mounier-Kuhn syndrome: a case report. Lung 2010;188:353–4.
60. Payandeh J, McGillivray B, McCauley G, et al. A clinical classification scheme for tracheobronchomegaly (Mounier-Kuhn Syndrome). Lung 2015;193:815–22.
61. Dunne MG, Reiner B. CT features of tracheobronchomegaly. J Comput Assist Tomogr 1988;12:388–91.
62. Brant WE, Helms CA, editors. Fundamentals of diagnostic radiology. 3rd edition. Philadelphia: Lippincott, Williams & Wilkins; 2007.
63. Schwartz M, Rossoff L. Tracheobronchomegaly. Chest 1994;106:1589–90.

Palliative Care in Chronic Obstructive Pulmonary Disease

Lubna Sorathia, MD*

KEYWORDS

- Palliative care • Chronic obstructive pulmonary disease • Dyspnea • Management

KEY POINTS

- Chronic obstructive pulmonary disease (COPD) is the fourth leading cause of mortality in the world.
- There may be similarities in symptoms of individuals with COPD and lung cancer, yet the care management is significantly different.
- Multiple comorbidities exist, which can worsen functional decline in COPD.
- Conventional therapies fall short in providing adequate symptom control with advancing disease.
- Early incorporation of palliative care with an interdisciplinary approach can improve the quality of life and alleviate suffering regardless of prognosis.

BACKGROUND

Advanced chronic obstructive pulmonary disease (COPD), is characterized by high morbidity and mortality. Patients with COPD and their families experience a range of stresses and suffering from a variety of sources throughout the disease's progression. So far conventional therapy is unable to alleviate patient suffering or maximize the quality of life. However, an interdisciplinary palliative care approach can improve the quality of life and alleviate suffering for those living with this serious illness, regardless of prognosis.

COPD is the fourth leading cause of death in the world.[1] It exists as a significant contributor to global morbidity and mortality,[2,3] and it results in substantial economic and social burden.[4,5] Globally, the prevalence of COPD and its burden is projected to increase in the following decades due to the increase in smoking rates, the reduced mortality from other previously common causes of death (eg, ischemic heart disease,

Disclosure Statement: Dr L. Sorathia has neither commercial or financial conflicts of interest nor any relevant funding sources.
Innovage Greater CO PACE, Denver, CO, USA
* 13635 East Weaver Place, Englewood, CO 80111.
E-mail address: lsorathia@myinnovage.com

Med Clin N Am 103 (2019) 517–526
https://doi.org/10.1016/j.mcna.2018.12.010
0025-7125/19/© 2019 Elsevier Inc. All rights reserved.

medical.theclinics.com

infectious diseases), and the changing age structure of the current world's population.[4,5]

In the United States, the estimated direct and indirect costs of COPD are approximately $29.5 billion and $20.4 billion, respectively.[6] As most would predict, there is a beautiful direct relationship between the severity of COPD, and it is a burden on the health care system in the form of COPD exacerbations, hospitalization, and ambulatory oxygen costs. This estimate of medical expenditures to society does not, however, take into consideration the hidden economic value of the care provided by the family members.

The Global Burden of Disease Study has formulated a method called "The Disability-Adjusted Life Year" (DALY).[4,7,8]. The DALYs for a specific condition are the sum of years lost due to premature mortality and the years of life lived with disability, which is adjusted in accordance with the severity of the disability. In 1990, COPD was the 12th leading cause of DALYs lost in the world. By 2030, COPD is expected to be the seventh leading cause of DALYs lost worldwide.[5]

COPD presents a significant public health challenge that is both preventable and treatable in most cases. Most national data suggest less than 6% of the adult population have been informed of this serious diagnosis,[9] which highlights the widespread underrecognition and underdiagnosis of COPD,[10,11] which in turn affects the accuracy of COPD mortality data.[12–14] Although this disease is often a primary cause of death, it is more likely to be listed as a contributory cause of death or often even omitted from the death certificate entirely.[15,16]

Many people suffer from this disease for years and eventually die prematurely from it or the substantial list of complications of COPD. The unpredictable course of the physical decline can be characterized as long-term deterioration with frequent exacerbations and often, without a distinct terminal phase.[12]

Taking into account that most health care resources are dedicated toward management and prevention of acute events, mortality following hospitalization for an acute exacerbation of COPD is falling[17]; it still varies between 23%[18] and 80%.[19] Progressive respiratory failure, cardiovascular diseases, malignancies, and other diseases remain the primary cause of death in patients with COPD hospitalized for a form of exacerbation.[19]

People with advanced COPD continue to report distressing physical and psychological symptoms comparable to those of patients with lung cancer,[20] often have limited insight into their disease, and often have infrequent discussions of care goals in a routine clinical setting. This is due in part to the significant lack of emphasis from physicians and researchers on both palliative and supportive care.[21] This may explain why patients with COPD are less likely to receive palliative care services compared with those with lung cancer.[22,23]

A particularly striking discovery is that COPD and lung cancer[12,24] affect multiple organ systems and are associated with[25] multimorbidity. This can occur in patients with mild, moderate, and severe airflow limitation[26] and can directly influence mortality and hospitalizations of the patients independently. Hence comorbidities should be actively looked for and treated appropriately, if present. Even when medical treatment is optimized for a patient with COPD, a large proportion of people with COPD still have symptom-related distress.[27]

In COPD, the line between curative and palliative therapies is quite blurred. However, the data on incidence, prevalence, the social, psychological, and economic burden are overwhelming and mandate the need for additional intervention. Palliative care expands the approach beyond the traditional disease-model medical treatment and toward the changing focus on therapeutic aims to reduce symptoms, improve function, enhance quality of life, help with decision-making about end-of-life care, and provide emotional and spiritual support to patients and their families regardless of the stage of disease or the need for other therapies.[28] In this approach, the person is put before the disease, quality of life is affirmed, and the patient's eventual death is seen as just that, eventual.

Both patient and caregiver outcomes can be improved by an early integration of palliative care based on complex symptomatology as opposed to the prognosis. The focus should be on primary and respiratory care along with rehabilitation services.

Palliative care teams are readily increasing in number and capacity for consultation of hospitalized patients.[29] Outpatient palliative care consultation is less commonly available, but when available, has been shown to relieve symptoms, improve quality of life, and even prolong survival for some patients, such as those with advanced lung cancer.[23] Clinicians caring for patients with COPD are responsible for helping identify patients who could benefit from palliative care services and identify the palliative care resources within their community that are available for these patients. For patients with the advanced or accelerated disease, the transition to hospice services may provide additional benefit and support. Hospice services are a Medicare-covered service with more defined enrollment criteria, with the focus on patients with severe disabilities or symptoms burden. These services offer a multidisciplinary approach tailored to patient's need in a multifaceted program, including services in various settings from the patient's home to dedicated hospice units, hospitals, and nursing homes. The National Hospice and Palliative Care Organization (http://www.nhpco.org) is a great resource in providing guidance for hospice services to those with noncancerous disease such as COPD.[22,23] These guidelines discuss the difficulties in accurately predicting the prognosis of patients with advanced COPD but recognize the appropriateness of providing hospice services for some of these patients.[28]

There is a substantial body of evidence supporting the use of palliative care in the early stages of the benign disease. In a systemic review and meta-analysis of more than 12,000 patients and more than 2400 caregivers,[30] palliative care was associated with improvements in both patient's symptom burden (standardized mean difference -0.66, 95% confidence interval [CI] -1.25 to -0.07) and quality of life at 1 to 3 months (0.46, $0.08-0.83$), and a consistent pattern of reduced health care use was recorded. More than 2 decades ago, the investigators of the SUPPORT study[31] of patients who were seriously ill due to complications with COPD who were admitted to the hospital advocated for earlier and enhanced palliative care, even for patients remaining open to life-sustaining treatments. Despite all these attempts, progress remains slow, and patients with COPD still face barriers to palliative care referral.

ASSESSMENT AND MANAGEMENT OF SYMPTOMS IN PALLIATIVE CARE

Patients with advanced COPD often experience a wide range of symptoms, the most common of them being breathlessness or dyspnea followed by any combination of anxiety, pain, depression, fatigue, insomnia, and anorexia.[6,32]

A study of patients referred to a palliative medicine program found that there were 10 symptoms for every one symptom that was reported by a patient.[33] The symptom analysis is critical to the diagnosis and treatment of symptoms; this missed opportunity was apparent after this study. A careful and comprehensive symptoms assessment, with a focus on common problems in palliative care practice, can define factors that are contributing to the symptom and may lead to a more successful treatment intervention that can subsequently improve quality of life.[34,35]

There are many validated symptom assessment tools available for use in palliative and hospice settings. These include "The Revised Edmonton Symptom Assessment Scale,"[36] "Memorial Symptom Assessment Scale-Short (MSAS)" and the more convenient version "Condensed MSAS,"[37–39] "MD Anderson Brief Symptom Inventory,"[40,41] and the "Symptom Distress Scale."[42] Besides, instruments are focusing specifically on single symptoms such as brief pain inventory.

The global strategy for the diagnosis, management, and prevention of COPD (GOLD) report recommends that all clinicians managing patients with COPD should be aware of the effectiveness of palliative approaches to symptom control and use them in their practice.[43] Palliative care is more than an end-of-life care; clinicians providing care to patients with the advanced respiratory disease would do well to consider the following quote from Dame Cicely Saunders, the founder of the modern hospice movement in the United Kingdom: "How people die remains in the memory of those who live on."[44]

SYMPTOM BURDEN

As COPD advances into its terminal stages, the care is often focused on preventing hospitalization, which can inadvertently neglect day-to-day symptoms resulting in patients living with high symptom burden.[45] The UK Regional Study of Care for the Dying indicated that the physical and psychological needs were as severe in patients with chronic lung disease at the end of life as patients with lung cancer.[46] Dyspnea or breathlessness was recorded in 94% followed by anorexia in 67% and constipation in 44% of cases. Other studies[47–51] have confirmed the prevalence of these symptoms along with providing information on other significant symptoms including fatigue, pain, anxiety and panic, poor sleep, and depression. A prospective study comparing patients with end-stage COPD and lung cancer[45] indicated that patients with COPD had significantly worse activities of daily living and physical, social, and emotional functioning than patients with lung cancer. In this study, 90% of patients with COPD suffered clinically relevant anxiety or depression. Sadly, none of the patients with COPD received specialist palliative care input.

MANAGING BREATHLESSNESS

Refractory dyspnea remains the most common and difficult symptom reported by the patient even when they are on optimal treatment with a combination of a long-acting beta agonist, an inhaled steroid, and a long-acting anticholinergic. Theophylline has fallen out of use due to narrow therapeutic index and multiple drug interactions.[52] Because of severe debility with advanced disease, pulmonary rehabilitation[53] may be of limited benefit due to difficulty attending these programs.[54] The use of a fan to ease the sensation of dyspnea may have some supporting evidence in normal subjects.[55] Relaxation techniques and humidification of air are some of the other nonpharmacologic interventions.

Oxygen and opioids remain the mainstays of palliative pharmacologic treatment. Oxygen is typically used with caution in patients with COPD because uncontrolled oxygen therapy can result in carbon dioxide narcosis, suppress respiratory derive, and ultimately result in respiratory arrest in some patients with COPD. On the other hand, long-term use of oxygen therapy for greater than 15 hours a day aims to improve survival in patients with COPD who have severe hypoxemia[56] as well as to reduce the incidence of complications including polycythemia and the progression of pulmonary hypertension and improve neuropsychological health. Short-term ambulatory oxygen use was associated with significant improvement in health-related quality of life of patients with COPD.[57]

The National Institute for Health and Care Excellence (NICE) guideline recommends short burst oxygen therapy be considered and continued for episodes of severe breathlessness in patients with COPD not relieved by other treatments, and they have documented relief in dyspnea following therapy. Caution and education is advised when using oxygen in individual who continues to smoke due to a real risk of fire, explosion, or facial burns.[6]

Association of Palliative Medicine working group recommends the use of oxygen be tailored to the individual needs and formal assessment be made to determine its efficacy for reducing breathlessness and improving quality of life for that person.[58] A systematic review[59] supported the use of both oral and parenteral opioids in the treatment of breathlessness with advanced disease. It also reassures that appropriate doses of opioids do not lead to respiratory depression. Another study[60] suggest sustained-release preparation of 20 mg of morphine sulfate given once daily provided significant symptomatic improvement in refractory dyspnea in the community setting. The usefulness of nebulized opioids remains unclear and may not be better than nebulized normal saline.

CACHEXIA

Decrease appetite and associated muscle wasting and weight loss are of grave concern to caregiver and patients alike. Unfortunately, pathophysiology is not completely understood.[61] Interventions including high calorie shakes and protein supplementation had limited success. A dietician advice may offer support even if it does not lead to actual weight gain.[62]

MANAGING DEPRESSION AND ANXIETY

Anxiety associated with dyspnea is quite distressing. Insomnia is commonly reported symptoms in COPD. Benzodiazepines are commonly prescribed in clinical practice, yet evidence for the safety and effectiveness of its use for palliation of these symptoms is lacking.[63]

Given the terminal nature of lung cancer, depression is very high, and it is considered a good practice to screen these patients actively and offer treatment when possible. The same practice is recommended for those suffering from COPD. Even in moderate stages of COPD, anxiety and depression are commonly noted in those who are hypoxic or severely dyspnoeic.[64] These disabling and distressing symptoms can have a downward spiral effect, leading to social isolation and anhedonia. The NICE guideline on COPD recommends treating patients suffering from COPD with anxiety and depression with conventional pharmacotherapy. Choice and route of drugs need to be taken into consideration with gradual functional decline, and the patient may need continuous subcutaneous infusion therapy via a syringe driver.

MANAGEMENT OF COMORBIDITIES AT THE END OF LIFE

Managing comorbidities also need special attention while caring for patients with advancing disease. Careful and passionate discussion is mandated regarding the question of whether or not to continue medication for risk stratification of conditions such as hypertension, hyperlipidemia, diabetes, osteoporosis, and continuation and monitoring of anticoagulation.

The Place of Complementary and Alternative Medicine

There is limited evidence for the use of complementary and alternative medicine in the management of dyspnoea.[65] Individual patients with severe COPD may benefit from the use of acupuncture, acupressure, and muscle relaxation with breathing retraining to relieve dyspnea.[66] Acupuncture has not demonstrated to be on any benefit in randomized controlled trial.[67] Given low-risk nature of these interventions, it is reasonable to consider these therapies on an individual basis based on patient request.

SUMMARY

With recent advances in medicine, more people are living longer, and fewer people are dying from chronic illnesses such as COPD. High-quality palliative care has a potential to have a significant impact on quality of life. Although it is appropriate for patients with advanced chronic illness to get palliative care, few patients get access to such care compared with a patient with cancer. Despite advances, much remains unknown regarding assessment, management, and prognostication in specific chronic nonmalignant lung diseases. It is difficult to predict less than 6 months survival in nonmalignant diseases such as COPD partially due to the unpredictable natural course of the disease. The multidisciplinary approach of palliative care helps patients with COPD navigate through the continuum of chronic disease management without giving up hope or treatment options. Highest quality of life, not necessarily the highest physiologic goals, with relief of physical and emotional suffering are most important to patients. Hospice care, the last phase of palliative care, can be offered to patients with COPD when their goal of care changes from life-prolonging therapies to comfort treatment.

REFERENCES

1. World Health Report. Geneva (Switzerland): World Health Organization; 2000. Available at: https://www.who.int/images/default-source/infographics/top-10-global-causes-of-deaths-2016.jpg?sfvrsn=56e8d56c_0.
2. Lozano R, Naghavi M, Foreman K, et al. Global and regional mortality from 235 causes of death for 20 age groups in 1990 and 2010: a systematic analysis for the Global Burden of Disease Study 2010. Lancet 2012;380:2095–128.
3. Murray CJL, Barber RM, Foreman KJ, et al. Global, regional, and national disability-adjusted life years (DALYs) for 306 diseases and injuries and healthy life expectancy (HALE) for 188 countries, 1990–2013: quantifying the epidemiological transition. Lancet 2015;386:2145–91.
4. Lopez AD, Shibuya K, Rao C, et al. Chronic obstructive pulmonary disease: current burden and future projections. Eur Respir J 2006;27:397–412.
5. Mathers CD, Loncar D. Projections of global mortality and burden of disease from 2002 to 2030. PLoS Med 2006;3:e442.
6. Solano JP, Gomes B, Higginson IJ. A comparison of symptom prevalence in far advanced cancer, AIDS, heart disease, chronic obstructive pulmonary disease and renal disease. J Pain Symptom Manage 2006;31(1):58.
7. Murray CJ, Lopez AD. Alternative projections of mortality and disability by cause 1990-2020: Global Burden of Disease Study. Lancet 1997;349:1498–504.
8. Murray CJL, Lopez AD, editors. The global burden of disease: a comprehensive assessment of mortality and disability from diseases, injuries and risk factors in 1990 and projected to 2020. Cambridge (MA): Harvard University Press; 1996.

9. Halbert RJ, Natoli JL, Gano A, et al. Global burden of COPD: systematic review and meta-analysis. Eur Respir J 2006;28:523–32.

10. van den Boom G, van Schayck CP, van Mollen MP, et al. Active detection of chronic obstructive pulmonary disease and asthma in the general population. Results and economic consequences of the DIMCA program. Am J Respir Crit Care Med 1998;158:1730–8.

11. Seymour J, Spruit M, Hopkinson N, et al. The prevalence of quadriceps weakness in COPD and the relationship with disease severity. Eur Respir J 2010;36:81–8.

12. Lunney JR, Lynn J, Foley DJ, et al. Patterns of functional decline at the end of life. JAMA 2003;289:2387–92.

13. Pena VS, Miravitlles M, Gabriel R, et al. Geographic variations in prevalence and underdiagnosis of COPD: results of the IBERPOC multicentre epidemiological study. Chest 2000;118:981–9.

14. Talamo C, de Oca MM, Halbert R, et al. Diagnostic labeling of COPD in five Latin American cities. Chest 2007;131:60–7.

15. Jensen HH, Godtfredsen N, Lange P, et al. Potential misclassification of causes of death from COPD in a Danish population study. Eur Respir J 2006;28:781–5.

16. McGarvey LP, Magder S, Burkhart D, et al. Cause-specific mortality adjudication in the UPLIFT® COPD trial: findings and recommendations. Respir Med 2012; 106(4):515–21.

17. Eriksen N, Vestbo J. Management and survival of patients admitted with an exacerbation of COPD: comparison of two Danish patient cohorts. Clin Respir J 2010; 4(4):208–14.

18. Groenewegen KH, Schols AM, Wouters EF. Mortality and mortality-related factors after hospitalization for acute exacerbation of COPD. Chest 2003;124:459–67.

19. Gudmundsson G, Ulrik CS, Gislason T, et al. Long-term survival in patients hospitalized for chronic obstructive pulmonary disease: a prospective observational study in the Nordic countries. Int J Chron Obstruct Pulmon Dis 2012;7:571–6.

20. Boland J, Martin J, Wells AU, et al. Palliative care for people with nonmalignant lung disease, summary of current evidence and future direction. Palliat Med 2013;27(9):811–6.

21. Taylor DR, Murray SA. Improving quality of care for end-stage respiratory disease: changes in attitude, changes in service. Chron Respir Dis 2018;15(1): 19–25.

22. Au DH, Udris EM, Fihn SD, et al. Differences in health care utilization at the end of life among patients with chronic obstructive pulmonary disease and patients with lung cancer. Arch Intern Med 2006;166(3):326–31.

23. Levy MH, Adolph MD, Back A, et al. Palliative care. J Natl Compr Canc Netw 2012;10(10):1284–309.

24. Lange P, Nyboe J, Appleyard M, et al. Ventilatory function and chronic mucus hypersecretion as predictors of death from lung cancer. Am Rev Respir Dis 1990; 141:613–7.

25. Yin HL, Yin SQ, Lin QY, et al. Prevalence of comorbidities in chronic obstructive pulmonary disease patients: a meta-analysis. Medicine 2017;96:e6836.

26. Agusti A, Calverley PM, Celli B, et al. Characterisation of COPD heterogeneity in the ECLIPSE cohort. Respir Res 2010;11:122.

27. Han MK, Martinez CH, Au DH, et al. Meeting the challenge of COPD care delivery in the USA: a multiprovider perspective. Lancet Respir Med 2016;4:473–526.

28. American Academy of Hospice and Palliative Medicine, Center to Advance Palliative Care, Hospice and Palliative Nurses Association, et al. National consensus

project for quality palliative care: clinical practice guidelines for quality palliative care, executive summary. J Palliat Med 2004;7(5):611–27.

29. Morrison RS, Maroney-Galin C, Kralovec PD, et al. The growth of palliative care programs in United States hospitals. J Palliat Med 2005;8(6):1127–34.

30. Kavalieratos D, Corbelli J, Zhang D, et al. Association between palliative care and patient and caregiver outcomes: a systematic review and meta-analysis. JAMA 2016;316:2104–14.

31. Claessens MT, Lynn J, Zhong Z, et al. Dying with lung cancer or chronic obstructive pulmonary disease: insights from SUPPORT. Study to understand prognoses and preferences for outcomes and risks of treatments. J Am Geriatr Soc 2000; 48(suppl 5):S146–53.

32. Reuben DB, Mor V, Hiris J. Clinical symptoms and length of survival in patients with terminal cancer. Arch Intern Med 1988;148(7):1586.

33. Homsi J, Walsh D, Rivera N, et al. Symptom evaluation in palliative medicine: patient report vs systematic assessment. Support Care Cancer 2006;14(5): 444.

34. Yennurajalingam S, Urbauer DL, Casper KL, et al. Impact of a palliative care consultation team on cancer-related symptoms in advanced cancer patients referred to an outpatient supportive care clinic. J Pain Symptom Manage 2011; 41(1):49.

35. Williams PD, Graham KM, Storlie DL, et al. Therapy-related symptom checklist use during treatments at a cancer center. Cancer Nurs 2013;36(3):245.

36. Watanabe SM, Nekolaichuk C, Beaumont C, et al. A multicenter study comparing two numerical versions of the Edmonton Symptom Assessment System in palliative care patients. J Pain Symptom Manage 2011;41(2):456–68.

37. Chang VT, Hwang SS, Feuerman M, et al. The memorial symptom assessment scale short form (MSAS-SF). Cancer 2000;89(5):1162.

38. Chang VT, Hwang SS, Kasimis B, et al. Shorter symptom assessment instruments: the Condensed Memorial Symptom Assessment Scale (CMSAS). Cancer Invest 2004;22(4):526.

39. Tranmer JE, Heyland D, Dudgeon D, et al. Measuring the symptom experience of seriously ill cancer and noncancer hospitalized patients near the end of life with the memorial symptom assessment scale. J Pain Symptom Manage 2003; 25(5):420.

40. Cleeland CS, Mendoza TR, Wang XS, et al. Assessing symptom distress in cancer patients: the M.D. Anderson Symptom Inventory. Cancer 2000;89(7):1634.

41. M D Anderson Sysmptom Assessment Scale. Available at: www.mdanderson. org/departments/prg/display.cfm?id=0EE78C60-6646-11D5-00508B603A14& pn=0EE78204-6646-11D5-812400508B603A14&method=displayfull. Accessed February 01, 2011.

42. McCorkle R. The measurement of symptom distress. Semin Oncol Nurs 1987; 3(4):248–56.

43. Vogelmeier CF, Criner GJ, Martinez FJ, et al. Global strategy for the diagnosis, management, and prevention of chronic obstructive lung disease 2017 report: GOLD executive summary. Eur Respir J 2017;49:1700214.

44. Saunders C. Pain and impending death. In: Wall PD, Melzak R, editors. Textbook of pain. 2nd ednition. Edinburgh (Scotland): Churchill Livingstone; 1989. p. 624–31.

45. Gore JM, Brophy CJ, Greenstone MA. How well do we care for patients with end stage chronic obstructive pulmonary disease (COPD)? A comparison of

palliative care and quality of life in COPD and lung cancer. Thorax 2000;55: 1000–6.

46. Jones I, Kirby A, Ormiston P, et al. The needs of patients dying of chronic obstructive pulmonary disease in the community. Fam Pract 2004;21:310–3.

47. Skilbeck J, Mott L, Page H, et al. Palliative care in chronic obstructive airways disease: a needs assessment. Palliat Med 1998;12:245–54.

48. Edmonds P, Karlsen S, Khan S, et al. A comparison of the palliative care needs of patients dying from chronic respiratory diseases and lung cancer. Palliat Med 2001;15:287–95.

49. Seamark DA, Blake SD, Seamark CJ, et al. Living with severe chronic obstructive pulmonary disease (COPD): perceptions of patients and their carers. An interpretative phenomenological analysis. Palliat Med 2004;18:619–25.

50. Elkington H, White P, Addington-Hall J, et al. The last year of life of COPD: a qualitative study of symptoms and services. Respir Med 2004;98:439–45.

51. Elkington H, White P, Addington-Hall J, et al. The healthcare needs of chronic obstructive pulmonary disease patients in the last year of life. Palliat Med 2005; 19:485–91.

52. Booth S, Silvester S, Todd C. Breathlessness in cancer and chronic obstructive pulmonary disease: using a qualitative approach to describe the experience of patients and carers. Palliat Support Care 2003;1:337–44.

53. Aronson JK, Hardman M, Reynolds DJ. ABC of monitoring drug therapy. Theophylline. BMJ 1992;305:1355–8.

54. British Thoracic Society Standards of Care Subcommittee on Pulmonary Rehabilitation. Pulmonary rehabilitation. Thorax 2001;56:827–34.

55. Ward JA, Akers G, Ward DG, et al. Feasability and effectiveness of a pulmonary rehabilitation programme in a community hospital setting. Br J Gen Pract 2002; 52:539–42.

56. Abernethy AP, Currow DC, Frith P, et al. Randomised, double blind, placebo controlled crossover trial of sustained release morphine for the management of refractory dyspnoea. BMJ 2003;327:523–8.

57. Swinburn CR, Mould H, Stone TN, et al. Symptomatic benefit of supplemental oxygen in hypoxemic patients with chronic lung disease. Am Rev Respir Dis 1991; 143:913–5.

58. Schwartzstein RM, Lahive K, Pope A, et al. Cold facial stimulation reduces breathlessness induced in normal subjects. Am Rev Respir Dis 1987;136: 53–61.

59. Booth S, Wade R, Johnson M, et al. The use of oxygen in the palliation of breathlessness. A report of the expert working group of the Scientific Committee of the Association of Palliative Medicine. Respir Med 2004;98:66–77.

60. Jennings AL, Davies AN, Higgins JP, et al. A systematic review of the use of opioids in the management of dyspnoea. Thorax 2002;57:939–44.

61. Wouters EF. Management of severe COPD. Lancet 2004;364:883–95.

62. Creutzberg EC, Wouters EF, Mostert R, et al. Efficacy of nutritional supplementation therapy in depleted patients with chronic obstructive pulmonary disease. Nutrition 2003;19:120–7.

63. Hirst A, Sloan R. Benzodiazepines and related drugs for insomnia in palliative care. Cochrane Database Syst Rev 2002;(4):CD003346.

64. van Manen JG, Bindels PJ, Dekker FW, et al. Risk of depression in patients with chronic obstructive pulmonary disease and its determinants. Thorax 2002;57: 412–6.

65. Pan CX, Morrison RS, Ness J, et al. Complementary and alternative medicine in the management of pain, dyspnea, and nausea and vomiting near the end of life. A systematic review. J Pain Symptom Manage 2000;20:374–87.

66. Corner J, Plant H, A'Hern R, et al. Non-pharmacological intervention for breathlessness in lung cancer. Palliat Med 1996;10:299–305.

67. Lewith GT, Prescott P, Davis CL. Can a standardized acupuncture technique palliate disabling breathlessness: a single-blind, placebo-controlled crossover study. Chest 2004;125:1783–90.

Sarcoidosis

Oscar Llanos, MD*, Nabeel Hamzeh, MD

KEYWORDS

- Sarcoidosis • Nonnecrotizing granuloma • Diagnosis • Organ involvement

KEY POINTS

- Sarcoidosis is a multisystemic granulomatous disease.
- A thorough evaluation to diagnosis, rule out other granulomatous disease, and evaluate extent of disease is essential.
- Treatment is indicated when there is symptomatic, progressive disease or critical organ involvement.

INTRODUCTION

Sarcoidosis was first described in 1877 by the dermatologist Jonathan Hutchinson who described violaceous skin lesions, which were called "sarcoid" by Caesar Boeck because of their histologic resemblance to sarcoma.[1] Sarcoidosis is a multisystemic disease that mostly affects the lungs (90% of cases), but can involve any organ in the body.[1]

EPIDEMIOLOGY

Sarcoidosis is a world-wide disease with variable prevalence and incidence depending on race and ethnicity.[2] In the United States, the reported incidence among African Americans is 35.5/100,000 compared with 10.9/100,000 in whites.[3] In Spain, it is about 1.3/100,000, Eastern Europe 3.7/100,000, and Japan 1/100,000.[4,5] The average age of presentation is 48 years.[6]

PATHOGENESIS

Sarcoidosis develops in genetically predisposed individuals after exposure to an environmental trigger.[7] Susceptibility and disease phenotype have been linked to several genes including HLA genes and various immune-related genes.[8] Sarcoidosis is a

Disclosure Statement: The authors have no potential conflicts of interest to disclose related to this article.
Division of Pulmonary, Critical Care and Occupational Medicine, University of Iowa College of Medicine, 200 Hawkins Drive, Iowa City, IA 52242, USA
* Corresponding author.
E-mail address: oscar-llanosulloa@uiowa.edu

Med Clin N Am 103 (2019) 527–534
https://doi.org/10.1016/j.mcna.2018.12.011
0025-7125/19/© 2019 Elsevier Inc. All rights reserved.

polygenic disease with no particular gene being predominantly responsible for the disease.[8] To date, genetic testing is not indicated for sarcoidosis in the United States.

The gene-environment interaction triggers a granulomatous inflammatory response that is driven by the interaction between antigen-presenting cells and T cells via the major histocompatibility complex II pathway.[9] After antigen presentation, T cells are activated and several cytokines and chemokines are secreted, including interferon-γ, tumor necrosis factor (TNF)-α, transforming growth factor-β, among others. The granuloma in sarcoidosis consists of a core that is composed of multinucleated giant cells, surrounded by CD4+ T cells and some CD8+ T cells (**Fig. 1**).[9] The granuloma in sarcoidosis is nonnecrotizing in most cases, although focal necrosis can sometimes be seen.

Although the triggers for sarcoidosis are still not elucidated, certain environmental factors have been associated with this disease. The ACCESS study (A Case Controlled Etiologic Study of Sarcoidosis), which recruited more than 700 incident cases of sarcoidosis and matched control subjects, did not show a clear cause, but suggested specific occupations and exposures that were more prevalent in patients with sarcoidosis. These included agricultural workers, health care, bird breeder, automotive industry, and middle/high school teachers. Exposures included insecticides, mildew, mold, musty odors, and home central air conditioning.[10] Among potential triggers are *Mycobacterium tuberculosis* and *Cutibacterium acnes* (*Propionibacterium acnes*) but sarcoidosis is not an active infectious disease.[11,12] Smokers have a lower incidence of sarcoidosis, and nicotine has been insinuated to have a protective role in sarcoidosis.[1]

CLINICAL PRESENTATION

Sarcoidosis has a variable clinical presentation that depends on organ involvement and the severity of involvement. The diagnosis is made based on history, physical examination, appropriate radiologic and pathologic findings, and the exclusion of other causes. Sarcoidosis is known as the great mimicker; as such, a thorough history, especially an exposure history, is crucial to exclude other causes of granulomatous disorders. Infectious agents, such as mycobacterium, fungi, and certain bacteria or parasites, can cause a granulomatous response.[13] Certain environmental or occupational exposures can cause granulomatous diseases, such beryllium (chronic beryllium disease),[14] or organic antigens (hypersensitivity pneumonitis). Several autoimmune diseases can also manifest with a granulomatous response, including

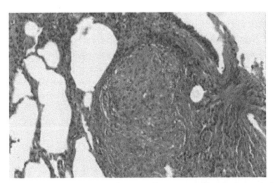

Fig. 1. Noncaseating granuloma in lung biopsy (hematoxylin-eosin, original magnification ×40).

granulomatous polyangiitis and Crohn disease, among others.[15] In addition, certain medications are associated with a granulomatous response, including immune checkpoint inhibitors (ie, pembrolizumab, nivolumab), antiretroviral therapy, interferons (α and β), and TNF-α inhibitors.[16]

Löfgren syndrome is an acute manifestation of sarcoidosis characterized by fever, uveitis, enlarged hilar lymph nodes, polyarthritis, and erythema nodosum. Its prognosis is often excellent.[17]

Pulmonary

The clinical presentation of pulmonary sarcoidosis is variable. Patients can be asymptomatic and diagnosed incidentally on chest imaging performed for unrelated reasons or can present with chronic nonspecific symptoms including cough, dyspnea on exertion, and fatigue.[1]

Chest radiograph abnormalities were graded by Scadding in 1950 (**Table 1**).[18] On computed tomography of the chest, common findings include bilateral hilar and/or mediastinal lymphadenopathy,[19] and parenchymal nodules in a peribronchovascular, subpleural, and/or interlobular distribution.[20]

Pulmonary function testing is variable. It can be normal, restrictive, or obstructive.[21] Diffusion capacity can also be impaired depending on the degree of pulmonary involvement. If diffusion capacity is disproportionately reduced to the extent of lung involvement, then further work-up for underlying pulmonary hypertension is warranted.[22]

The diagnosis of suspected sarcoidosis is accomplished by pathologic confirmation from the lymph nodes and/or parenchyma. Lymph nodes are sampled via endobronchial ultrasound with transbronchial needle aspiration with a high diagnostic yield obviating mediastinoscopy.[23] Bronchoalveolar lavage is not diagnostic for sarcoidosis but typical findings include bronchoalveolar lavage lymphocytosis and CD4/CD8 ratio more than 3.5. Cultures to exclude infectious causes of granulomatous lung disease are important.

Extrapulmonary Sarcoidosis

Skin

The skin is the second most common organ involved in sarcoidosis.[24] Cutaneous manifestations include maculopapular lesions, hypopigmented and hyperpigmented lesions, subcutaneous nodules, localized alopecia, ulcers, and pustules.[25] Lupus pernio consists of indurated facial lesions, seen more commonly in patients of African descent and usually associated with chronic disease and sinonasal disease.[26] Biopsy

Table 1 Scadding chest radiograph stages	
Scadding Stage	**Radiographic Description**
0	Normal
I	Bilateral hilar lymphadenopathy without parenchymal changes
II	Bilateral hilar lymphadenopathy with parenchymal changes
III	Parenchymal changes without hilar lymphadenopathy
IV	Pulmonary fibrosis, conglomerate mass formation

Data from Scadding JG. Sarcoidosis, with special reference to lung changes. Br Med J 1950;1(4656):745–53.

of sarcoidosis skin lesions reveals noncaseating granulomas. Sarcoidosis tends to affect scars and tattoos for unclear reasons.[27] Erythema nodosum, which is seen in Löfgren syndrome, does not exhibit granulomas on biopsy.

Eyes

Approximately one-third of patients have eye involvement, being more common in African Americans and women.[24] It can be the first manifestation of sarcoidosis with these patients' initially presenting to an ophthalmologist. Any part of the globe can be involved. The most frequent manifestation is anterior uveitis and symptoms include acute eye pain, redness, photophobia, and increased lacrimation. Posterior uveitis can have a more subacute course and cause vision impairment. The conjunctiva can also be involved.[28] Lacrimal gland swelling can also be seen in sarcoidosis and a lacrimal gland biopsy can reveal evidence of granulomatous inflammation. Ophthalmic involvement in sarcoidosis requires urgent attention and management because it can lead to irreversible vision impairment.

Gastrointestinal

Granulomas are frequently detected in the liver of patients with sarcoidosis.[24,29] Liver involvement can cause a wide spectrum of manifestations, from asymptomatic to jaundice, abdominal pain, pruritus, with elevated alkaline phosphatase being more common abnormal liver function test then elevated aminotransferases.[29,30] Hepatomegaly is present in approximately 50% of patients.[29] Hepatic involvement can lead to cirrhosis. Sarcoidosis can affect any part of the gastrointestinal tract, but involvement remains rare.[29]

Nervous system

Neurologic involvement is seen in 10% of cases.[31] Isolated neurosarcoidosis is rare and approximately 90% of patients have other organ involvement by the time of diagnosis.[32] The cranial nerves and spinal cord are the sites most frequently affected with facial and optic nerves among the most commonly involved cranial nerves.[33] Parenchymal brain disease can present with headaches, cognitive/behavioral disorders, and seizures.[34]

Cerebrospinal fluid analysis is nonspecific, but usually exhibits a lymphocytic pattern with elevated protein and negative cultures.[35] MRI findings include intraparenchymal lesions, leptomeningeal and cranial nerve enhancement in T1-weighted images.[36]

Diagnostic criteria for neurosarcoidosis have been proposed and characterize it as definite, probable and possible sarcoidosis.[37] Definite requires clinical presentation suggestive of neurosarcoidosis; other causes are excluded; supportive nervous system pathology; or in the absence of nervous system pathology, a beneficial response to immunotherapy over 1 year. For probable, patients have similar characteristics as definite but lack nervous system pathology or response to therapy over 1 year. For possible, the presentation suggests sarcoidosis but there is no confirmation of an overall diagnosis of sarcoidosis.[37] Consultation with a neurologist with expertise in neurosarcoidosis is essential.

Endocrine

Hypercalcemia occurs in about 5% to 10% of patients with sarcoidosis patients, and hypercalciuria (>300 mg/d) is more common, occurring three times more than hypercalcemia. The macrophages in the granuloma express 1α-hydroxylase, converting 25-hydroxycholecalciferol into 1,25-dihydroxycholecalciferol, the active form of vitamin

D, which increases blood calcium levels.[38] Symptoms of hypercalcemia include lethargy, mental status changes, constipation, nephrolithiasis, and renal dysfunction.

Additional monitoring and caution should be taken when considering vitamin D supplementation in patients with sarcoidosis because this could precipitate the development of hypercalcemia and subsequent renal dysfunction. Persistent hypercalciuria can lead to stone formation. Overall management includes ruling out other causes of hypercalcemia/hypercalciuria, avoiding excessive sun exposure, avoiding excessive dairy intake, and avoiding vitamin D supplementation. In cases of persistent hypercalcemia or hypercalciuria, immunosuppressive therapy (IST) may be needed.

Cardiac

Cardiac sarcoidosis is associated with significant morbidity and mortality. It is under-recognized and can be subclinical. It is detected clinically in 5% of patients but in autopsies it has been detected in up to 40% of cases.[39]

Cardiac sarcoidosis can be asymptomatic, or present with arrhythmias, conduction defects, heart failure, or rarely sudden cardiac death. Screening for asymptomatic disease includes history, physical examination, and 12-lead electrocardiogram. The role of echocardiogram and/or Holter monitor in screening is yet unknown.[40] Diagnostic modalities include cardiac MRI with gadolinium, which can detect scar formation (delayed enhancement). Cardiac fluorodeoxyglucose PET can detect active myocarditis but needs to be performed at specialized centers familiar with the cardiac sarcoidosis protocol. In confirmed cases of cardiac sarcoidosis, electrophysiologic assessment is important in assessing risk of fatal arrhythmias, need for an automated implantable cardiac defibrillator, and managing ongoing arrhythmias.[41]

IST can minimize further cardiac damage and potentially reverse existing damage caused by active myocarditis but has no impact on existing scar tissue.

Musculoskeletal

Sarcoidosis can involve the joints, bones, and/or muscles. Bone involvement is usually asymptomatic and is detected incidentally on imaging for other indications. It can affect any bone. Radiographic findings include osteolysis in the small bones of the hands and feet and osteosclerosis in the long bones and vertebrae. Bone scans and fluorodeoxyglucose PET scans can detect increased activity in the involved bones. Acute arthritis is reactive in nature and commonly manifests as part of Löfgren syndrome. Chronic arthritis is uncommon. Muscle involvement in sarcoidosis is rare and presents as chronic myopathy, nodules, or masses.[42]

MANAGEMENT

The cornerstone of treatment in sarcoidosis is IST. Not all patients with sarcoidosis need to be treated and a thorough assessment of organ involvement and dysfunction is needed before initiating IST. IST is indicated when there is vital organ involvement (ocular, nervous system, cardiac) or when there are symptoms, organ dysfunction, and/or progressive disease. Consultation with a sarcoidosis center of excellence is advised before contemplating empiric therapy.

Various agents are used in the management of sarcoidosis and include corticosteroids, hydroxychloroquine, steroid-sparing agents (methotrexate, azathioprine, leflunomide, mycophenolate mofetil), and anti-TNF-α inhibitors (infliximab and adalimumab).[43] Hydroxychloroquine is typically used for hypercalcemia/hypercalciuria, skin involvement, and some cases of fatigue.[44,45] Corticosteroids are fast-acting agents but are fraught with numerous side effects limiting their long-term use. They are useful when there is critical organ involvement (ocular, nervous system, and cardiac), symptomatic organ involvement, and in the setting of symptomatic hypercalcemia.[46] Steroid-sparing agents are used for the long-term management of sarcoidosis. Their onset of action is delayed but they are associated with less side effects than corticosteroids.[47] Anti-TNF-α agents are used in cases that are unresponsive to steroid-sparing agents and occasionally as first-line therapy in neurologic involvement.[48]

REFERENCES

1. Statement on sarcoidosis. Am J Respir Crit Care Med 1999;160(2):736–55.
2. Sharma OP. Sarcoidosis around the world. Clin Chest Med 2008;29(3):357–63.
3. Rybicki BA, Major M, Popovich J, et al. Racial differences in sarcoidosis incidence: a 5-year study in a health maintenance organization. Am J Epidemiol 1997;145(3):234–41.
4. Sharma S, Ghosh B, Sharma SK. Association of TNF polymorphisms with sarcoidosis, its prognosis and tumour necrosis factor (TNF)-alpha levels in Asian Indians. Clin Exp Immunol 2008;151(2):251–9.
5. Morimoto T, Azuma A, Abe S, et al. Epidemiology of sarcoidosis in Japan. Eur Respir J 2008;31(2):372–9.
6. Erdal BS, Clymer BD, Yildiz VO, et al. Unexpectedly high prevalence of sarcoidosis in a representative U.S. metropolitan population. Respir Med 2012;106(6): 893–9.
7. Culver DA, Newman LS, Kavuru MS. Gene-environment interactions in sarcoidosis: challenge and opportunity. Clin Dermatol 2007;25(3):267–75.
8. Fingerlin TE, Hamzeh N, Maier LA. Genetics of sarcoidosis. Clin chest Med 2015; 36(4):569–84.
9. Gerke AK, Hunninghake G. The immunology of sarcoidosis. Clin chest Med 2008; 29(3):379–90, vii.
10. Newman LS, Rose CS, Bresnitz EA, et al. A case control etiologic study of sarcoidosis: environmental and occupational risk factors. Am J Respir Crit Care Med 2004;170(12):1324–30.
11. Gupta D, Agarwal R, Aggarwal AN, et al. Molecular evidence for the role of mycobacteria in sarcoidosis: a meta-analysis. Eur Respir J 2007;30(3):508–16.
12. Nishiwaki T, Yoneyama H, Eishi Y, et al. Indigenous pulmonary propionibacterium acnes primes the host in the development of sarcoid-like pulmonary granulomatosis in mice. Am J Pathol 2004;165(2):631–9.
13. Zumla A, James DG. Granulomatous infections: etiology and classification. Clin Infect Dis 1996;23(1):146–58.
14. Muller-Quernheim J, Gaede KI, Fireman E, et al. Diagnoses of chronic beryllium disease within cohorts of sarcoidosis patients. Eur Respir J 2006;27(6):1190–5.
15. Timmermans WM, van Laar JA, van Hagen PM, et al. Immunopathogenesis of granulomas in chronic autoinflammatory diseases. Clin Transl Immunology 2016;5(12):e118.
16. Chopra A, Nautiyal A, Kalkanis A, et al. Drug-induced sarcoidosis-like reactions. Chest 2018;154(3):664–77.
17. Keary PJ, Palmer DG. Benign self-limiting sarcoidosis with skin and joint involvement. N Z Med J 1976;83(560):197–9.
18. Scadding JG. Sarcoidosis, with special reference to lung changes. Br Med J 1950;1(4656):745–53.

19. Reich JM. Mortality of intrathoracic sarcoidosis in referral vs population-based settings: influence of stage, ethnicity, and corticosteroid therapy. Chest 2002; 121(1):32–9.

20. Criado E, Sanchez M, Ramirez J, et al. Pulmonary sarcoidosis: typical and atypical manifestations at high-resolution CT with pathologic correlation. Radiographics 2010;30(6):1567–86.

21. Sharma OP, Johnson R. Airway obstruction in sarcoidosis. A study of 123 nonsmoking black American patients with sarcoidosis. Chest 1988;94(2):343–6.

22. Rapti A, Kouranos V, Gialafos E, et al. Elevated pulmonary arterial systolic pressure in patients with sarcoidosis: prevalence and risk factors. Lung 2013;191(1): 61–7.

23. Tremblay A, Stather DR, MacEachern P, et al. A randomized controlled trial of standard vs endobronchial ultrasonography-guided transbronchial needle aspiration in patients with suspected sarcoidosis. Chest 2009;136(2):340–6.

24. Judson MA, Boan AD, Lackland DT. The clinical course of sarcoidosis: presentation, diagnosis, and treatment in a large white and black cohort in the United States. Sarcoidosis Vasc Diffuse Lung Dis 2012;29(2):119–27.

25. Mana J, Marcoval J, Graells J, et al. Cutaneous involvement in sarcoidosis. Relationship to systemic disease. Arch Dermatol 1997;133(7):882–8.

26. Baughman RP, Judson MA, Teirstein A, et al. Chronic facial sarcoidosis including lupus pernio: clinical description and proposed scoring systems. Am J Clin Dermatol 2008;9(3):155–61.

27. Marchell RM, Judson MA. Chronic cutaneous lesions of sarcoidosis. Clin Dermatol 2007;25(3):295–302.

28. Baughman RP, Lower EE, Kaufman AH. Ocular sarcoidosis. Semin Respir Crit Care Med 2010;31(04):452–62.

29. Ebert EC, Kierson M, Hagspiel KD. Gastrointestinal and hepatic manifestations of sarcoidosis. Am J Gastroenterol 2008;103(12):3184–92 [quiz: 3193].

30. Cremers J, Drent M, Driessen A, et al. Liver-test abnormalities in sarcoidosis. Eur J Gastroenterol Hepatol 2012;24(1):17–24.

31. Ungprasert P, Matteson EL. Neurosarcoidosis. Rheum Dis Clin North Am 2017; 43(4):593–606.

32. Ungprasert P, Carmona EM, Utz JP, et al. Epidemiology of sarcoidosis 1946-2013: a population-based study. Mayo Clin Proc 2016;91(2):183–8.

33. Ferriby D, de Seze J, Stojkovic T, et al. Long-term follow-up of neurosarcoidosis. Neurology 2001;57(5):927–9.

34. Stern BJ, Aksamit A, Clifford D, et al. Neurologic presentations of sarcoidosis. Neurol Clin 2010;28(1):185–98.

35. Joseph F, Scolding NJ. Neurosarcoidosis: a study of 30 new cases. J Neurol Neurosurg Psychiatry 2008;80(3):297–304.

36. Smith JK, Matheus MG, Castillo M. Imaging manifestations of neurosarcoidosis. AJR Am J Roentgenol 2004;182(2):289–95.

37. Terushkin V, Stern BJ, Judson MA, et al. Neurosarcoidosis: presentations and management. Neurologist 2010;16(1):2–15.

38. Baughman RP, Janovcik J, Ray M, et al. Calcium and vitamin D metabolism in sarcoidosis. Sarcoidosis Vasc Diffuse Lung Dis 2013;30(2):113–20.

39. Mehta D, Lubitz SA, Frankel Z, et al. Cardiac involvement in patients with sarcoidosis: diagnostic and prognostic value of outpatient testing. Chest 2008;133(6): 1426–35.

40. Hamzeh NY, Wamboldt FS, Weinberger HD. Management of cardiac sarcoidosis in the United States: a Delphi study. Chest 2012;141(1):154–62.

41. Birnie DH, Sauer WH, Bogun F, et al. HRS expert consensus statement on the diagnosis and management of arrhythmias associated with cardiac sarcoidosis. Heart Rhythm 2014;11(7):1305–23.
42. Zisman DA, Shorr AF, Lynch JP 3rd. Sarcoidosis involving the musculoskeletal system. Semin Respir Crit Care Med 2002;23(6):555–70.
43. Wijsenbeek MS, Culver DA. Treatment of sarcoidosis. Clin chest Med 2015;36(4): 751–67.
44. Jones E, Callen JP. Hydroxychloroquine is effective therapy for control of cutaneous sarcoidal granulomas. J Am Acad Dermatol 1990;23(3 Pt 1):487–9.
45. Adams JS, Diz MM, Sharma OP. Effective reduction in the serum 1,25-dihydroxyvitamin D and calcium concentration in sarcoidosis-associated hypercalcemia with short-course chloroquine therapy. Ann Intern Med 1989;111(5):437–8.
46. Grutters JC, van den Bosch JM. Corticosteroid treatment in sarcoidosis. Eur Respir J 2006;28(3):627–36.
47. Baughman RP, Lower EE. Steroid-sparing alternative treatments for sarcoidosis. Clin chest Med 1997;18(4):853–64.
48. Sodhi M, Pearson K, White ES, et al. Infliximab therapy rescues cyclophosphamide failure in severe central nervous system sarcoidosis. Respir Med 2009; 103(2):268–73.

Occupational Lung Disease

David M. Perlman, MD[a], Lisa A. Maier, MD, MSPH[b,c,*]

KEYWORDS

- Occupational lung disease • Pneumoconiosis • Work-related asthma and COPD
- Lung cancer • Mesothelioma

KEY POINTS

- Occupational exposures are a significant source of lung disease and disability worldwide.
- Occupational exposures can cause a broad range of types of lung disease, including obstructive airways disease, interstitial lung disease, and malignancy.
- A detailed and complete history is critical to the diagnosis of occupational lung disease.
- Clinicians need to be familiar with common types of disease causing occupational exposure and should be vigilant in evaluating for potential exposures in patients presenting with lung disease.

INTRODUCTION

Occupational and environmental exposures can cause most categories of lung diseases described in this issue of the *Medical Clinics of North America*, including airways diseases, interstitial lung diseases (ILDs), and cancers. It is important to define these diseases because they have implications for public health, including workers or other individuals that may be exposed and at risk of developing disease. In addition, when a diagnosis of an occupational lung disease is made, this finding has implications for the patient/worker's ability to continue work and eligibility for compensation programs and other benefits.[1] The key to defining occupational lung diseases is to consider them in the differential diagnosis of patients being evaluated for respiratory complaints, and to ask some simple but important questions about the patient's current and past occupations, home environment, hobbies, and potential for second-hand or paraoccupational exposures (**Table 1**). In addition, focusing the history of the present illness around the timing of symptoms can also be helpful, because some diseases result in symptoms with temporality to exposures. The key elements

[a] Division of Pulmonary and Critical Care Medicine, University of Minnesota, MMC # 276, 420 Delaware Street Southeast, Minneapolis, MN 55045, USA; [b] Division of Environmental and Occupational Health Sciences, National Jewish Health, 1400 Jackson Street, G212, Denver, CO 80206, USA; [c] Division of Pulmonary and Critical Care Sciences, Environmental Occupational Health Department, School of Medicine, Colorado School of Public Health, University of Colorado, Denver, CO, USA
* Corresponding author. National Jewish Health, 1400 Jackson Street, G212, Denver, CO 80206.
E-mail address: LisaMaier@NJHealth.org

Med Clin N Am 103 (2019) 535–548
https://doi.org/10.1016/j.mcna.2018.12.012
0025-7125/19/© 2019 Elsevier Inc. All rights reserved.

Table 1
Key elements of the occupational history and features with different types of occupational lung disease

History Element	Obstructive	ILD

Nature of exposure
  Detailed job history of current and past occupations including type of industry and nature of activities.
  Detailed exposures outside of work, including hobbies, potential for second hand exposure (eg, laundering spouses clothing)
  Types of possible exposure
  Dusts, gases, and vapors
  Particulate, including diesel
  Elongate mineral particles
  Metals
  Chemicals, including pesticides, insecticides, herbicides, isocyanates, solvents and organic chemicals
  Animal, plant, or food antigens and or bioaerosols
	OA and HP
	  HMW exposures
	  Plant, animal, and fish
	  Mold (many possible exposures)
	  Manufacturing (organic/bioaerosol exposure, metal working fluids)
	  Farming
	  Food workers
	  LMW exposures
	  Chemicals (Isocyanates, acid anhydrides, persulfates)
	  Metal salts
	COPD
	  Dust
	  Gases/fumes
	  Particulate/diesel
		Pneumoconiosis
		  Dust: Coal, silica, mixed
		  Elongate mineral particles
		  Metal-induced lung disease
		Can be manufacturing, manipulating or using the material
		Risk for bystander exposure (near someone working with material)
		Second-hand exposure well-documented for asbestos, beryllium

Duration of exposure
  Overall duration (years of employment)
  Single exposure vs ongoing
  Continuous vs intermittent
  Percent of time at work with exposure
  Route of exposure
	Exposure can be brief in the case of IIA/WEA
	Sensitizer induced OA requires initial sensitization and ongoing exposure
		History is typically longer term exposure owing to long latency in dust-induced ILD
		Duration of employment tends to correlate with risk for pneumoconiosis

Intensity of exposure
  Intermittent high level vs low level chronic
  Method of exposure
    Spraying
    Fume inhalation
    Ambient dust
  Mitigating factors
    Personal protective equipment
    Industrial hygiene
	Low level exposures can cause both OA and IIA/WEA
	Higher intensity exposures can lead to higher risk of WRA
	Can have single, high-level exposure lead to ongoing symptoms (RADS)
		History is typically longer term exposure
		Higher cumulative exposure tends to correlate with risk of pneumoconiosis
		Latency is less clear in sensitizer-induced ILD (eg, CBD or HP)

(continued on next page)

Table 1 (continued)		
History Element	**Obstructive**	**ILD**

Timing or temporality
  Temporal relationship with exposure
  Improvement in symptoms on weekends or during vacation
	Sensitizer induced OA typically has period of latency before the onset of symptoms
	Timing can vary in OA with immediate period or delay of several hours
	IIA/WRA tend to have more rapid onset of symptoms after exposure and resolve more quickly when exposure is removed
		Patients are often asymptomatic during the exposure
		May have some respiratory symptoms if irritant induced airways disease is present

Abbreviations: CBD, chronic beryllium disease; COPD, chronic obstructive pulmonary disease; HMW, high molecular weight; HP, hypersensitivity pneumonitis; IIA, irritant-induced asthma; ILD, interstitial lung disease; LMW, low molecular weight; OA, occupational asthma; RADS, reactive airways dysfunction syndrome; WEA, work-exacerbated asthma; WRA, work-related asthma.

of an occupational exposure history are reviewed in **Table 1**. Once specific exposures are identified, the diagnosis of occupational and environmental lung disease is similar to evaluation for nonoccupational and environmental lung disease, with a basis in lung function testing and chest radiography (**Fig. 1**). Because many of the pneumoconioses are diagnosed based on the clinical radiographic manifestations, sometimes lung biopsy is not needed, although in some cases it is the foundation of diagnosis. We provide an overview of the major classes of occupational lung diseases as well as specific examples and a diagnostic outline and testing that can be used to confirm specific diseases. Once a diagnosis is made of occupational lung disease, it is often medically prudent to remove the patient/worker from ongoing exposure, especially in the case of exposure to sensitizers and fibrogenic agents; ongoing exposure can result in progressive disease without the chance for remission or improvement. In general, other treatment recommendations are similar to those of the nonoccupational forms of the lung disease, or in some cases, like coal workers pneumoconiosis, silicosis, and asbestosis, removal from exposure, prevention of infections (eg, mycobacterial disease, common in silicosis and coal workers' pneumoconiosis, or routine respiratory infections) and treatment with oxygen, are the only real options for treatment.

OCCUPATIONAL AIRWAYS DISEASES
Work-Related Asthma

The current prevalence of asthma in the United States among adults is 8% to 9% (according to the Centers for Disease Control and Prevention), and it is estimated that work related exposures account for as much as 15% to 25% of the asthma burden in the United States,[2] however, occupational exposures may be underreported.[3] Work-related asthma (WRA) is associated with significant levels of functional impairment and disability[4,5] and tends to cause more severe disease when compared with the general asthma population.[6] When new cases of asthma are identified in adults without other clear precipitation, WRA should be considered.

In general, WRA is divided into 2 categories: asthma caused by work, generally termed occupational asthma (OA) and preexisting asthma that is exacerbated by

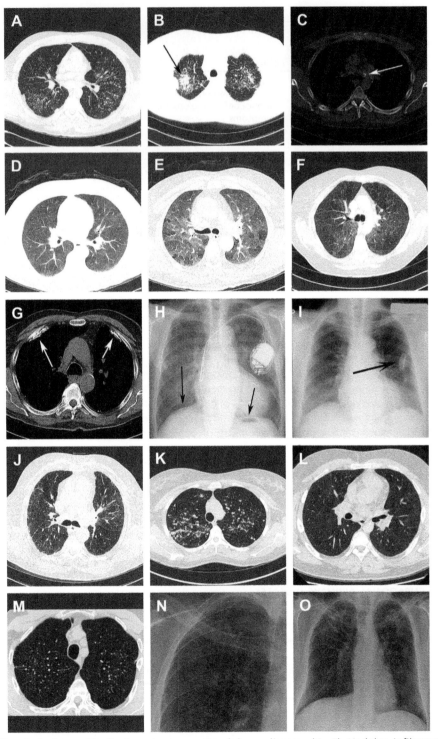

Fig. 1. Radiographic findings in occupational lung disease. (*A*, *B*) Nodular infiltrates in silicosis. (*B*) *Arrow* shows the area of conglomeration representing early progressive

working conditions, or work-exacerbated asthma. The OA can be further subdivided into those that are sensitizer induced, in which an immune response to a specific antigen is present, and irritant-induced asthma (IIA), in which the airway inflammation is due to exposure to an irritant without specific sensitization.[7,8]

Sensitizer-Induced Occupational Asthma

Sensitizer-induced asthma can have many causes; antigens are usually divided into high-molecular weight (HMW) and low-molecular weight (LMW) categories. The HMW antigens consist of animal and plant proteins, fungi, and other large organic molecules. The LMW antigens consist of chemicals and some metal salts.[7] More than 350 workplace antigens that can cause both sensitizer-induced asthma and IIA have been identified.[9] Some of the more common causes of both types of OA are shown in **Table 1**. The immunologic mechanism of sensitizer induced OA for most HMW antigens involves the development of IgE-specific antibodies produced by exposure to the antigen. In the cases of LMW that are IgE mediated (most notably platinum and other hard metal salts and acid anhydrides), the chemicals react with other proteins (endogenous or exogenous) to create an antigen capable of producing an allergic response.[7,10] Most chemical sensitizers are organic molecules with reactive side chains, suggesting that the ability to cross-link proteins may be important in the immune mechanism of LMW OA[11]; however, the mechanism of OA owing to LMW causes in many cases is unclear. Other mechanisms such as cell mediated immunity and T helper 2 type innate responses have been proposed.[12] In the case of toluene diisocyanate, one of the most well-described LMW causes of OA, specific IgE antibodies are detected in some cases, although other data suggest an IgE-independent response.[13] The phenotype of airway response is different in LMW versus HMW OA, and LMW-induced OA may have a tendency to be more severe compared with HMW agents.[14,15] HMW OA can often be associated with a late or dual phase reaction compared with LMW, which may result in greater difficulty in making a diagnosis of work relatedness.

Irritant-Induced Asthma

Although most cases of OA involve sensitization and an immune response, IIA may comprise up to 15% to 20% of OA cases.[16] IIA consists of a spectrum of disease from prolonged symptoms owing to a single large exposure, referred to a reactive airways dysfunction syndrome,[17] to asthma induced by long-term, low-level exposure to irritant chemicals.[7] The mechanism of inflammation in IIA is thought to involve the breakdown of the epithelial barrier in the lung owing to injury.[12] IIA usually has a short

---

massive fibrosis (PMF). (*C*) Egg shell calcification of lymph node seen in silicosis. (*D–F*) Hypersensitivity pneumonitis (HP). (*D*) Diffuse ground glass opacities with expiratory views showing (*E*) mosaic attenuation and (*F*) a case of HP owing to hot tub exposure showing a more nodular infiltrate. (*G–I*) Pleural plaque seen in asbestos exposure. (*G*) Calcified pleural plaque (*arrows*) on high-resolution computed tomography, (*H*) diaphragmatic plaques (*arrows*) on chest radiographs and (*I*) an en-face plaque (*arrow*). (*J*) Mixed dust/silica exposure in a stone cutter showing a more interstitial pattern in the mid lungs. (*K*) Nodular infiltrates in chronic beryllium disease (CBD), similar to sarcoidosis and (*L*) ground glass opacities in (CBD), similar to those seen in HP. (*M–O*) Radiographs of coal workers pneumoconiosis with (*M*) computed tomography changes of simple coal workers' pneumoconiosis (CWP), as shown in (*N*) a close up chest radiograph. (*O*) Progression to CWP in the same individual years later.

latency period when compared with OA,[18] particularly in cases of a high level of exposure. Studies of first responders and recovery workers after the World Trade Center Collapse demonstrated that asthma can persist long after a single, high-level exposure.[19] Conversely, long-term, low-level exposure has been shown to be associated with asthma, notably in cleaning products.[20] In the latter cases, genetic susceptibility may play a role,[21] and there is likely overlap with work-exacerbated asthma because the mechanisms for work-exacerbated asthma and IIA are similar.[22]

Diagnosis of Work-Related Asthma

The diagnosis of WRA can be challenging, and hinges on demonstrating a relationship between workplace exposures and the development or worsening of asthma. Specific inhalational challenge tests are considered the gold standard for the diagnosis of OA; a negative test in the setting of otherwise good evidence does not exclude a diagnosis of OA and can occur if the testing occurs after extended removal from exposure.[23] Although specific inhalational challenge tests can diagnose all LMW and HMW OA, and the level of response correlates with bronchial reactivity on methacholine challenge tests, these tests are expensive to carry out and are not available in most clinical settings.[24] In the case of OA, skin or serologic immunologic testing can be performed for most HMW and some LMW antigens; however, these tests lack specificity, because exposed workers without symptoms may test positive as well.[25] As a result, these tests are a measure of exposure and cannot be used alone to diagnose IIA or non–IgE-mediated OA; a diagnosis of asthma is also needed in conjunction with exposure, with a demonstration of airways responsiveness on spirometry and/or methacholine challenge responsivity. Serial peak flow measurement, another method of linking worsening of asthma to the workplace, is considered to have good sensitivity and specificity for the diagnosis of WRA (although the evidence is limited); however, it cannot distinguish between OA and IIA and requires good adherence for accurate results.[25] Preshift and postshift spirometry can be used to link asthma to the workplace and or an exposure, although this information is not always feasible to obtain clinically.

Occupational Chronic Obstructive Pulmonary Disease and Bronchiolitis

Other obstructive lung diseases, such as chronic obstructive pulmonary disease (COPD) and bronchiolitis, are also associated with occupational exposures. About 15% of COPD cases have been attributed to occupational exposures, even in smokers. Multiple exposures have been identified of various types including vapors, gas, dust, and fumes.[26] Studies of nonsmokers with COPD have demonstrated strong associations with exposure, with organic dust showing the strongest associations.[27] Because many of the exposures in the vapors, gas, dust, and fumes category can cause OA and pneumoconioses, there is likely significant overlap among all these conditions. Several studies have demonstrated an association of coal dust exposure[28] and the presence of pneumoconiosis[29] with COPD. This is also noted in the absence of pneumoconiosis and has been called chronic airways obstruction owing to coal and silica. Similarly, there is a recognized OA/COPD overlap syndrome, with recent data suggesting a distinct clinical phenotype.[30] Exposure-related obstructive bronchiolitis may have multiple histologic patterns of bronchiolitis, and several types of exposures that have been identified.[31] One of the most well-described syndromes is popcorn workers lung, which may be caused by diacetyl, a butter flavoring or other chemical used in the production of microwave popcorn and flavorings.[32]

OCCUPATIONAL INTERSTITIAL LUNG DISEASES

The occupational pneumoconioses can present with a number of patterns, all of which can be similar to other nonoccupational ILD (**Table 2**). Thus, it is critical in the evaluation of all patients with ILD that a detailed occupational and exposure history is obtained including the nature, intensity, and duration of the exposure, to help distinguish exposure-related ILD from other causes. Other than the history, the pattern seen on chest radiograph and/or high-resolution computed tomography can help to classify occupational ILD.

Coal, Silica, and Mixed Dust

Exposure to coal and silica dust are well-described causes of ILD[33,34] and have similar clinical presentations. They both typically cause opacities consisting of small nodules that can coalesce to form progressive massive fibrosis.[35] The term mixed dust is not well-defined, but generally refers to dust consisting of a mix of crystalline silica and nonfibrous silicates and can present with a similar pattern.[36] Although nodular infiltrates are common on chest radiographs or computed tomography scans, pneumoconiosis can also present with a more fibrotic interstitial pneumonia in a pattern that may be similar to usual interstitial pneumonia.[37] The pneumoconioses are clinically characterized by restrictive pulmonary physiology, although obstruction may be present in many cases, especially those with airways disease as noted, or mixed obstructive and restrictive physiology. There is no proven therapy for the dust-induced pneumoconioses; the treatment of obstructive disease if present may improve symptoms. Additional clinical concerns with silica include an increased risk of tuberculosis in people with silica exposure, and an increased risk for the development of autoimmune diseases. Although cases of coal workers' pneumoconiosis were thought to be on the decline, rapidly progressive cases of coal workers' pneumoconiosis have been found in younger miners recently, primarily in the eastern United States. This finding has been attributed to changes in work practices, exposure to coal with high

---

Table 2
High-resolution computed tomography findings in exposure and non–exposure-related disease

High-Resolution Computed Tomography Pattern	Exposure Related	Non–Exposure Related
Nodular infiltrates	Silicosis Coal workers pneumoconiosis Some HP (more ground glass nodules) CBD	Sarcoidosis Miliary tuberculosis Desquamative interstitial pneumonitis Vasculitis Infection
Interstitial fibrosis (UIP)	Mixed dust Asbestosis	Idiopathic pulmonary fibrosis Nonspecific interstitial pneumonitis
Ground glass infiltrates	HP Some CBD	Organizing pneumonia Infection Vasculitis
Mosaic attenuation	HP	Small airways disease Pulmonary hypertension

Abbreviations: CBD, chronic beryllium disease; HP, hypersensitivity pneumonitis; UIP, usual interstitial pneumonia.

silica content.[38] Similarly, silicosis cases have been attributed to newer exposures, including sandblasting jeans and work with artificial stone (eg, making countertops).

Asbestos and Elongate Mineral Particles

The term asbestos refers to a group of naturally occurring minerals that can cleave to form long thin particles that are in the larger category of elongate mineral particles (EMP), previously referred to as fibers. Most types of asbestos are classified as amphibole asbestos, which is felt to be more pathogenic than the serpentine type of asbestos.[39] The toxicity of amphibole asbestos has been well-documented. It is a known carcinogen that can also cause pleural and parenchymal disease and may cause obstructive lung disease in some cases.[40] Asbestos-related disease tends to have a very long (>25 years) latency from exposure to onset of disease. Asbestos exposure typically causes interstitial pulmonary fibrosis, often in a usual interstitial pneumonia pattern and can cause pleural disease, including effusions, plaques, and diffuse thickening.[41] The mechanism by which asbestos causes disease is not well-defined. The toxicity is felt to be related to its shape and durability, making it difficult for the immune system to clear and causing persistent inflammation and potentially activating other signaling pathways. EMP can have other sources other than naturally occurring asbestos, such as cleavage fragments, and the toxicity of nonasbestiform EMP is not well-defined.[39,42,43] Recently, an association between EMP exposure and pleural abnormalities on chest radiographs was found in a population of iron ore miners in northern Minnesota.[44]

Metal-Induced Interstitial Lung Disease

In addition to causing OA, metal exposure can cause ILD. The effects of various types of metal exposure are varied and distinct histopathologic patterns have been described.[45] Exposure to hard metals, mainly tungsten and cobalt, is best known to cause a giant cell interstitial pneumonitis, although other histologic patterns have been described, with imaging typically showing ground glass opacities.[46,47] Both obstructive and restrictive lung disease have been associated with indium, with manifestations including pulmonary alveolar proteinosis and fibrotic lung disease.[48–50] Cadmium, in addition to being a potential carcinogen, has been linked in small studies to ILD as well as the potential to induce autoimmunity.[46] ILD caused by aluminum is rare, but it can cause both fibrotic and granulomatous disease.[51]

Granulomatous Disease

Granulomatous diseases can result from a number of exposures. Hypersensitivity pneumonitis may result from exposure to biologic agents and less commonly nonorganic LMW agents. A number of metals may cause granulomatous lung disease, including beryllium, causing chronic beryllium disease (CBD), aluminum, titanium, copper, and potentially zirconium.

Occupational Hypersensitivity Pneumonitis

Numerous HMW/organic and LWM antigens have been identified as causes of occupational hypersensitivity pneumonitis (see **Table 1**).[52,53] In the occupational setting, it typically presents in the acute or subacute pattern of hypersensitivity pneumonitis. Acute symptoms such as fever, chills, myalgias, and shortness of breath are associated with exposures and usually result in ground glass nodular opacities and mosaic attenuation on high-resolution computed tomography. Chronic hypersensitivity pneumonitis presents with a more interstitial pattern on high-resolution computed tomography and without a clear exposure–symptom response relationship, and can be more difficult to establish the connection to a workplace exposure with variable exposure latency. The typical histopathology consists of peribronchiolar inflammation (bronchiolitis) with lymphoid aggregates and loosely formed noncaseating granulomas as well as organizing pneumonia.[54] Acute and subacute hypersensitivity pneumonitis can have a restrictive and/or obstructive physiology. Given that many of the same antigens that cause occupational hypersensitivity pneumonitis are also implicated in OA, there is likely some overlap; not surprisingly, positive methacholine challenge may be seen in hypersensitivity pneumonitis. Chronic hypersensitivity pneumonitis tends to have more of a restrictive pattern, although airway involvement can be seen in these patients as well. Precipitins, a blood test measuring IgG response to specific antigens, are not usually helpful in the diagnosis of hypersensitivity pneumonitis. The test is not well-standardized and the presence of antibodies demonstrates exposure but does not prove causation. The presence of positive bird precipitins in the setting of the right clinicoradiographic presentation is a useful marker of hypersensitivity pneumonitis owing to birds. Treatment for hypersensitivity pneumonitis is focused on antigen identification, removal from exposure, and immunosuppression with prednisone and/or steroid-sparing agents.

Chronic Beryllium Disease

CBD occurs in 2% to 10% of those exposed to beryllium in the workplace. Exposure to respirable beryllium occurs in the manufacture of beryllium and in other industries where beryllium is smelted, cast, machined, or otherwise manipulated to produce a respirable particulate, including the aerospace, automotive, electronics, jewelry, military, nuclear energy, recycling, and telecommunications industries.[55,56] Unfortunately, many workers still do not know if they are or have been exposed to beryllium. As a result, work with metals in someone with sarcoidosis or granulomatous lung disease should prompt a consideration of CBD and additional evaluation. The diagnosis of CBD relies on the demonstration of a beryllium-specific immune response, or beryllium sensitization with a beryllium lymphocyte proliferation test.[57] This test is usually obtained on blood cells and is used to screen workers for health effects, but can be obtained on bronchoalveolar lavage cells and is an indication for bronchoscopy. The presence of an abnormal blood and/or bronchoalveolar lavage beryllium lymphocyte proliferation test in conjunction with granulomatous inflammation on biopsy not only provides a diagnosis of CBD, but also differentiates it from other granulomatous lung diseases like hypersensitivity pneumonitis and sarcoidosis. The associated radiographic and lung function abnormalities are similar to those found in hypersensitivity pneumonitis or sarcoidosis. The treatment approach is also similar to that used for these diseases.

OCCUPATIONAL LUNG CANCER

Occupational exposure to carcinogens is a significant contributor to the overall incidence of cancer, and lung cancer is the most common type of occupational cancer.[58,59] It is estimated that up to 25% of lung cancer cases occur in lifetime nonsmokers. Although it is difficult to assess the fraction of lung cancer attributable to occupational exposures, owing mainly to the overlap with smoking and difficulty obtaining accurate exposure data, it is likely that occupational exposure contributes significantly to the burden of lung cancer. Numerous occupational exposures, including chemicals, metals, minerals, fumes, and radiation, have been shown to have been linked to risk of lung cancer.[60] Of note, some studies have shown a synergistic effect of asbestos and tobacco smoke to increase the risk of lung cancer[61]; however, the data are somewhat mixed and the interaction between tobacco smoke and other carcinogens in lung cancer risk is less well-understood.[62]

Lung Cancer

Adenocarcinoma is the most common form of lung cancer in never smokers and is the most common type in asbestos exposure; however, other types of lung cancer have been seen with occupational exposures. Radon exposure, seen in uranium miners, is one of the leading causes of exposure-related lung cancer in nonsmokers and has been associated with small cell lung cancer.[63] In addition to asbestos, silica is another mineral where there is a strong association between exposure and lung cancer.[64] Similarly, beryllium has been classified as a carcinogen and can cause lung cancer. Arsenic, a naturally occurring metal, is well-documented as a potent carcinogen and cause of lung cancer. The ingestion of arsenic-contaminated water is the most common form of exposure, but it may also occur via inhalation.[65] Occupational exposure of arsenic has been documented in many occupations, notably copper smelters and in workers exposed to pesticides and insectisides.[66] Squamous cell lung cancer and small cell lung cancer are the most common types of lung cancer associated with arsenic exposure. Numerous metals, including cadmium, nickel, chromium, and aluminum, have been implicated as potential causes of occupational lung cancer, but the data are limited.[67] Painters have been shown to be at increased risk for lung cancer,[68] which may be due to metal-based pigments in the paint; the use of solvents has also been implicated.[67,69] Multiple types of exposure have been demonstrated in the rubber manufacturing industry, including chemicals, dusts, and fumes, and there is evidence for increased risk for lung cancer in this industry.[70]

Mesothelioma

Malignant mesothelioma is a cancer of serosal surfaces, most commonly pleural and peritoneal, that has a poor prognosis.[71] Mesothelioma is strongly associated with exposure to amphibole asbestos (particularly in males) and it is felt that most of the risk for mesothelioma worldwide is attributable to exposure to asbestos.[72] The vast majority of the asbestos-related mesothelioma is likely caused by exposure to amphibole asbestos; however, the risk of mesothelioma owing to exposures to other EMP such as cleavage fragments is not clear. Most evidence suggests that the risk of these exposures is negligible or at least much lower than amphibole asbestos.[39] Other nonasbestos causes have been suggested; carbon nanotubes and the SV40 virus have been shown to induce mesothelioma in animal models, but there are no data to support a contribution to disease in humans.[73] The mechanism by which asbestos causes mesothelioma is not well-defined. It is likely a multifactorial process, including ongoing inflammation owing to the inability of the lung to clear the asbestos particles. In addition, asbestos fibers can penetrate mesothelial cells causing DNA mutations, the production of free radicals and abnormal cell proliferation owing to interference with protooncogenes.[74]

SUMMARY

Occupational exposures can cause a wide spectrum of lung disease and are a significant contributor to disease and disability worldwide. It is incumbent on the clinician to be familiar with potential exposures and have a high suspicion for the possibility of occupational lung disease in the proper setting. A detailed history of occupational exposures and symptoms is crucial to raise the potential of these diseases and help to determine diagnosis because other testing can be supportive, but is often impractical or not definitive.

REFERENCES

1. Cowl CT. Occupational asthma: review of assessment, treatment, and compensation. Chest 2011;139(3):674–81.
2. Blanc PD, Toren K. How much adult asthma can be attributed to occupational factors? Am J Med 1999;107(6):580–7.
3. Baur X, Bakehe P, Vellguth H. Bronchial asthma and COPD due to irritants in the workplace - an evidence-based approach. J Occup Med Toxicol 2012;7(1):19.
4. Vandenplas O, Toren K, Blanc PD. Health and socioeconomic impact of work-related asthma. Eur Respir J 2003;22(4):689–97.
5. White GE, Mazurek JM, Moorman JE. Work-related asthma and employment status–38 states and District of Columbia, 2006-2009. J Asthma 2013;50(9): 954–9.
6. Dodd KE, Mazurek JM. Asthma medication use among adults with current asthma by work-related asthma status, Asthma Call-back Survey, 29 states, 2012-2013. J Asthma 2018;55(4):364–72.
7. Tarlo SM, Lemiere C. Occupational asthma. N Engl J Med 2014;370(7):640–9.
8. Tarlo SM, Balmes J, Balkissoon R, et al. Diagnosis and management of work-related asthma: American College Of Chest Physicians Consensus Statement. Chest 2008;134:1S–41S.
9. Baur X. A compendium of causative agents of occupational asthma. J Occup Med Toxicol 2013;8(1):15.
10. Maestrelli P, Boschetto P, Fabbri LM, et al. Mechanisms of occupational asthma. J Allergy Clin Immunol 2009;123(3):531–42 [quiz: 543–4].
11. Jarvis J, Seed MJ, Elton R, et al. Relationship between chemical structure and the occupational asthma hazard of low molecular weight organic compounds. Occup Environ Med 2005;62(4):243–50.
12. Lummus ZL, Wisnewski AV, Bernstein DI. Pathogenesis and disease mechanisms of occupational asthma. Immunol Allergy Clin North Am 2011;31(4):699–716, vi.
13. Daniels RD. Occupational asthma risk from exposures to toluene diisocyanate: a review and risk assessment. Am J Ind Med 2018;61(4):282–92.
14. Meca O, Cruz MJ, Sanchez-Ortiz M, et al. Do low molecular weight agents cause more severe asthma than high molecular weight agents? PLoS One 2016;11(6): e0156141.
15. Dufour MH, Lemiere C, Prince P, et al. Comparative airway response to high-versus low-molecular weight agents in occupational asthma. Eur Respir J 2009; 33(4):734–9.
16. Chatkin JM, Tarlo SM, Liss G, et al. The outcome of asthma related to workplace irritant exposures. CHEST 1999;116(6):1780–5.
17. Brooks SM, Weiss MA, Bernstein IL. Reactive airways dysfunction syndrome (RADS). Persistent asthma syndrome after high level irritant exposures. Chest 1985;88(3):376–84.
18. Brooks SM, Bernstein IL. Irritant-induced airway disorders. Immunol Allergy Clin North Am 2011;31(4):747–68, vi.
19. Banauch GI, Alleyne D, Sanchez R, et al. Persistent hyperreactivity and reactive airway dysfunction in firefighters at the World Trade Center. Am J Respir Crit Care Med 2003;168(1):54–62.

20. Arif AA, Delclos GL. Association between cleaning-related chemicals and work-related asthma and asthma symptoms among healthcare professionals. Occup Environ Med 2012;69(1):35–40.
21. Holgate ST, Davies DE, Powell RM, et al. Local genetic and environmental factors in asthma disease pathogenesis: chronicity and persistence mechanisms. Eur Respir J 2007;29(4):793–803.
22. Brooks SM, Hammad Y, Richards I, et al. The spectrum of irritant-induced asthma: sudden and not-so-sudden onset and the role of allergy. Chest 1998; 113(1):42–9.
23. Vandenplas O, Suojalehto H, Aasen TB, et al. Specific inhalation challenge in the diagnosis of occupational asthma: consensus statement. Eur Respir J 2014; 43(6):1573–87.
24. Ortega HG, Weissman DN, Carter DL, et al. Use of specific inhalation challenge in the evaluation of workers at risk for occupational asthma: a survey of pulmonary, allergy, and occupational medicine residency training programs in the United States and Canada. Chest 2002;121(4):1323–8.
25. Stenton SC. Occupational and environmental lung disease: occupational asthma. Chron Respir Dis 2010;7(1):35–46.
26. Omland O, Wurtz ET, Aasen TB, et al. Occupational chronic obstructive pulmonary disease: a systematic literature review. Scand J Work Environ Health 2014;40(1):19–35.
27. Wurtz ET, Schlunssen V, Malling TH, et al. Occupational COPD among Danish never-smokers: a population-based study. Occup Environ Med 2015;72(6): 456–9.
28. Santo Tomas LH. Emphysema and chronic obstructive pulmonary disease in coal miners. Curr Opin Pulm Med 2011;17(2):123–5.
29. Peng Y, Li X, Cai S, et al. Prevalence and characteristics of COPD among pneumoconiosis patients at an occupational disease prevention institute: a cross-sectional study. BMC Pulm Med 2018;18(1):22.
30. Ojanguren I, Moullec G, Hobeika J, et al. Clinical and inflammatory characteristics of Asthma-COPD overlap in workers with occupational asthma. PLoS One 2018;13(3):e0193144.
31. Krefft SD, Cool CD, Rose CS. The emerging spectrum of exposure-related bronchiolitis. Curr Opin Allergy Clin Immunol 2018;18(2):87–95.
32. Kreiss K, Gomaa A, Kullman G, et al. Clinical bronchiolitis obliterans in workers at a microwave-popcorn plant. N Engl J Med 2002;347(5):330–8.
33. Petsonk EL, Rose C, Cohen R. Coal mine dust lung disease. New lessons from old exposure. Am J Respir Crit Care Med 2013;187(11):1178–85.
34. Leung CC, Yu IT, Chen W. Silicosis. Lancet 2012;379(9830):2008–18.
35. Satija B, Kumar S, Ojha UC, et al. Spectrum of high-resolution computed tomography imaging in occupational lung disease. Indian J Radiol Imaging 2013;23(4): 287–96.
36. Honma K, Abraham JL, Chiyotani K, et al. Proposed criteria for mixed-dust pneumoconiosis: definition, descriptions, and guidelines for pathologic diagnosis and clinical correlation. Hum Pathol 2004;35(12):1515–23.
37. Arakawa H, Johkoh T, Honma K, et al. Chronic interstitial pneumonia in silicosis and mix-dust pneumoconiosis: its prevalence and comparison of CT findings with idiopathic pulmonary fibrosis. Chest 2007;131(6):1870–6.
38. Cohen RA, Petsonk EL, Rose C, et al. Lung pathology in U.S. coal workers with rapidly progressive pneumoconiosis implicates silica and silicates. Am J Respir Crit Care Med 2016;193(6):673–80.

39. Mossman BT. Assessment of the pathogenic potential of asbestiform vs. nonas-bestiform particulates (cleavage fragments) in in vitro (cell or organ culture) models and bioassays. Regul Toxicol Pharmacol 2008;52(1 Suppl):S200–3.
40. Antonescu-Turcu AL, Schapira RM. Parenchymal and airway diseases caused by asbestos. Curr Opin Pulm Med 2010;16(2):155–61.
41. Peacock C, Copley SJ, Hansell DM. Asbestos-related benign pleural disease. Clin Radiol 2000;55(6):422–32.
42. Addison J, McConnell E. A review of carcinogenicity studies of asbestos and non-asbestos tremolite and other amphiboles. Regul Toxicol Pharmacol 2008; 52(1, Supplement):S187–99.
43. Gamble JF, Gibbs GW. An evaluation of the risks of lung cancer and mesotheli-oma from exposure to amphibole cleavage fragments. Regul Toxicol Pharmacol 2008;52(1 Suppl):S154–86.
44. Perlman D, Mandel JH, Odo N, et al. Pleural abnormalities and exposure to elon-gate mineral particles in Minnesota iron ore (taconite) workers. Am J Ind Med 2018;61(5):391–9.
45. Nemery B. Metal toxicity and the respiratory tract. Eur Respir J 1990;3(2):202–19.
46. Assad N, Sood A, Campen MJ, et al. Metal-induced pulmonary fibrosis. Curr En-viron Health Rep 2018;5(4):486–98.
47. Mizutani RF, Terra-Filho M, Lima E, et al. Hard metal lung disease: a case series. J Bras Pneumol 2016;42(6):447–52 [in English, Portuguese].
48. Choi S, Won YL, Kim D, et al. Interstitial lung disorders in the indium workers of Korea: an update study for the relationship with biological exposure indices. Am J Ind Med 2015;58(1):61–8.
49. Amata A, Chonan T, Omae K, et al. High levels of indium exposure relate to pro-gressive emphysematous changes: a 9-year longitudinal surveillance of indium workers. Thorax 2015;70(11):1040–6.
50. Wyman AE, Hines SE. Update on metal-induced occupational lung disease. Curr Opin Allergy Clin Immunol 2018;18(2):73–9.
51. Taiwo OA. Diffuse parenchymal diseases associated with aluminum use and pri-mary aluminum production. J Occup Environ Med 2014;56(5 Suppl):S71–2.
52. Quirce S, Vandenplas O, Campo P, et al. Occupational hypersensitivity pneumo-nitis: an EAACI position paper. Allergy 2016;71(6):765–79.
53. Seed MJ, Enoch SJ, Agius RM. Chemical determinants of occupational hyper-sensitivity pneumonitis. Occup Med (Lond) 2015;65(8):673–81.
54. Selman M, Pardo A, King TE Jr. Hypersensitivity pneumonitis: insights in diag-nosis and pathobiology. Am J Respir Crit Care Med 2012;186(4):314–24.
55. Balmes JR, Abraham JL, Dweik RA, et al. An official American Thoracic Society statement: diagnosis and management of beryllium sensitivity and chronic beryl-lium disease. Am J Respir Crit Care Med 2014;190(10):e34–59.
56. Mayer AS, Mroz PM, Maier LA. Beryllium and related granulomatous responses. In: Taylor AN, Cullinan P, Blanc P, et al, editors. Parkes' occupational lung disor-ders. 4th edition. Boca Raton (FL): Taylor & Francis Group; 2017. p. 299–316.
57. Hines SE, Pacheco K, Maier LA. The role of lymphocyte proliferation tests in as-sessing occupational sensitization and disease. Curr Opin Allergy Clin Immunol 2012;12(2):102–10.
58. Marant Micallef C, Shield KD, Baldi I, et al. Occupational exposures and cancer: a review of agents and relative risk estimates. Occup Environ Med 2018;75(8): 604–14.
59. Driscoll T, Nelson DI, Steenland K, et al. The global burden of disease due to occupational carcinogens. Am J Ind Med 2005;48(6):419–31.

60. Loomis D, Guha N, Hall AL, et al. Identifying occupational carcinogens: an update from the IARC monographs. Occup Environ Med 2018;75(8):593–603.
61. Ngamwong Y, Tangamornsuksan W, Lohitnavy O, et al. Additive synergism between asbestos and smoking in lung cancer risk: a systematic review and meta-analysis. PLoS One 2015;10(8):e0135798.
62. El Zoghbi M, Salameh P, Stucker I, et al. Absence of multiplicative interactions between occupational lung carcinogens and tobacco smoking: a systematic review involving asbestos, crystalline silica and diesel engine exhaust emissions. BMC Public Health 2017;17(1):156.
63. Roscoe RJ, Steenland K, Halperin WE, et al. Lung cancer mortality among nonsmoking uranium miners exposed to radon daughters. JAMA 1989;262(5): 629–33.
64. Poinen-Rughooputh S, Rughooputh MS, Guo Y, et al. Occupational exposure to silica dust and risk of lung cancer: an updated meta-analysis of epidemiological studies. BMC Public Health 2016;16(1):1137.
65. Hubaux R, Becker-Santos DD, Enfield KS, et al. Arsenic, asbestos and radon: emerging players in lung tumorigenesis. Environ Health 2012;11:89.
66. Enterline PE, Day R, Marsh GM. Cancers related to exposure to arsenic at a copper smelter. Occup Environ Med 1995;52(1):28–32.
67. Spyratos D, Zarogoulidis P, Porpodis K, et al. Occupational exposure and lung cancer. J Thorac Dis 2013;5(Suppl 4):S440–5.
68. Guha N, Merletti F, Steenland NK, et al. Lung cancer risk in painters: a meta-analysis. Cien Saude Colet 2011;16(8):3613–32.
69. Ramanakumar AV, Parent ME, Richardson L, et al. Exposures in painting-related occupations and risk of lung cancer among men: results from two case-control studies in Montreal. Occup Environ Med 2011;68(1):44–51.
70. Boniol M, Koechlin A, Boyle P. Meta-analysis of occupational exposures in the rubber manufacturing industry and risk of cancer. Int J Epidemiol 2017;46(6): 1940–7.
71. Robinson BW, Lake RA. Advances in malignant mesothelioma. N Engl J Med 2005;353(15):1591–603.
72. Spirtas R, Heineman EF, Bernstein L, et al. Malignant mesothelioma: attributable risk of asbestos exposure. Occup Environ Med 1994;51(12):804–11.
73. Attanoos RL, Churg A, Galateau-Salle F, et al. Malignant mesothelioma and its non-asbestos causes. Arch Pathol Lab Med 2018;142(6):753–60.
74. Bianco A, Valente T, De Rimini ML, et al. Clinical diagnosis of malignant pleural mesothelioma. J Thorac Dis 2018;10(Suppl 2). S253–s261.

Pulmonary Embolism

Eno-Obong Essien, MD[a], Parth Rali, MD[b],*,
Stephen C. Mathai, MD, MHS[c]

KEYWORDS

- Pulmonary embolism (PE) • Pulmonary embolism response team
- Deep vein thrombosis (DVT) • Venous thromboembolism (VTE)

KEY POINTS

- Diagnostic work up of pulmonary embolism (PE) should be based on well-described clinical prediction scores (Wells score, Geneva score, and so forth). Every patient with a high likelihood of having PE should be started on prompt anticoagulation if there is no absolute contraindication for it.
- Newer oral anticoagulants are the preferred agent of choice over vitamin K antagonists, except in cancer patients and patients with antiphospholipid antibody syndrome.
- Patients with submassive or massive PE should ideally be managed in a multidisciplinary setting and care of such patients should be individualized.

INTRODUCTION

Venous thromboembolism (VTE) includes pulmonary embolism (PE) and deep vein thrombosis (DVT). PE is third most common cause of cardiovascular death worldwide after stroke and heart attack. Management of PE has evolved recently with availability of local thrombolysis; mechanical extraction devices; hemodynamic support devices like extracorporeal membrane oxygenation; and surgical embolectomy. There has been development of multidisciplinary PE response teams (PERTs) nationwide to optimize the care of patients with VTE. This review describes the epidemiology of PE, discusses diagnostic strategies and current and emerging treatments for VTE, and considers post-PE follow-up care.

Disclosure Statement: None of the listed authors have any commercial or financial conflicts of interest and any funding sources pertaining to topic in discussion.
[a] Division of Internal Medicine Residency Program, Temple University Hospital, 3401 North Broad Street, Philadelphia, PA 19140, USA; [b] Division of Thoracic Surgery and Medicine, Pulmonary Embolism Response Team (PERT), Temple University Hospital, 3401 North Broad Street, Philadelphia, PA 19140, USA; [c] John Hopkins Hospital, 830 East Monument Street, 1830 Building 5th Floor Pulmonary, Baltimore, MD 21287, USA
* Corresponding author.
E-mail address: parth.rali@tuhs.temple.edu

Epidemiology

The exact prevalence of VTE is unknown due to absence of surveillance methods.[1] Most PEs originate from DVTs of lower extremities, and approximately 50% of DVTs may lead to silent PE.[2] In the United States, the incidence is 300,000 to 600,000 annually, similar to the incidence in parts of Europe.[3] Necroscopic review shows PE accounts for death in approximately 5% to 10% of hospitalized patients.[4] When untreated, VTE can have a mortality up to 25% but decreases to 1% to 5% with treatment.[5] Despite treatment of VTE, the short-term mortality at 3 months ranges from 15% to 30%.[6,7] This high mortality, however, is often attributed to patient comorbidities, such as underlying malignancy, heart failure, chronic obstructive pulmonary disease (COPD), and older age.[7] VTE incidence also varies with gender and race. A recent Canadian study showed VTE may be more prevalent in men than in women and that recurrence rate may also be higher in men.[8] Black men also have a higher likelihood of developing VTE than white men.[9]

VTE also has a significant economic burden, with $2 billion to $10 billion spent annually.[10] Patients with VTE often also have advanced cardiopulmonary disease or malignancy that also may contribute to excessive health care resource utilizations. Costs are not just related to initial hospital encounters, because the rate of VTE occurrence remains high in the immediate post–hospital discharge period.[11] As such, there has been a focus not only on inpatient but also on postdischarge VTE prophylaxis.[12]

Pulmonary Embolism Definition and Pathophysiology

Anything that obstructs the pulmonary arteries (clot, tumor, fat, or air) can be considered PE. Most commonly in clinical practice, PE refers to a blood clot that lodges into pulmonary circulation. The pathophysiology of VTE was described by Virchow in the nineteenth century and still holds true. Stasis, endothelial disruption, and hypercoagulability are the foundations of understanding the pathophysiology of VTE.[13]

PE induces several pathophysiologic derangements that can lead to significant hemodynamic compromise, particularly if the clot burden is high. The most important determinant of outcomes in PE is the impact on and response of the right ventricle (RV) to the PE. The RV is a thin-walled structure that, in the normal state, pumps against a low-pressure and low-resistance pulmonary circulation. Pulmonary vascular resistance is regulated by several factors, including oxygen-sensing mechanisms. Thus, in the setting of a PE and obstruction of the vasculature, RV afterload can be acutely increased not only by the mechanical obstruction but also by hypoxic vasoconstriction.[14–16] Additionally, inflammatory mediators, such as thromboxane A2 and histamine, released in response to clot further increase vasoconstriction.[17] The ability of the RV to adapt to acute increases in pulmonary vascular resistance is limited, particularly compared with the left ventricle (LV).[18] RV failure ensues not only as a result of increased pulmonary vascular resistance but also as a consequence of decreased contractility from RV myocardial ischemia and increased RV preload. These processes lead to RV dilation that cause bowing of the interventricular septum into the LV, decreased LV filling, and obstructive shock.[19]

Genetic/Primary Risk Factors

There have been well-described genetic mutations that increase the risk of VTE. These include factor V Leiden, activated protein C resistance, prothrombin (factor

II) G20210A mutation, protein S deficiency, and antithrombin deficiency. Factor V and protein C are the most common, occurring in approximately 5% of the population; prothrombin gene mutation occurs in approximately 2% of the population.[20] In patients diagnosed with VTE, one of these mutations can be found in up to 20% to 52%.[21,22] These mutations encode for factors involved in the coagulation cascade. Inability to produce these factors results in a hypercoagulable state predisposing to clot formation. These mutations occur more commonly in white populations but overall incidence of VTE remains higher in blacks.[23] Genetic mutation increases the risk of first VTE occurrence but not necessarily subsequent episodes. Thus, hypercoagulable work-up is not recommended in every patient with VTE.[24–26] On the other hand, identifying a genetic mutation may help identify relatives who are at increased VTE risk. Screening for the antiphospholipid antibody syndrome (APS) may be indicated in appropriate patients, such as young female patients with history of arterial and venous thrombosis and/or recurrent miscarriages.[27,28]

Acquired/Secondary Risk Factors

Major acquired or secondary risk factors include postoperative states, pregnancy, malignancy, and age.[22] In keeping with the Virchow triad, these states often result from stasis and endothelial injury, creating a thrombophilic state. Comorbid conditions play a significant role in determining patient-related outcomes in VTE and should be addressed when deciding type of treatment of VTE. Approximately 85% of patients who develop VTE have chronic comorbid conditions. Specific comorbidities may be more commonly associated with PE. For example, PE should be in the differential for repeated COPD exacerbations. In a recent meta-analysis, 16.1% of unexplained acute COPD exacerbations were due to PE and may contribute to higher mortality in this population.[29] In comparison, patients without comorbid conditions have less than 2% mortality at 12 months.[30] **Table 1** summarizes acquired and hereditary risk factors for development of VTE.

Table 1 Risk factors for venous thromboembolism	
Hereditary/genetic	Family history
	Factor V Leiden
	Prothrombin G20210A
	Protein C deficiency
	Antithrombin deficiency
	Sickle cell trait
	Protein S deficiency
Acquired	Pregnancy
	Oral contraceptives pills or hormonal therapy
	Hospitalization
	Surgery
	Trauma
	Immobilization
	Antiphospholipid antibodies
	Active malignancy
	Chronic cardiopulmonary disease
	Long travel (>4–6 h)
	History of previous VTE
	Advanced age

CLASSIFICATION OF PULMONARY EMBOLISM

PE can be classified based on clot location or hemodynamic compromise. Saddle PE refers to a clot located in the main PA or bifurcation. Saddle PE does not necessarily translate into a massive PE (defined later). Mortality rate related to saddle PE is close to 5%.[31] Likewise, lobar, segmental, and subsegmental PE describe clot location in the pulmonary arterial branches corresponding to the anatomic lung lobe, segment, or subsegment respectively. Terms, such as nonmassive PE and major PE, are being phased out and their use in scientific literature is no longer encouraged. Appropriate classification of PE has implications in the management, such as selecting reperfusion strategies or anticoagulation only.[19]

The following definitions are obtained from American Heart Association (AHA) and American College of Chest Physicians (ACCP) guidelines[19]:

- Massive PE is defined as persistent hypotension of systolic blood pressure (SBP) less than 90 mm Hg lasting more than 15 minutes or requiring inotropic support, pulselessness, or bradycardia less than 40 beats per minutes.
- Submassive PE is a PE without systemic hypotension (SBP >90 mm Hg) but with RV dysfunction. RV dysfunction is based on either imaging (CT pulmonary angiogram [CTPA] or transthoracic echocardiogram) or elevated biomarkers (brain natriuretic peptide [BNP], N-terminal pro-BPN [NT-proBNP], or elevated troponin).
- Low-risk PE is an acute PE without hemodynamic instability and without RV dysfunction.

DIAGNOSIS AND EVALUATION

Diagnosis of PE can be challenging because symptoms are nonspecific. Nonetheless, the classic presenting symptoms are pleuritic chest pain (39%) and dyspnea at rest (50%).[29] Hemoptysis also is a common presenting complaint due to pulmonary infarction. Hemoptysis can be seen in up to 20% of patients with PE. Hemoptysis in setting of PE is not an absolute indication to stop anticoagulation. Syncope can be an initial presentation of hemodynamically significant PE. It is also important to elicit history for the aforementioned risk factors in **Table 1** because this assists in determination of the pretest probability of PE.

The physical examination, in particular, the cardiovascular examination, is of utmost importance. Patients with a PE may have tachycardia and/or hypoxia with a new or increasing oxygen requirement from baseline. Low-grade fever and white blood cell count also have been reported but are less common. Elevated jugular venous pressure with a hepatojugular reflex, RV heave, or a loud P2 may be noted if there is significant right heart failure. Lung sounds are often unremarkable; however, the patient may appear to be in respiratory distress. Homans sign has been reported in the past but is now widely accepted as having limited sensitivity and specificity for diagnosing DVT.[32]

Risk Prediction Tools

Risk prediction tools have been developed to help clinicians both identify patients with VTE and stratify the risk of short-term morbidity and mortality in patients with VTE. The most common tools for prediction of VTE include Wells score, revised Geneva score, and Pulmonary Embolism Rule-out Criterion (PERC) score. Each aims to provide an objective method for estimating pretest probability of having PE into low, intermediate, and high categories. These tools help encourage the practice of evidence-based medicine, rather than ordering unnecessary studies, such as a CTPA. Of these scores, Wells is one of the most extensively studied and well validated and thus used more frequently. Prevalence of PE was only 1.3% in low-risk category based on Wells score.[25]

Prediction of short-term morbidity and mortality is also an important clinical concern. The PE severity index (PESI) and simplified PESI (sPESI) are most commonly use to predict short-term morbidity and mortality with PE. These scores were derived from 11 patient factors associated with a 30-day mortality (**Table 2**). Based on these scores, patients are risk stratified and management strategies are tailored to the risks of adverse outcomes. These tools have been extensively validated[33,34] and found to have a high sensitivity and negative predictive value of 95% to 99% for predicting short-term outcomes.[35] **Table 2** highlights the PESI and sPESI scores. Multiple studies have demonstrated that patients with low PESI scores (group I) had mortality less than 1% compared with high PESI group (group V) with 24% 30-day mortality.[33–35]

LABORATORY TESTING
D-Dimer

D-dimer is a fibrin degradation product. It is used as a surrogate marker of fibrinolysis and is expected to be elevated during a thrombotic event. Measured using ELISA, a normal level is less than 500 ng/mL in most laboratories. D-dimer can be elevated in various conditions, such as pregnancy, postoperative state, and malignancy, which lowers its specificity. It is also known to have levels that increase with age and thus the levels are adjusted for this parameter.[36] In combination with a low pretest probability for PE, a normal D-dimer has been shown to rule out PE due to its high sensitivity (80%–100%) and negative predictive value up to 100%.[19] Age adjusted D-dimer

Table 2
Original and simplified pulmonary embolism severity indexes

Parameter	Original Pulmonary Embolism Severity Index Points	Simplified Pulmonary Embolism Severity Index Points
Age	Age in years	1 point (if aged >80 y)
Male gender	+10 points	N/A
History of cancer	+30 points	1 point
History of chronic lung disease[a]	+10 points	1 point
History of heart failure[a]	+10 points	
HR >110 beats/min	+20 points	1 point
SBP <100 mm Hg	+30 points	1 point
Respiratory rate >30 breaths/min	+20 points	N/A
Temperature <36°C	+20 points	N/A
Altered mental status	+60 points	N/A
Oxygen saturation <90%	+20 points	1 point

Abbreviations: HR, heart rate; N/A, not applicable.

[a] In sPESI scoring, 1 point is given for history of chronic cardiopulmonary disease (history of chronic lung disease, or history of heart failure, or history of both).

From Rali PM, Criner GJ. Submassive pulmonary embolism. Am J Respir Crit Care Med 2018;198(5):590; with permission.

(patient age [in years over 50]) × 10 µg/L (fibrinogen equivalent units) can further reduce false-positive results, particularly in older patients.[37]

Cardiac Troponin

Elevated cardiac troponins suggest myocardial injury. During PE, the myocardium can become ischemic and thus release troponins. In combination with the BNP, the troponin has found a useful marker of RV dysfunction. Some studies have shown elevated cardiac troponin associated with increased short-term mortality risk of 1% to 10%.[38] Using cardiac markers in combination with other imaging and clinical assessment tools can be useful in risk stratification. Using them in isolation, however, is not ideal because there may be other etiologies for elevated cardiac troponin.[38,39]

Brain Natriuretic Peptide

BNP is released by ventricular myocytes when they are stretched, which typically occurs in volume overload. Both products of cleaved proBNP, BNP (active portion) and NT-proBNP (inactive portion), can be used to measure ventricular stretch. Like cardiac troponin, BNP can represent RV strain and also aid in stratification of PE. NT-proBNP has been found to have a sensitivity and negative predictive value of nearly 100% for detecting RV dysfunction whereas troponin has a sensitivity of 73%.[40] BNP alone cannot be used to diagnose PE but, used in conjunction with RV/LV measurements on CTPA imaging, it has been found to increase diagnostic accuracy.[40]

IMAGING
Venous Ultrasound Duplexes

Ultrasound of the lower extremity is useful when evaluating a patient for PE. It is relatively quick and does not require radiation. The goal is to find noncompressible veins, suggesting vessel occlusion. Ultrasonography is not used alone, however; rather, it supplements the diagnosis of PE by identifying a source. A negative venous ultrasound does not rule out the possibility of PE.

Echocardiography

Transthoracic echocardiography is commonly used in evaluating a patient with suspected PE. Echocardiography does not diagnose PE; rather, it aids risk stratification, which in turn has an impact on urgent management decisions. McConnell sign (decreased RV free wall function with apical sparing) is specific for PE.[41] Tricuspid annular plane systolic excursion less than 18 mm, lack of inferior vena cava (IVC) collapsibility, and elevated RV systolic pressure have been associated with increased mortality.[42] RV free wall thickness may help differentiate acute or chronic RV failure. Data suggest that RV hypokinesis on echocardiography correlates closely with RV diameter/LV diameter dilatation seen on CTPA imaging, with a negative predictive value of approximately 94%.[43]

CT Pulmonary Angiography

CTPA has largely replaced the tradition gold standard, pulmonary angiography. It is less invasive and quick and readily available in most institutions. Even when it is negative, it can be helpful in identifying other etiologies responsible for hypoxic respiratory failure, such as interstitial lung disease, pneumonia, or effusion. It is not without its risks, however, which include contrast-induced nephropathy, particularly in patients with chronic renal insufficiency, such as the elderly; anaphylaxis; and exposure to radiation. The Prospective Investigation of Pulmonary Embolism Diagnosis study showed sensitivity of CTPA of sensitivity of approximately 80% with a specificity of

95%.[44] The sensitivity of CTPA can be impacted by appropriate timing of contrast injection, motion artifact, and reader accuracy. When CTPA was compared with conventional pulmonary angiography in a meta-analysis, the rate of VTE diagnosis after a negative CTPA was no different from that of conventional pulmonary angiography.[45] Thus, CTPA has adequately replaced the need for conventional pulmonary angiography. CTPA not only is useful in diagnosing PE but also provides additional data for prognostication and risk stratification. CTPA-based prognostication, including septum position, RV/LV ratio, and IVC reflux contrast, correlates with echocardiographic findings of RV strain. CTPA gives first insight into RV dysfunction due to acute PE; echocardiography, in particular point-of-care echocardiography, can be used in real time to assess the treatment responses. Both imaging modalities are complementary in risk stratification and managing patients with PE.

Ventilation-Perfusion Scintigraphy

Commonly known as a ventilation-perfusion (V/Q) scan, V/Q scintigraphy also can be used to evaluate acute PE with a high sensitivity and high specificity. Its use is typically reserved for patients with contraindication to CTPA. Sometimes indeterminate results leave treating physicians in a dilemma as to whether or not to treat patients for acute PE. V/Q scan remains, however, the imaging modality of choice for diagnosing chronic thromboembolism in the evaluation of chronic thromboembolic pulmonary hypertension (CTEPH).[46] V/Q scan is more sensitive in diagnosing chronic PE than CTA (97.4% vs 51%).[47] Other benefits of V/Q scan are less radiation exposure and avoidance of contrast injections. Findings of chronic PE on CTA are subtle and need expertise, making V/Q scan the imaging of choice for evaluating patients with CTEPH. A normal or low-probability V/Q scan can effectively rule out CTEPH whereas a high-probability and indeterminate scan requires further diagnostic work-up.[48]

MANAGEMENT OF PULMONARY EMBOLISM

All patients with high pretest probability or confirmed PE should be initiated on anticoagulation. Empiric early anticoagulation has been associated with decreased mortality for patients with acute PE.[49,50] Mainstay therapy for patients being admitted is unfractionated heparin that is administered as an 80 U/kg bolus followed by an infusion at 18 U/kg/h bolus or a weight-based dosing for low-molecular-weight heparin (LMWH), such as enoxaparin. Studies have shown there is no difference between using either of these, but LMWH is favored due to ease of monitoring.[51] In a patient who may require interventions beyond anticoagulation and in patients with poor renal function (creatine clearance <30 mL/min), however, unfractionated heparin is preferred. When initiating anticoagulation, the risks and benefits should be weighed, particularly in those with high bleeding risk, such as unexplained anemia, recent hemorrhagic stroke, advanced age, liver disease, and severe thrombocytopenia.

Other supportive therapies may be provided. Supplemental oxygen is recommended when patients are hypoxic. If a patient is borderline hypotensive, caution must be exercised with fluid resuscitation because excessive preload can worsen RV dysfunction. If a patent is hypotensive, vasopressors or inotropic support can be initiated promptly along with reperfusion therapies. Other RV support therapies, such as inhaled nitric oxide, should be considered with expert consultation. Massive PE and submassive PE patients with comorbidities should be managed in ICU setting. **Box 1** provides a list of conditions where expert pulmonary consultation should be obtained in comanaging patients with PE.

Box 1
Triggers for pulmonary consultation

CTPA evidence of right heart strain

Unable to perform CTA but PE is highly likely

PE with
  Complex medical problems (ie, CHF, COPD, and malignancy)
  Contraindication to systemic lysis/anticoagulation
  DVT
  Echo evidence of right heart strain
  Positive troponin/BNP
  Risk of bleeding with A/C
  Risk of decompensation
  Recent surgery
  Shock
  Thrombocytopenia

Recurrent PE

Acute or chronic PE

Abbreviations: CHF, congestive heart failure; A/C, anticoagulation.

Managing patients with acute PE requires physicians from varied specialties. It also needs coordination of care in time sensitive manner. This has led to the concept of development of institutionally based multidisciplinary PERT.[52] A PERT team explores all possible treatment options, weighs in against bleeding risk, and offers comprehensive care of patients with acute PE in real time. As a multidisciplinary model, PERT can make team-based decisions rather than individualized decisions that can take longer, delaying appropriate care. Members of the PERT team also can follow patients in outpatient setting once discharged, which may reduce short-term and long-term complications.[11,52]

Low-Risk Pulmonary Embolism

Choice of treatment of low-risk PE patients is anticoagulation only. Patients with low-risk PE should be considered for early discharge and may not need admission. Decision to admit or not should also rely on how immediately patient would have access to newer oral anticoagulants or LMWH once discharged. Novel oral anticoagulants (NOACs) are the preferred agent of choice over vitamin K antagonists (VKAs) in general.[53,54] In patients with extremes of weight or with the APS syndrome, VKA remains the agent of choice. Rivaroxaban and apixaban do not require bridging whereas edoxaban and dabigatran need bridging with unfractionated heparin or LMWH. In cancer-associated VTE, LMWH remains the agent of choice, even though there has been a growing role of NOACs in cancer-associated VTE. Edoxaban is currently approved for treating cancer-related VTE and has been established to be noninferior to LMWH.[55] In patients with small segmental PE without DVT and no risk factors for recurrence, a decision may be to hold anticoagulation based on recent ACCP 2016 VTE guidelines.[54]

The first provoked VTE should be treated for 3 months with anticoagulation. The first unprovoked PE should be treated for at least 3 months if there is high risk of bleeding. If a patient is deemed a low risk for bleeding, the duration should extend beyond 3 months. Longer duration of therapy should be considered in certain patients after 3 months of anticoagulation based on several studies demonstrating increased risk of subsequent VTE in men[56] and in patients with elevated D-dimer levels after 3 months of anticoagulation.[57–59] For a second VTE episode (provoked or unprovoked), long-term anticoagulation should be considered after weighing in risk of bleeding on an ongoing basis. Bleeding risk should be evaluated annually to guide dose, duration, and type of anticoagulation. The availability of andexanet alfa (Andexxa, South San Francisco, California), a reversal agents for factor Xa inhibitors (rivaroxaban, apixaban, and edoxaban), and of idarucizumab (Praxbind, Praxbind Burlington, Ontario, Canada), a reversal agent for dabigatran, has added to safety profile for NOACs, thus making them preferred options.

Submassive and Massive Pulmonary Embolism

For patients who present with cardiac arrest or hemodynamic instability, it is widely accepted that reperfusion strategies should be initiated. Tissue plasminogen activator (tPA) cleaves plasminogen to plasmin. Plasmin itself plays a role in causing thrombolysis. Currently approved thrombolytics for PE include alteplase (tPA), urokinase, and streptokinase. Systemic thrombolysis, however, is not without risk; the International Cooperative Pulmonary Embolism Registry shows a 20% risk of major bleeding events and a 3% risk of intracranial hemorrhage after receiving thrombolytics.[7] The Food and Drug Administration–approved dose of systemic tPA is 100 mg over 2 hours over peripheral infusion. **Box 2** lists universally accepted absolute and relative contraindications for systemic thrombolysis.

After determining a patient has a submassive PE based on echocardiographic findings, RV/LV changes on CTPA, and biomarkers, in addition to initiating anticoagulation (discussed previously), further risk stratification for an adverse outcome should be assessed using PESI or sPESI scores. According to European Society of Cardiology (ESC) guidelines, patients can be categorized into low-intermediate risk and high-intermediate risk based on clinical data.[60] Low-intermediate risk is when RV strain is established either by imaging or by the presence of biomarkers. High-intermediate risk is when both RV stain and elevated biomarkers are present. One of the main advantages of using ESC classification compared with AHA/ACCP is ability provide conservative approach in low-risk intermediate PE and aggressive approach in high-risk intermediate PE.[19,54,60] The decision to pursue reperfusion strategies, which include half-dose systemic thrombolysis and catheter-directed thrombolysis, currently remains controversial in these patients. A multicenter randomized controlled trial assessed 1005 patients with submassive PE treated with

---

Box 2
Contraindication of systemic thrombolysis

Absolute contraindications to thrombolysis
　History of prior intracranial hemorrhage
　Structural intracranial cerebrovascular disease (arteriovenous malformation)
　Intracranial malignancy
　Active bleeding or bleeding diathesis
　Recent surgery in spinal canal or brain
　Ischemic stroke within 3 mo
　Recent Closed head injury or facial trauma with radiographic evidence of brain injury

Relative contraindications
　Age >75 y
　Puncture of a noncompressible vessel
　Traumatic or prolonged cardiopulmonary resuscitation (>10 min)
　Internal bleeding (within 2–4 wk)
　History of chronic poorly controlled hypertension or severe uncontrolled hypertension on presentation
　History of ischemic stroke >3 mo

unfractionated heparin who were randomized to tenecteplase versus placebo. The trial showed a decrease in the primary outcome of all-cause mortality or hemodynamic decompensation in the tenecteplase arm. The observed difference between arms, however, was attributed solely to improvement in hemodynamics because there was no survival benefit.[61] The incidence of extracranial bleeding was 6.3% in the tPA group compared with 1.7% in the placebo group; similarly, the risk of stroke at 7 days was increased in the tPA group versus the placebo group (2.4% vs 0.2%). Furthermore, a long-term 3-year follow-up study did not show a difference in mortality or incidence of CTEPH between arms.[62] There is enough evidence to recommend against full-dose systemic thrombolysis in every patient with submassive PE.[63] Nevertheless, current ACCP guidelines suggest consideration of systemic thrombolytics in patients with clinical decline and low bleeding risk.[54]

ACCP 2016 VTE guidelines recommend considering bleeding risk in patients with acute PE. Bleeding risk helps in determining type of treatment offered. Patients who are deemed a high bleeding risk should be considered for a more conservative approach. Total duration of anticoagulation and type of anticoagulation should be individualized based on bleeding risk profile of a patient. Bleeding risk assessment should be done annually, particularly in the elderly population, to determine the need for ongoing anticoagulation.[54]

Due to the risks of major bleeding with systemic thrombolysis, catheter-based techniques are quickly gaining popularity. Catheter-directed thrombolytic therapies (CDTs) are indicated if urgent revascularization is warranted. Ideally, they should be ideally in an experienced center.[64] There are 2 categories of catheter interventions: Conventional catheter-directed thrombolysis, which involves local application of thrombolytics via catheters placed in pulmonary artery, and catheter thrombectomy, which involves mechanical clot removal. Pharmacomechanical ultrasound-facilitated CDT involves placing a catheter directly in the thrombus, with administration of a thrombolytic and the use of ultrasound to enhance clot fragmentation. An advantage of CDT that the dose of the tPA administered is much lower and the duration of the tPA infusion is much longer. Thus, this combination of modalities may lead to fewer bleeding complications.[65] CDT procedures are performed in interventional radiology or cardiac catheterization laboratory. Patient should be clinically stable for the transport when such modalities are considered. Ideal patient selection along with dose and duration for CDT remains controversial and should be decided based on local expertise and multidisciplinary settings.[11]

A meta-analysis showed a pooled success rate of approximately 86% with CDT; however, there are few randomized controlled trials comparing CDT to systemic thrombolysis.[66]

Surgical embolectomy should be considered in massive PE patients and selected subgroup of submassive PE patients who are not candidates for systemic thrombolysis. Patients who are considered for surgery, however, also need to be able to tolerate systemic anticoagulation. Cumulative surgical mortality rates for patients with massive PE have dropped significantly from 1968 to 2008 (35% vs 19%).[67] Age greater than 80 years is associated with significant operative mortality compared with age range 60 years to 80 years in hemodynamically stable patients undergoing surgical embolectomy. The case fatality rate of unstable patients undergoing surgical embolectomy, however, is approximately 40% compared with 24% in hemodynamically stable patients.[67,68]

Role of Inferior Vena Cava Filters

Routine use of IVC filter in patients with PE who can tolerate anticoagulation is not recommended irrespective of whether they have concomitant DVT or not. IVC filters should only be considered when there is absolute contraindication to anticoagulation.[54] The Prevention du Risque d'Embolie Pulmonaire par Interruption Cave (PREPIC) and PREPIC2 trials showed no benefit of IVC filters in patients with acute PE or DVT to prevent future recurrent VTE events. The IVC filter itself can be thrombogenic if not removed. The current ACCP recommendation is to use retrievable filter rather than permanent filters. Every attempt should be made to remove IVC filter when no longer indicated.[69,70]

POST–PULMOMARY EMBOLISM DISCHARGE

Every patient with VTE should have close outpatient follow-up.[71] An attempt should be made to determine the etiology of PE, which sometimes can be difficult in the inpatient setting. Hypercoagulable work-up should be considered on individualized basis and after discussing with patients. Age-appropriate cancer screening should be performed. Modifiable risk factors for VTE like smoking cessation and weight reduction can be addressed on outpatient follow-up visits.[72] It is also of paramount importance to determine if patients are adherent to prescribed regimen and are achieving therapeutic levels of anticoagulation. Interactions of anticoagulants with other coadministered medications and appropriate dose adjustments in overweight patients and in those with renal impairment should be made. The duration of anticoagulation and bleeding risk should be assessed annually, and regimens should be individualized accordingly. Ultimately, patients with abnormal echocardiograms who remain symptomatic after 3 months of uninterrupted anticoagulation should be screened for CTEPH. A follow-up echocardiogram and V/Q scan should be obtained in such patients. If abnormal, patients should be referred to an expert CTEPH center for further evaluation. CTEPH occurs in approximately 3.2% of patients after acute PE, but it is believed underdiagnosed.[73] It is also important to screen patients for CTEPH, because it is the only potentially curable form of pulmonary hypertension (group IV).[11,67,73]

SUMMARY

The authors conclude this review with the following salient points for readers:

1. The authors recommend using predictive score (Wells, Geneva, or PERC) for VTE before ordering CTPA.
2. CTPA remains the gold standard for diagnosis of PE.
3. High pretest probabilities for PE and low bleeding risk should prompt empiric anticoagulation while waiting for confirmative testing.
4. Treatment decisions for PE should be based on hemodynamic impact, not merely a clot location and risk stratification.
5. Echocardiography, troponin, BNP/proBNP, and PESI score should be used to risk-stratify patients with PE. Low-risk PE patients should be considered for early discharge.
6. NOACs are preferred agent of choice over VKA, except in morbidly obese patients, patients with renal failure, or patients with APS syndrome.
7. In cancer-associated VTE, LMWH is still the preferred agent of choice. The role of NOACs is still evolving.
8. Hypercoagulable work-up is not mandated in every patient with PE and should be undertaken on an individual basis.
9. Catheter-directed thrombolysis seems safe and effective compared with systemic thrombolysis, but candidacy of such therapy over simple anticoagulation ideally should be assessed in a multidisciplinary setting.

10. Routine use of IVC filter is not recommended in patients with PE.
11. Abnormal echocardiogram and persistent symptoms after 3 months of uninter-rupted anticoagulation after an acute PE should prompt screening and referral to a CTEPH center for further evaluation.

REFERENCES

1. Beckman MG, Hooper WC, Critchley SE, et al. Venous thromboembolism. A public health concern. Am J Prev Med 2010. https://doi.org/10.1016/j.amepre.2009.12.017.
2. Meignan M, Rosso J, Gauthier H, et al. Systematic lung scans reveal a high frequency of silent pulmonary embolism in patients with proximal deep venous thrombosis. Arch Intern Med 2000. https://doi.org/10.1001/archinte.160.2.159.
3. Cohen AT, Agnelli G, Anderson FA, et al. Venous thromboembolism (VTE) in Europe - The number of VTE events and associated morbidity and mortality. Thromb Haemost 2007. https://doi.org/10.1160/TH07-03-0212.
4. Alikhan R, Peters F, Wilmott R, et al. Fatal pulmonary embolism in hospitalised patients: a necropsy review. J Clin Pathol 2004;57(12):1254–7.
5. Barritt DW, Jordan SC. Anticoagulant drugs in the treatment of pulmonary embolism. A controlled trial. Lancet 1960;275(7138):1309–12.
6. Heit JA, Silverstein MD, Mohr DN, et al. Predictors of survival after deep vein thrombosis and pulmonary embolism: a population-based, cohort study. Arch Intern Med 1999;159(5):445–53.
7. Goldhaber SZ, Visani L, De Rosa M. Acute pulmonary embolism: clinical outcomes in the International Cooperative Pulmonary Embolism Registry (ICOPER) [see comment]. Lancet 1999;353(9162):1386–9.
8. Heit JA, Crusan DJ, Ashrani AA, et al. Effect of a near-universal hospitalization-based prophylaxis regimen on annual number of venous thromboembolism events in the US. Blood 2017. https://doi.org/10.1182/blood-2016-12-758995.
9. Deitelzweig SB, Lin J, Johnson BH, et al. Venous thromboembolism in the US: does race matter? J Thromb Thrombolysis 2011. https://doi.org/10.1007/s11239-010-0503-3.
10. Park B, Messina L, Dargon P, et al. Recent trends in clinical outcomes and resource utilization for pulmonary embolism in the United States findings from the nationwide inpatient sample. Chest 2009. https://doi.org/10.1378/chest.08-2258.
11. Rali PM, Criner GJ. Submassive pulmonary embolism. Am J Respir Crit Care Med 2018. https://doi.org/10.1164/rccm.201711-2302CI.
12. Cohen AT, Harrington RA, Goldhaber SZ, et al. Extended thromboprophylaxis with betrixaban in acutely ill medical patients. N Engl J Med 2016. https://doi.org/10.1056/NEJMoa1601747.
13. Bagot CN, Arya R. Virchow and his triad: a question of attribution. Br J Haematol 2008;143(2):180–90.
14. Burrowes KS, Clark AR, Wilsher ML, et al. Hypoxic pulmonary vasoconstriction as a contributor to response in acute pulmonary embolism. Ann Biomed Eng 2014. https://doi.org/10.1007/s10439-014-1011-y.
15. Mizera R. Pathophysiology of development of pulmonary hypertension after acute pulmonary embolism. Cesk Fysiol 2012;61(1):4–8 [in Czech].
16. Delcroix M, Melot C, Vermeulen F, et al. Hypoxic pulmonary vasoconstriction and gas exchange in acute canine pulmonary embolism. J Appl Physiol 1996;80(4):1240–8.

17. Elliott CG. Pulmonary physiology during pulmonary embolism. Chest 1992; 101(4):163S–71S.
18. Wiedemann HP, Matthay RA. Heart disease : a textbook of cardiovascular medicine. In: Braunwald E, editor. Heart disease: a textbook of cardiovascular medicine. 5th edition. Philadelphia : Saunders; 1997. p. 1604–25.
19. Jaff MR, McMurtry MS, Archer SL, et al. Management of massive and submassive pulmonary embolism, iliofemoral deep vein thrombosis, and chronic thromboembolic pulmonary hypertension: a scientific statement from the american heart association. Circulation 2011. https://doi.org/10.1161/CIR.0b013e318214914f.
20. Blom JW, Doggen CJM, Osanto S, et al. Malignancies, prothrombotic mutations, and the risk of venous thrombosis. J Am Med Assoc 2005. https://doi.org/10.1001/jama.293.6.715.
21. Seligsohn U, Lubetsky A. Genetic susceptibility to venous thrombosis. N Engl J Med 2001. https://doi.org/10.1056/NEJM200104193441607.
22. Goldhaber SZ. Risk factors for venous thromboembolism. J Am Coll Cardiol 2010; 56(1):1–7.
23. Buckner TW, Key NS. Venous thrombosis in blacks. Circulation 2012;125(6): 837–9.
24. Murin S, Marelich GP, Arroliga AC, et al. Hereditary thrombophilia and venous thromboembolism. Am J Respir Crit Care Med 1998;158(5):1369–73.
25. Coppens M, Reijnders JH, Middeldorp S, et al. Testing for inherited thrombophilia does not reduce the recurrence of venous thrombosis. J Thromb Haemost 2008; 6(9):1474–7.
26. Middeldorp S, Van Hylckama Vlieg A. Does thrombophilia testing help in the clinical management of patients? Br J Haematol 2008;143(3):321–35.
27. Connors JM. Thrombophilia testing and venous thrombosis. N Engl J Med 2017. https://doi.org/10.1056/NEJMra1700365.
28. Carroll BJ, Piazza G. Hypercoagulable states in arterial and venous thrombosis: When, how, and who to test? Vasc Med 2018;23(4):388–99.
29. Pollack CV, Schreiber D, Goldhaber SZ, et al. Clinical characteristics, management, and outcomes of patients diagnosed with acute pulmonary embolism in the emergency department: Initial report of EMPEROR (multicenter emergency medicine pulmonary embolism in the real world registry). J Am Coll Cardiol 2011. https://doi.org/10.1016/j.jacc.2010.05.071.
30. Kroep S, Chuang L-H, Cohen A, et al. The impact of co-morbidity on the disease burden of VTE. J Thromb Thrombolysis 2018. https://doi.org/10.1007/s11239-018-1732-0.
31. Sardi A, Gluskin J, Guttentag A, et al. Saddle pulmonary embolism: Is it as bad as it looks? A community hospital experience. Crit Care Med 2011. https://doi.org/10.1097/CCM.0b013e31822571b2.
32. Ambesh P, Obiagwu C, Shetty V. Homan's sign for deep vein thrombosis: a grain of salt? Indian Heart J 2017;69(3):418–9.
33. Aujesky D, Obrosky DS, Stone RA, et al. Derivation and validation of a prognostic model for pulmonary embolism. Am J Respir Crit Care Med 2005;172(8):1041–6.
34. Aujesky D. Validation of a model to predict adverse outcomes in patients with pulmonary embolism. Eur Heart J 2005;27(4):476–81.
35. Jiménez D, Yusen RD, Otero R, et al. Prognostic models for selecting patients with acute pulmonary embolism for initial outpatient therapy. Chest 2007; 132(1):24–30.
36. Righini M, Van Es J, Den Exter PL, et al. Age-adjusted D-dimer cutoff levels to rule out pulmonary embolism: the ADJUST-PE study. JAMA 2014;311(11):1117–24.

37. Barth BE, Waligora G, Gaddis GM. Rapid systematic review: age-adjusted D-Dimer for ruling out pulmonary embolism. J Emerg Med 2018. https://doi.org/10.1016/j.jemermed.2018.07.003.
38. Becattini C, Vedovati MC, Agnelli G. Prognostic value of troponins in acute pulmonary embolism a meta-analysis. Circulation 2007. https://doi.org/10.1161/CIRCULATIONAHA.106.680421.
39. Jiménez D, Uresandi F, Otero R, et al. Troponin-based risk stratification of patients with acute nonmassive pulmonary embolism. Chest 2009;136(4):974–82.
40. Henzler T, Roeger S, Meyer M, et al. Pulmonary embolism: CT signs and cardiac biomarkers for predicting right ventricular dysfunction. Eur Respir J 2012. https://doi.org/10.1183/09031936.00088711.
41. Fields JM, Davis J, Girson L, et al. Transthoracic echocardiography for diagnosing pulmonary embolism: a systematic review and meta-analysis. J Am Soc Echocardiogr 2017;30(7):714–23.e4.
42. Khemasuwan D, Yingchoncharoen T, Tunsupon P, et al. Right ventricular echocardiographic parameters are associated with mortality after acute pulmonary embolism. J Am Soc Echocardiogr 2015;28(3):355–62.
43. Rang Park J, Chang S-A, Yi Jang S, et al. Evaluation of right ventricular dysfunction and prediction of clinical outcomes in acute pulmonary embolism by chest computed tomography: comparisons with echocardiography. Int J Cardiovasc Imaging 2012;28:979–87.
44. Stein PD, Fowler SE, Goodman LR, et al. Multidetector computed tomography for acute pulmonary embolism. N Engl J Med 2006;354:2317–27. Available at: www.nejm.org.
45. Moores LK, Jackson WL, Shorr AF, et al. Meta-analysis: outcomes in patients with suspected pulmonary embolism managed with computed tomographic pulmonary angiography. Ann Intern Med 2004;141(11):866–74. Available at: www.annals.org.
46. Hitchen S, James J, Thachil J. Ventilation perfusion scan or computed tomography pulmonary angiography for the detection of pulmonary embolism? Eur J Intern Med 2016;32:e26–7.
47. Tunariu N, Gibbs SJR, Win Z, et al. Ventilation-perfusion scintigraphy is more sensitive than multidetector CTPA in detecting chronic thromboembolic pulmonary disease as a treatable cause of pulmonary hypertension. J Nucl Med 2007;48(5):680–4.
48. Memon HA, Lin CH, Guha A. Chronic thromboembolic pulmonary hypertension: pearls and pitfalls of diagnosis. Methodist Debakey Cardiovasc J 2016;12(4):199–204.
49. Smith SB, Geske JB, Maguire JM, et al. Early anticoagulation is associated with reduced mortality for acute pulmonary embolism. Chest 2010;137(6):1382–90.
50. Willoughby L, Adams DM, Evans RS, et al. Preemptive anticoagulation in patients with a high pretest probability of pulmonary embolism. Chest 2018;153(5):1153–9.
51. Findik S, Erkan ML, Selcuk MB, et al. Low-molecular-weight heparin versus unfractionated heparin in the treatment of patients with acute pulmonary thromboembolism. Respiration 2002;69(5):440–4.
52. Kabrhel C, Rosovsky R, Channick R, et al. A multidisciplinary pulmonary embolism response team. Chest 2016;150(2):384–93.
53. Van Es N, Coppens M, Schulman S, et al. Direct oral anticoagulants compared with vitamin K antagonists for acute venous thromboembolism: evidence from phase 3 trials. Blood 2014. https://doi.org/10.1182/blood-2014-04.

54. Kearon C, Akl EA, Ornelas J, et al. Antithrombotic therapy for VTE disease: CHEST guideline and expert panel report. Chest 2016. https://doi.org/10.1016/j.chest.2015.11.026.

55. Raskob GE, van Es N, Verhamme P, et al. Edoxaban for the treatment of cancer-associated venous thromboembolism. N Engl J Med 2017;378(7):615–24.

56. Douketis J, Tosetto A, Marcucci M, et al. Risk of recurrence after venous thromboembolism in men and women: patient level meta-analysis. BMJ 2011;342: d813. Available at: http://www.bmj.com/content/342/bmj.d813.abstract.

57. Douketis J, Tosetto A, Marcucci M, et al. Patient-level meta-analysis: Effect of measurement timing, threshold, and patient age on ability of d-dimer testing to assess recurrence risk after unprovoked venous thromboembolism. Ann Intern Med 2010;153(8):523–31.

58. Kearon C, FA S, O'Keeffe D, et al. D-dimer testing to select patients with a first unprovoked venous thromboembolism who can stop anticoagulant therapy: a cohort study. Ann Intern Med 2015;162(1):27–34.

59. Palareti G, Cosmi B, Legnani C, et al, DULCIS (D-dimer and ULtrasonography in Combination Italian Study) Investigators. D-dimer to guide the duration of anticoagulation in patients with venous thromboembolism: a management study. Blood 2014;124(2):196. Available at: http://www.bloodjournal.org/content/124/2/196.abstract.

60. Torbicki A, Linhart A, Spyropoulos AC, et al. 2014 ESC Guidelines on the diagnosis and management of acute pulmonary embolism: The Task Force for the Diagnosis and Management of Acute Pulmonary Embolism of the European Society of Cardiology (ESC) Endorsed by the European Respiratory Society (ERS). Eur Heart J 2014;35(43):3033–69k.

61. Meyer G, Vicaut E, Danays T, et al. Fibrinolysis for patients with intermediate-risk pulmonary embolism. N Engl J Med 2014. https://doi.org/10.1056/NEJMoa1302097.

62. Konstantinides SV, Vicaut E, Danays T, et al. Impact of thrombolytic therapy on the long-term outcome of intermediate-risk pulmonary embolism. J Am Coll Cardiol 2017;69(12):1536–44.

63. Konstantinides S, Geibel A, Heusel G, et al. Heparin plus alteplase compared with heparin alone in patients with submassive pulmonary embolism. N Engl J Med 2002. https://doi.org/10.1056/NEJMoa021274.

64. Engelberger RP, Kucher N. Catheter-based reperfusion treatment of pulmonary embolism. Circulation 2011. https://doi.org/10.1161/CIRCULATIONAHA.111.023689.

65. Kuo WT, Van Den Bosch MAAJ, Hofmann LV, et al. Catheter-directed embolectomy, fragmentation, and thrombolysis for the treatment of massive pulmonary embolism after failure of systemic thrombolysis. Chest 2008. https://doi.org/10.1378/chest.07-2846.

66. Kuo WT, Gould MK, Louie JD, et al. Catheter-directed therapy for the treatment of massive pulmonary embolism: systematic review and meta-analysis of modern techniques. J Vasc Interv Radiol 2009. https://doi.org/10.1016/j.jvir.2009.08.002.

67. Samoukovic G, Malas T, de Varennes B. The role of pulmonary embolectomy in the treatment of acute pulmonary embolism: a literature review from 1968 to 2008. Interact Cardiovasc Thorac Surg 2010;11(3):265–70.

68. Stein PD, Matta F. Pulmonary embolectomy in elderly patients. Am J Med 2014; 127(4):348–50.

69. PREPIC Study Group. Eight-year follow-up of patients with permanent vena cava filters in the prevention of pulmonary embolism: the PREPIC (Prevention du

Risque d'Embolie Pulmonaire par Interruption Cave) randomized study. Circulation 2005. https://doi.org/10.1161/CIRCULATIONAHA.104.512834.

70. Mismetti P, Laporte S, Pellerin O, et al. Effect of a retrievable inferior vena cava filter plus anticoagulation vs anticoagulation alone on risk of recurrent pulmonary embolism: a randomized clinical trial. JAMA 2015. https://doi.org/10.1001/jama.2015.3780.

71. Rosovsky R, Borges J, Kabrhel C, et al. Pulmonary embolism response team: inpatient structure, outpatient follow-up, and is it the current standard of care? Clin Chest Med 2018;39(3):621–30.

72. Heit JA, Silverstein MD, Mohr DN, et al. Risk factors for deep vein thrombosis and pulmonary embolism: a population-based case-control study. Arch Intern Med 2000;160(6):809–15.

73. Ende-Verhaar YM, Cannegieter SC, Vonk Noordegraaf A, et al. Incidence of chronic thromboembolic pulmonary hypertension after acute pulmonary embolism: a contemporary view of the published literature. Eur Respir J 2017;49(2) [pii:1601792]. Available at: http://erj.ersjournals.com/content/49/2/1601792.abstract.

Pulmonary Function Testing and Cardiopulmonary Exercise Testing: An Overview

Katherine Krol, MD[a], Mary Anne Morgan, MD[a], Sandhya Khurana, MD[b],*

KEYWORDS

- Pulmonary function test • Cardiopulmonary exercise test • Spirometry
- Diffusing capacity

KEY POINTS

- Common pulmonary function tests include spirometry, lung volumes, and diffusing capacity for carbon monoxide (DLCO). These tests are complementary and help inform the characteristics of underlying lung pathophysiology.
- Spirometry assesses airflow limitation. Diffusing capacity for carbon monoxide provides information on the health of alveolar-capillary membrane. Lung volume testing evaluates for restriction or hyperinflation.
- Bronchoprovocation testing gauges airway reactivity. Methacholine challenge has a high negative predictive value in a symptomatic patient and can be used to "rule out" asthma.
- Integrated cardiopulmonary exercise testing (CPET) is a complex procedure but can be invaluable when evaluating unexplained exertional dyspnea.
- Understanding the indications, limitations, and basics of test performance and interpretation will assist in selecting the appropriate test.

INTRODUCTION

Respiratory symptoms, including dyspnea and cough, are common reasons for patients to seek medical care and contribute significantly to the use of health care resources.[1] Identifying the underlying etiology of a respiratory symptom is key to its management, yet pinpointing the cause can be challenging. Familiarity with the tools

Disclosure Statement: None.
[a] Pulmonary and Critical Care Medicine, University of Rochester School of Medicine, University of Rochester Medical Center, 601 Elmwood Avenue, Box 692, Rochester, NY 14642, USA;
[b] Pulmonary and Critical Care Medicine, Mary Parkes Center for Asthma & Pulmonary Care, University of Rochester School of Medicine, University of Rochester Medical Center, 601 Elmwood Avenue, Box 692, Rochester, NY 14642, USA
* Corresponding author.
E-mail address: sandhya_khurana@urmc.rochester.edu

Med Clin N Am 103 (2019) 565–576
https://doi.org/10.1016/j.mcna.2018.12.014
0025-7125/19/© 2018 Elsevier Inc. All rights reserved.

medical.theclinics.com

available to help discern between the various contributing etiologies is crucial in guiding the next steps in management. In conjunction with a thorough history and physical examination, assessment of pulmonary function can provide an objective measure to guide diagnosis and therapy.

This article will review key points of pulmonary function evaluation, highlighting indications and contraindications, fundamentals of interpretation, and the limitations of each individual component.

Spirometry

Spirometry is an accessible, reproducible, non-invasive, and relatively simple means of measuring lung function. Although best at identifying airflow obstruction, it may suggest the presence of restrictive lung disease. It can also allow objective assessment of therapeutic response and disease progression. Minimal required training, availability of clear and concise standards for interpretation, and reproducibility across health care settings are some strengths of this test.[2,3]

Indications

- Evaluate pulmonary symptoms
- Measure severity of airflow obstruction
- Monitor disease and response to treatment
- Assess pre-operative pulmonary risk

Contraindications[4]

- Recent myocardial infarction (<4 weeks) or unstable angina
- Ascending aortic aneurysm
- Recent thoracic, abdominal, or ophthalmologic surgery
- Recent pneumothorax

Procedure

Following full inspiration, the patient exhales forcefully into a closed system for a minimum of 6 seconds. The test is repeated at least three times to ensure repeatability. The patient's performance is reported as a comparison with "predicted" values, and helpful flow-versus-volume and volume-versus-time graphs are generated.

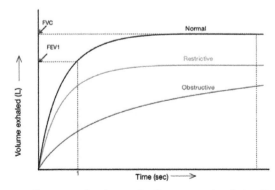

Fig. 1. Volume-versus-time graph demonstrating normal, obstructive, and restrictive pattern.

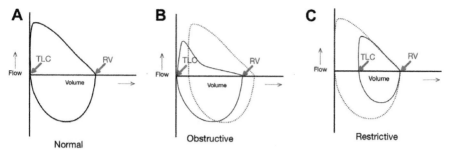

Fig. 2. Typical shape of flow-versus-volume loops in normal (*A*) spirometry, (*B*) obstruction, and (*C*) restriction.

Acceptability and repeatability

- All trials should produce similarly shaped flow-volume curves. Cough or glottic closure in the first second of exhalation renders the test unacceptable.
- Examine the volume-versus-time graph. Effort is manifested by a sharp rise in volume on exhalation, by a minimum of 6-second exhalation forced expiratory time (FET), and by plateauing of respiratory effort at the end of exhalation.
- To demonstrate consistency (here termed repeatability), the two largest measurements of forced expiratory volume in 1 second (FEV_1) and the two largest measurements of forced vital capacity (FVC) should be within 150 mL of each other.[3]

Interpretation

The most useful parameters measured by spirometry are FEV_1, FVC, and the calculated ratio of the two (FEV_1/FVC) (**Fig. 1**).[2,5] For interpretation, these individual tests are compared with population-derived reference values matched for similar age, gender, height, and race.[6,7]

- The flow-volume loop can help differentiate an obstructive from a restrictive process (**Fig. 2**), as well as hint at the presence of central airway obstruction (**Fig. 3**).

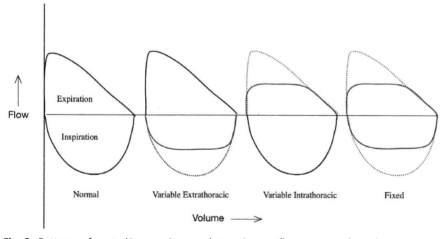

Fig. 3. Patterns of central/upper airways obstruction on flow-versus-volume loop.

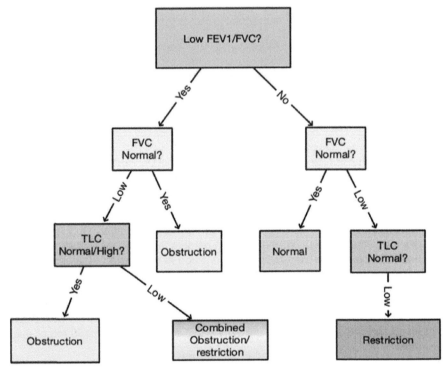

Fig. 4. Basic algorithm to assist spirometry interpretation.

- Analyze and compare patient's results to the normalized reference ranges. **Fig. 4** provides a simplified algorithm for interpretation of spirometry results.
  - An FEV_1/FVC that falls below the lower limit of the confidence interval suggests obstruction. Severity of obstruction is defined by the percent predicted of FEV_1 (**Table 1**).
  - Low FVC suggests a possible restrictive process but can also be low in severe obstructive disease. Lung volume measurements are needed for confirmation of restriction.

Table 1 Determining severity of obstructive lung disease based on percent predicted FEV_1	
% Predicted FEV_1	**Severity**
>70	Mild
60–69	Moderate
50–59	Moderately severe
35–49	Severe
<35	Very severe

Of note, mild only applies if given result is outside the reference range.

Reproduced from Pellegrino R, Viegi G, Brusasco V, et al. Interpretative strategies for lung function tests. Eur Respir J 2005;26(5):948–68. © ERS 2018; with permission.

Limitations and caveats

- Spirometry identifies obstructive pulmonary physiology but cannot diagnose a specific cause of airflow obstruction.
- A low FVC can be seen in very severe obstructive lung disease and should not be interpreted as co-existing restrictive disease without a confirmatory lung volume study.
- The quality of spirometry depends on a patient's ability to understand and follow instructions, as well as the ability of the testing personnel to guide the patient and determine the adequacy of results.
- Results can be affected by use of an inhaler, smoking, or even eating. Patients are asked to avoid smoking for one hour prior and eating for two hours prior to the test. They are advised to wear comfortable loose-fitting clothes for testing. The test should be performed with the subject seated as syncope can occur, more commonly in older subjects or those with severe airflow limitation.
- Using "normal" reference values to identify abnormalities may result in simplistic interpretations, particularly if results border the confidence interval.

Bronchodilator Challenge

In patients with suspected or confirmed obstructive lung disease, bronchodilator challenge is often used to assess for reversibility of airflow obstruction.

Procedure
The patient undergoes routine spirometry to establish a baseline. After a gentle and incomplete exhalation, four sequential doses of a short-acting beta agonist (SABA) are given at 30-second intervals via a spacer device. After waiting 15 minutes, repeat spirometry is performed and compared with the baseline.[3] It is recommended that patients not use a rescue inhaler (SABA) for 4 hours, a long-acting beta agonist (LABA) for 12 hours, or a long-acting anti-muscarinic antagonist (LAMA) for 24 hours before testing.

Interpretation
Baseline spirometry is interpreted as described above. An improvement in FEV_1 or FVC by 12% *and* 200 mL from baseline is considered a "significant" bronchodilator response.[2]

Limitations and caveats

- Presence or lack of a bronchodilator response does not predict or preclude a clinical response to therapy, respectively.
- Bronchodilator challenge has traditionally been used to distinguish asthma from chronic obstructive pulmonary disease (COPD); however, it has become increasingly evident that a significant portion of patients with COPD demonstrate a positive bronchodilator response.[8]

Lung Volume Testing

Lung volume measurement is technically more challenging and requires specialized equipment. It remains a useful non-invasive and reproducible tool to assess common pulmonary symptoms.

Indications

- Confirm restrictive lung physiology from any underlying disease process
- Assess for hyperinflation or air-trapping

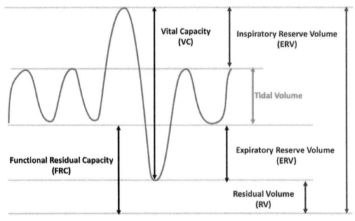

Fig. 5. Lung volumes and capacities.

- Sort out more complex physiologic derangements (ie, coexistent restriction and obstruction)

Procedure

Lung volume testing measures functional residual capacity (FRC) and vital capacity (VC) directly, and residual volume (RV) and total lung capacity (TLC) indirectly (**Fig. 5**). Testing is performed by one of three methods: helium dilution, nitrogen washout, or whole body plethysmography. Although plethysmography is the gold standard for lung volume measurement, gas dilution/washout methods are often used as they are simple to perform and the equipment is less expensive. Details on the three methods can be found in the 2005 ATS/ERS taskforce paper.[9]

Interpretation

- Similar to spirometry, a patient's results should be compared with the normalized reference ranges based on the patient's demographics.
- TLC below the reference range/confidence interval suggests a restrictive process.
- The severity of restriction is defined by the percent predicted of FEV_1.
- Air-trapping is indicated by elevated RV and RV/TLC (>120% predicted). Hyperinflation is indicated by elevated TLC (>120% predicted). These findings are typically observed with obstructive lung disease and are a strong driver of exercise intolerance.

Limitations and caveats

- Gas dilution and washout methods may underestimate lung volumes in patients with unequal distribution of ventilation, particularly in severe obstructive lung disease.

DLCO

Diffusing capacity for carbon monoxide (also called transfer factor) assesses the exchange of gas across the very thin alveolar-capillary interface, a process that occurs by passive diffusion. As such, gas exchange depends on the surface area and integrity of both the alveolar membrane and the pulmonary vasculature, as well as on carrying capacity (hemoglobin). Processes that interfere with diffusion cause impaired gas transfer. Examples include diseases marked by thickening of the membrane (fibrosis or scarring), by excess fluid in the interstitium (pulmonary edema, pneumonia), or by reduction in surface area/integrity of the alveoli (emphysema) or vascular bed (pulmonary vascular disease).

Indications

- Evaluate diseases causing reduced oxygenation
- Assess for drug or exposure toxicity
- Inform pre-operative risk

Procedure

Diffusing capacity for carbon monoxide is determined by measuring the diffusion of carbon monoxide across the alveolar-capillary membrane after a single breath-hold.[10,11] Wearing nose clips and breathing through a mouth piece with a tight seal, the patient exhales completely (to RV) before quickly and completely inhaling a composite gas composed of 21% oxygen, nitrogen, an inert tracer, and 0.3% carbon monoxide (to TLC). A 10-second breath-hold is essential for equilibration. The content of carbon monoxide measured in the exhaled gas is used to calculate the diffusion capacity. Carbon monoxide is customarily used because it is diffusion−not perfusion−limited, and therefore is independent of cardiac function. The test is repeated twice or until two results are within 2 mL/min/mm Hg of each other.

Interpretation

- DLCO is abnormal (generally reduced) if it falls outside the reference range, and severity is based on the degree to which it is reduced (**Table 2**).
- DLCO is adjusted for changes in hemoglobin (anemia/polycythemia) and carboxyhemoglobin (smoking).
- An abnormal DLCO value should be interpreted in the context of contemporaneously performed spirometry and lung volume studies.
  - A low DLCO with restrictive physiology can indicate interstitial lung disease
  - Reduced DLCO with obstructive pattern usually suggests emphysema
  - An isolated reduction in DLCO should raise concern for pulmonary vascular disorders such as chronic pulmonary embolism or pulmonary hypertension
- DLCO may be elevated in pulmonary hemorrhage, asthma, polycythemia, mild left heart failure, and obesity.[12]

Limitations and caveats

- Patients must inhale to at least 85% of their VC for the test to be reliable.
- Adjustment of DLCO for lung volume (DLCO/VA) is controversial as their relationship is non-linear and clinical utility has not been established.

Table 2	
Determining severity of diffusion impairment based on percent predicted DLCO	
% Predicted DLCO	**Severity**
>60	Mild
40–60	Moderate
<40	Severe

Of note, mild only applies if DLCO value is outside the reference range.

Reproduced from Pellegrino R, Viegi G, Brusasco V, et al. Interpretative strategies for lung function tests. Eur Respir J 2005;26(5):948–68. © ERS 2018; with permission.

- Accidentally performing a Valsalva or Mueller maneuver (exhaling or inspiring against a closed glottis) during the breath-hold alters pulmonary capillary blood flow and therefore affects the measurement.
- This test has the most variability of all of the pulmonary function tests.[13] With high-quality studies, a change greater than 4 mL/min/mm Hg is considered significant.[14]

Bronchoprovocation Testing

Bronchoprovocation testing is used to assess airway hyper-responsiveness, defined as excessive narrowing of the airways (bronchoconstriction) in response to a stimulus.[15] Based on the type of stimulus, they can be categorized as direct (methacholine, histamine) or indirect (exercise, eucapnic hyperventilation, osmolar agent). Methacholine stimulates muscarinic receptors on airway smooth muscle causing airway constriction. Methacholine wears off quickly and reverses with beta agonist treatment, making it a safe means of assessing bronchial reactivity.

Indications

- Confirm a diagnosis of asthma when spirometry is normal
- Evaluate occupational or other stimulant-specific asthma
- "Rule out" asthma in individuals with low pretest probability of disease

Contraindications

- Baseline moderate-to-severe airflow limitation (FEV_1 <60% for methacholine challenge test and <75% for indirect challenge)
- Cardiovascular diseases including uncontrolled hypertension, recent myocardial infarction/stroke, or known aneurysm
- Pregnancy and lactation
- Use of cholinesterase inhibitor medication
- Inability to perform acceptable and repeatable spirometry maneuvers

Procedure

Methacholine challenge test After performing baseline spirometry, the patient inhales incrementally increasing doses of methacholine with spirometry repeated after each dose. If the FEV_1 drops by 20%, the test is terminated and the patient is given a bronchodilator. If there is no drop, the patient inhales to a maximum total dose before bronchodilation.

Exercise challenge test Following baseline spirometry, the patient exercises on a treadmill or stationary cycle ergometer, achieving target heart rate in the first 2 to 4 minutes and maintaining it for 4 to 6 minutes. Spirometry is performed at 5, 10, 15, and 30 minutes after stopping.[16]

Interpretation

Methacholine challenge test If the FEV_1 drops by 20% (from baseline) at any administered dose of methacholine, the result is considered positive. The dose of methacholine inducing the drop in FEV_1 defines the degree of airway reactivity (**Table 3**).

Exercise challenge A decline in FEV_1 of 10% or greater is considered positive, with severity of exercise-induced bronchoconstriction classified based on FEV_1 decline from baseline (see **Table 3**).

Table 3		
Determining the degree of airway reactivity for exercise and methacholine challenge test		
Exercise Challenge Test [a]Decrease in FEV_1 (%) from Baseline	Methacholine Challenge Test [b]PC_{20} mg/ml (PD_{20} μg)	Severity [a]EIB or [b]AHR
<10	>16 (>400) 4–16 (100–400)	Normal Borderline
10–25	1–4 (25–100)	Mild
25–50	0.25–1 (6–25)	Moderate
>50	<0.25 (<6)	Severe

Abbreviations: AHR, airway hyper-reactivity; EIB, exercise-induced bronchoconstriction; PC_{20}, provocative concentration causing 20% drop in FEV_1; PD_{20}, provocative dose causing 20% drop in FEV_1.

Modified from Coates AL, Wanger J, Cockcroft DW, et al. ERS technical standard on bronchial challenge testing: general considerations and performance of methacholine challenge tests. Eur Respir J 2017;49(5)1601526; with permission.

Limitations and caveats

- Methacholine challenge has a better negative than positive predictive value for diagnosing asthma because airway hyper-responsiveness is not specific to asthma. False-positive results may be seen with allergic rhinitis, cystic fibrosis, COPD, and bronchitis.
- Patients must be instructed not to use bronchodilators before testing: SABA 6 hours, LABA 36 to 48 hours, ipratropium 12 hours, LAMA greater than 168 hours, and theophylline 12 to 24 hours. Continuing to use medications can result in false-negative test results.
- If paradoxic vocal fold motion is a concern, careful assessment of inspiratory and expiratory flow-volume loops with sequential methacholine dose may reveal flattening consistent with inducible laryngeal obstruction.

Cardiopulmonary Exercise Testing

Cardiopulmonary exercise testing is an important tool for the global assessment of exercise capacity and in particular unexplained dyspnea. It is a dynamic measure of the entire oxygen transport system, integrating evaluation of pulmonary, cardiovascular, and musculoskeletal function and their relative contributions to the exercise response. Results may indicate limitation caused by cardiovascular disease, pulmonary disease, deconditioning, obesity, or any combination. Cardiopulmonary exercise testing (CPET) is performed in a specialized laboratory under the auspices of trained personnel.[17]

Indications

- Assess exertional dyspnea after unrevealing initial work-up
- Evaluate relative contributions of heart and/or lung disease to exercise intolerance in patients with co-existing disease, guiding further diagnostics and/or directed therapies
- Assess perioperative risk of cardiopulmonary complications from major surgery, especially lung resection
- Allow for more directed exercise prescription, especially in cardiopulmonary rehabilitation
- Provide integrated assessment of fitness for organ transplant evaluation

Contraindications

- Active cardiovascular disease: acute myocardial infarction, unstable angina, or significant rhythm or valvular dysfunction
- Acute pulmonary embolism
- Mental or physical conditions limiting ability to cooperate
- Baseline resting hypoxemia (oxygen saturation <85%)

Procedure

The patient exercises on a stationary bicycle or a treadmill while wearing a variety of sensors, including a mouthpiece with a non-rebreathing valve (airflow or volume transducer, gas analyzer). As the workload increases, heart rate, blood pressure, respiratory rate, exhaled CO_2, and oximetry are monitored. The test is continued until the patient reaches maximum exercise ability (or peak oxygen consumption, VO_2) or develops intolerable symptoms (electrocardiogram changes, drop in blood pressure, or significant oxygen desaturation).

Interpretation

An impressive number of variables are measured and/or calculated during CPET. The ATS/ERS recommends an "integrated approach to CPET interpretation", incorporating factors such as the clinical indication for testing and known patient variables (medications, diagnoses, and results of past testing) into a final assessment of the CPET-generated results, rather than relying on a specific algorithm for interpretation. Assessment of test adequacy based on effort expended is crucial, as sub-maximal effort will muddy interpretation considerably. Test performance patterns can help distinguish between various causes of exercise intolerance, although caution against over-reliance on these algorithms is recommended, given often overlapping etiologic factors.[17]

Limitations and caveats

- Patient effort is critical in the utility of CPET as a tool for identifying reasons for exercise intolerance
- No standardized exercise protocols exist; therefore, reproducibility of results may be limited
- Significant training for the personnel performing the test and for those interpreting results is required

SUMMARY

- Respiratory complaints are among the most common symptoms reported in primary care offices, affecting a large proportion of chronically ill individuals and becoming more frequent with age. Elucidating the causes can be complex, given the many overlapping disease states affecting perception of dyspnea and/or respiratory limitation.
- Knowledge of the array of pulmonary function testing available will help inform the health care provider on how best to identify, manage, and follow patients with respiratory complaints. **Fig. 6** offers a basic algorithm for pulmonary disease assessment.
- Understanding the indications, shortcomings, and basics of test performance and interpretation will assist in selection of appropriate test and judicious use of health resources.

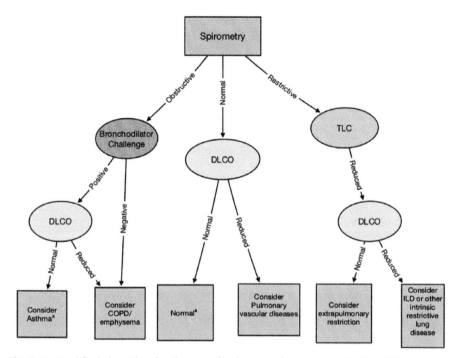

Fig. 6. A simplified algorithm for the use of pulmonary function tests in identifying certain pulmonary disorders. [a]Spirometry may be normal in asthma. If clinical concern, consider bronchoprovocation testing.

REFERENCES

1. Khan AA, Khan A, Harezlak J, et al. Somatic symptoms in primary care: etiology and outcome. Psychosomatics 2003;44(6):471–8.
2. Pellegrino R, Viegi G, Brusasco V, et al. Interpretative strategies for lung function tests. Eur Respir J 2005;26(5):948–68.
3. Miller MR, Hankinson J, Brusasco V, et al. Standardisation of spirometry. Eur Respir J 2005;26(2):319–38.
4. Cooper BG. An update on contraindications for lung function testing. Thorax 2011;66(8):714–23.
5. Culver BH, Graham BL, Coates AL, et al. Recommendations for a standardized pulmonary function report. An Official American Thoracic Society Technical Statement. Am J Respir Crit Care Med 2017;196(11):1463–72.
6. Hankinson JL, Odencrantz JR, Fedan KB. Spirometric reference values from a sample of the general U.S. population. Am J Respir Crit Care Med 1999; 159(1):179–87.
7. Quanjer PH, Stanojevic S, Cole TJ, et al. Multi-ethnic reference values for spirometry for the 3-95-yr age range: the global lung function 2012 equations. Eur Respir J 2012;40(6):1324–43.
8. Calverley PM, Albert P, Walker PP. Bronchodilator reversibility in chronic obstructive pulmonary disease: use and limitations. Lancet Respir Med 2013;1(7): 564–73.
9. Wanger J, Clausen JL, Coates A, et al. Standardisation of the measurement of lung volumes. Eur Respir J 2005;26(3):511–22.

10. Graham BL, Brusasco V, Burgos F, et al. 2017 ERS/ATS standards for single-breath carbon monoxide uptake in the lung. Eur Respir J 2017;49(1) [pii: 1600016].
11. Macintyre N, Crapo RO, Viegi G, et al. Standardisation of the single-breath determination of carbon monoxide uptake in the lung. Eur Respir J 2005;26(4):720–35.
12. Saydain G, Beck KC, Decker PA, et al. Clinical significance of elevated diffusing capacity. Chest 2004;125(2):446–52.
13. Hathaway EH, Tashkin DP, Simmons MS. Intraindividual variability in serial measurements of DLCO and alveolar volume over one year in eight healthy subjects using three independent measuring systems. Am Rev Respir Dis 1989;140(6): 1818–22.
14. Robson AG, Innes JA. Short term variability of single breath carbon monoxide transfer factor. Thorax 2001;56(5):358–61.
15. Coates AL, Wanger J, Cockcroft DW, et al. ERS technical standard on bronchial challenge testing: general considerations and performance of methacholine challenge tests. Eur Respir J 2017;49(5) [pii:1601526].
16. Parsons JP, Hallstrand TS, Mastronarde JG, et al. An official American Thoracic Society clinical practice guideline: exercise-induced bronchoconstriction. Am J Respir Crit Care Med 2013;187(9):1016–27.
17. ATS/ACCP Statement on cardiopulmonary exercise testing. Am J Respir Crit Care Med 2003;167(2):211–77.

Pulmonary Rehabilitation in the Management of Chronic Lung Disease

Sharon D. Cornelison, RCP, RRT-NPS[a], Rodolfo M. Pascual, MD[b],*

KEYWORDS

• Pulmonary • Rehabilitation • Education • Training • Functioning • Self-management

KEY POINTS

- Patients with chronic lung disease often suffer from significant exercise and functional limitation due to multi-factorial causes. The increased work of breathing imposed on patients with chronic lung disease leads to a maladaptive reduction in activity levels.
- Patients with chronic lung disease experience high rates of anxiety and depression. Poor physical and psychosocial functioning is associated with morbidity and mortality and use of health care resources.
- PR improves physical and psychosocial functioning in patients with a variety of chronic lung diseases.
- Evidence-based standardization ensures that PR programs are staffed by trained providers, that appropriate patients are enrolled, that programs have medical supervision. and that all facets of the patient's disability are addressed.
- Although PR is efficacious, cost effective, and safe it is an underused therapy.

INTRODUCTION

Pulmonary rehabilitation (PR) is a central component in the long-term management of patients with chronic obstructive pulmonary disease (COPD) and other non-obstructive respiratory diseases. It has been shown to help reduce symptoms, improve functional and exercise capacity, improve overall quality of life (QOL), and decrease health care use and associated costs. Given these outcomes, PR has now become the standard of care in most COPD treatment plans as per guidelines, including the 2018 Global Initiative for Chronic Obstructive Lung Disease (GOLD).[1]

---

[a] Department of Pulmonary and Cardiac Rehabilitation, J. Paul Sticht Center on Aging and Rehabilitation, Wake Forest Baptist Medical Center, Medical Center Boulevard, Winston Salem, NC 27157, USA; [b] Department of Internal Medicine, Section on Pulmonary Medicine, Critical Care, Allergy and Immunologic Diseases, Wake Forest Baptist Medical Center, Medical Center Boulevard, Winston Salem, NC 27157, USA
* Corresponding author.
E-mail address: rpascual@wakehealth.edu

Med Clin N Am 103 (2019) 577–584
https://doi.org/10.1016/j.mcna.2018.12.015
0025-7125/19/© 2019 Elsevier Inc. All rights reserved.
medical.theclinics.com

Despite significant evidence of its efficacy, PR is underused and remains inaccessible to patients, especially those in rural or remote locations.[2] The aim of this review is to provide an increased knowledge of how to use PR in the management of patients with chronic lung disease. In addition, it will provide the reader with an understanding of the patient selection process, the components of a PR program, and the expected benefits for enrolled patients.[3]

DEFINITION

The 2006 American Thoracic Society and European Respiratory Society statement on pulmonary rehabilitation defines PR as: an evidence-based, multidisciplinary, and comprehensive intervention for patients with chronic respiratory diseases who are symptomatic and often have decreased daily life activities. Integrated into the individualized treatment of the patient, PR is designed to reduce symptoms, optimize functional status, increase participation, and reduce health care costs by stabilizing or reversing systemic manifestations of the disease.[4]

Ideally, PR programs should be certified by the American Association of Cardiovascular and Pulmonary Rehabilitation and should include the following components *individualized* to each patient: entry assessment/goal setting, disease management education, exercise training/physical conditioning, psychosocial intervention/support, nutrition/pharmacologic support, and an outcomes assessment at program completion.[5] Pulmonary rehabilitation programs usually meet in an outpatient setting and vary from 6 to 12 weeks in length. Patients attend 3 days per week for 1.5 to 4 hours per session, which includes exercise training, education components, and psychosocial support.

RATIONALE: EXERCISE AND FUNCTIONAL LIMITATION

Patients with chronic lung disease experience worsening shortness of breath initially with exertion and then at rest as their disease progresses. Much of our knowledge of the physiology explaining physical impairment and evidence of efficacy in the area of physical training comes from the study of patients with COPD. Currently, most patients referred for PR have COPD. Patients with COPD and other chronic lung diseases have higher ventilation requirements during exercise due to more work required for breathing, increased dead space ventilation, and gas exchange abnormalities. This leads to decreased activity levels, which, over time, can result in progressive, peripheral muscle weakness and worsening physical deconditioning.[6,7] These derangements can be reversed at least in part by exercise training. A variety of types of training including constant-load endurance, interval, resistance/strength, and inspiratory muscle and transcutaneous neuromuscular electrical stimulation have demonstrated efficacy. Details about these modes is beyond the scope of this article but have been reviewed elsewhere.[8] Patients with COPD tend to be frail and experience high rates of falls owing in part to reductions in skeletal muscle mass and strength.[9,10] In addition, as their functional status declines, many patients begin to suffer from anxiety, isolation, and depression. If left untreated, these symptoms lead to significant disability and increased health care use for patients.[11]

EVIDENCE OF EFFICACY

Globally, PR has been shown to help decrease shortness of breath, increase functional and exercise capacity, reduce handicap, and improve overall QOL.[12] There is new, emerging evidence that it also helps decrease healthcare use and associated costs.[13] Pulmonary rehabilitation compared favorably with monotherapy maintenance inhalers in terms of cost per quality-adjusted life-year and was more cost effective than the use of multiple inhaled medications from 3 drug classes or so-called "triple therapy" in one analysis.[14] Although PR does not improve these outcomes by directly increasing lung function (ie, FEV_1, FVC), it is thought to do so by identifying, addressing, and treating the systemic and psychosocial conditions associated with lung disease, such as obesity, deconditioning, anxiety, depression, peripheral muscle weakness, suboptimal self-management skills, sedentary lifestyle, and low health literacy.[15,16] As stated above, although most of the science in the field comes from the study of COPD patients, other patient populations can also benefit from PR.

PATIENT SELECTION CRITERIA FOR OUTPATIENT PULMONARY REHABILITATION

Comprehensive PR can be effectively delivered in outpatient, inpatient, and community-based settings. There have been many clinical trials supporting the use of PR in patients with COPD. New, emerging evidence supports the use and benefits of the program in other chronic respiratory diseases, such as idiopathic pulmonary fibrosis, interstitial lung disease, and others listed in **Table 1**. Selecting appropriate patients for PR is important to ensure positive outcomes and that the patient's goals are achieved. The following points should be considered by providers referring patients to a PR program:

1. *When referring patients with a diagnosis of COPD* (ICD 10 code J44.9), many insurance carriers require a pre/post bronchodilator spirometry pulmonary function test (PFT) documenting a post bronchodilator FEV1/FVC ratio less than 0.70 and an FEV1 less than 80% thus meeting the GOLD guidelines for stage II-IV airway obstruction. Pulmonary function testing, as per GOLD guidelines, is the definitive method for diagnosing COPD.[27] Without PFTs documenting GOLD II-IV obstruction, insurance coverage for PR can be quite difficult to obtain.

Table 1
Pulmonary rehabilitation for chronic respiratory diseases

Patient Population	Outcomes
Acute exacerbation of COPD (AECOPD)	Multiple randomized clinical trials (RCT), improves health-related QOL, 6-min walk distance (6MWD)[17]
Asthma	Improved asthma symptoms, QOL, anxiety and depression[18]
Bronchiectasis	Improved walk distance and endurance when inspiratory muscle training was combined with whole-body exercise training[19]
COPD (stable)	Multiple RCT, improves health-related QOL, 6MWD, and exercise capacity[20]
Cystic fibrosis (CF)	Improved exercise capacity, studies small[21]
Interstitial lung disease (ILD)	Short-term improvement in 6MWD, dyspnea, and QOL[22]
Lung cancer	Increased exercise tolerance and endurance, studies small[23]
Lung transplantation	Improved exercise capacity[24]
Lung volume reduction surgery	Improved exercise capacity, 6MWD, QOL[25]
Pulmonary hypertension	Improved 6MWD, QOL, functional class[26]

Adapted from Spruit MA, Singh SJ, Garvey C, et al. An official American Thoracic Society/European Respiratory Society statement: key concepts and advances in pulmonary rehabilitation. Am J Respir Crit Care Med 2013;188(8):e13–64; with permission.

2. *When referring patients with a diagnosis of COPD and the post bronchodilator PFT shows a ratio less than 0.70 and an FEV1 greater than 80%,* consider an alternative qualifying diagnosis, when possible. Computed tomographic scan evidence of emphysema, chronic bronchitis, or bronchiectasis are acceptable alternatives. Whereas a diagnosis of dyspnea on exertion or shortness of breath is acceptable in some instances, given the specificity of the new ICD 10 coding system, it is strongly recommended to avoid referring under these 2 diagnoses if an acceptable alternative can be used.

3. *PFTs are generally not required when referring patients to PR with non-COPD respiratory diseases.* However, providing baseline PFTs to the PR team helps quantify the degree of lung impairment, and thus assists the team when designing an individualized exercise and education treatment plan for the patient.

4. *A referral to PR should be considered* when the symptoms of chronic lung disease become persistent and interfere with the patient's daily life, when QOL is impaired, when the patient's functional status and exercise tolerance are decreasing, or the patient's health care resource use is increasing (ie, unscheduled hospital admissions, emergency department visits, and physician office visits owing to worsening respiratory symptoms).[3]

5. *Patients with chronic lung disease frequently have known comorbidities* or other diseases that could potentially place them at risk for serious and sometimes life-threatening complications during PR exercise training. These conditions should be stabilized or corrected before patient referral. Examples of these issues include unstable angina, critical aortic stenosis, severe and poorly controlled pulmonary arterial hypertension, and unstable coronary artery disease.

6. *Patients who continue to abuse tobacco are often excluded from entry* in some PR programs as it is believed that these patients will be less motivated to quit and unreceptive to tobacco cessation education. There is no evidence to support this notion. Rather, active smokers who are willing to make a good faith attempt to quit should be referred to PR. For these patients, tobacco cessation education and support will be a central component of their individualized treatment program. It should be noted that lung function, particularly FEV_1, in patients who continue to abuse tobacco declines significantly faster than in those who have successfully maintained cessation.[28,29]

7. *For patients who have been admitted to the hospital for an acute exacerbation of COPD,* there are new, evidence-based data recommending that patients be referred to a PR program on discharge, and these patients should begin the program within the following 3 weeks.[3,7]

COMPONENTS OF A PULMONARY REHABILITATION PROGRAM

There are 6 essential components of an American Association of Cardiovascular and Pulmonary Rehabilitation-certified PR program: entry assessment and goal setting, education and disease self-management strategies, exercise training and physician conditioning, psychosocial intervention and support, nutritional and pharmacologic intervention, and outcomes assessment.[3] The following is a brief description of each component:

1. *Entry assessment and goal setting:* on entering a program, patients undergo an intake history and physical examination, set personal rehab goals, perform a pulmonary fitness test such as a 6-minute walk distance, shuttle walk, or maximal effort cardiopulmonary exercise test (CPET), and complete detailed, written assessments of pain, nutritional status, psychosocial issues such as anxiety and

depression, exercise capability, and educational needs. Patients enter PR with different degrees of physical, emotional and functional impairment, and variable knowledge about their disease and how it is managed. This initial assessment is important for tailoring the program to the individual patient, which is emphasized in guidelines.

2. *Education and disease self-management strategies:* common topics covered for COPD and non-COPD diseases include breathing techniques, nutrition, energy conservation, exacerbation management, respiratory medications, advanced directives, home exercise, chronic lung disease, airway clearance, and stress management. Although the patient is learning about these topics there is an emphasis on the promotion of collaborative self-management. In particular, attention is paid to the development of strategies for self-management of chronic respiratory disease, including action plans for the early recognition and treatment of COPD exacerbations because this can reduce health care utilization and subsequent costs.[30]

3. *Exercise training and physical conditioning:* patients receive an individualized exercise plan using high- and low-intensity aerobic training; upper- and lower-extremity strength training; balance, flexibility, and proper body mechanics training; and respiratory muscle strength training. There are several different modalities that can be used for conditioning the muscles and to improve cardiorespiratory fitness. Most often constant-load endurance training is used; however, for some patients, low-intensity or interval training is used to improve tolerance. Resistance training including upper limb training can be used to improve performance of activities of daily living and household tasks.

4. *Psychosocial intervention and support:* participants receive intervention and support related to issues with depression, anxiety, panic, cognitive impairment, and other concerns such as poor coping skills, ongoing tobacco dependence, and the need for stress management techniques. Up to 40% of patients with COPD have depression or anxiety symptoms, with evidence showing that PR can reduce the symptoms.[31] Pulmonary rehabilitation is also an opportunity to engage patients in advanced care planning, which is important because many patients overestimate their life expectancy, whereas others have concerns about dying but do not discuss them with their clinician.

5. *Nutritional and pharmacologic intervention:* this domain addresses issues related to poor nutritional intake, cachexia, obesity, alcohol consumption, high blood pressure, elevated cholesterol, sodium and fluid management, and any issues related to meal preparation and food insecurity. Patients with chronic lung disease often have abnormalities of body composition with reductions in lean body mass. Weight loss and underweight status,[32] are associated with increased mortality, whereas underweight patients who are able to gain weight may have a reduction in mortality risk.

6. *Outcomes assessment:* patients will undergo pulmonary fitness testing and other written outcome measurements at program completion to evaluate changes in exercise capacity, daily symptoms, and overall health-related QOL.

PROGRAM LENGTH AND MAINTAINING THE BENEFITS OF PULMONARY REHABILITATION

As stated previously, PR programs can vary in length from 4 to 12 weeks. It has been demonstrated in prior studies that shorter courses of PR (4–7 weeks) are not as effective, and patients do not gain the same overall benefit as they would when completing an 8- to 12-week program.[33] Research has shown that it takes an average of 66 days (range 18–254 days) to establish new, healthy habits such as exercise, mindful eating,

---

Box 1
Benefits gained from outpatient pulmonary rehabilitation

Decreased dyspnea

Improvements in a 6-minute walk distance, shuttle walk test and/or CPET

Improvements in overall health-related QOL

Reduction in depression and anxiety symptoms

Reduction in health care resource utilization and associated costs

Adapted from Carlin BW. Pulmonary rehabilitation and chronic lung disease: opportunities for the respiratory therapist. Respir Care 2009;54(8):1095; with permission.

---

tobacco cessation, and stress-reduction techniques.[34] For patients with chronic lung disease, adopting new, healthy habits are key components of their PR program. It could be extrapolated that lengthier courses of PR could afford this population the time necessary to firmly establish the lifestyle changes they need to maintain health-related QOL and exercise-related physical strength and endurance after completing an initial course of PR. Therefore, longer courses of PR (>8 weeks) may be more efficacious in many patients.

The short-term benefits of PR in those with COPD are thoroughly documented in the literature, and are found in **Box 1**. However, once the patient completes the initial PR program, these gained benefits start to decline over the following 6 to 12 months, especially if they do not maintain some type of endurance and strength training.[35] Studies have shown, however, that, despite this decline, some patients may continue to experience benefits, such as improved exercise capacity and health-related QOL, for up to 2 years after completing PR if they continue with some type of exercise training.[36]

So, should patients continue with maintenance therapy post PR program completion to help maintain QOL and exercise-related gains in physical endurance and strength? The evidence suggests yes, if clinicians and patients expect to maintain the benefits gained from an initial course of PR for at least an additional 12 months.[37] There are many options available for those who want to continue therapy after initial PR completion, including on-site, medically supervised, maintenance phase programs, online, web-based programs, specialty programs such as Silver Sneakers, and exercising at home.

SUMMARY

Pulmonary rehabilitation has been shown to improve exercise capacity and physical functioning, to alleviate anxiety and depression, and to improve QOL for patients with many types of chronic lung disease especially COPD. PR is cost effective and, if well planned and executed, can provide durable benefits and reduce health care use. Despite the wealth of evidence of efficacy and guidelines stating that PR is a key element in the management of most chronic lung diseases it is not prescribed for or used by many eligible patients. Further efforts are needed to improve the use, implementation, and delivery of this valuable therapy.

REFERENCES

1. Global Initiative for Chronic Obstructive Lung Disease. Pocket guide to COPD diagnosis, management, and prevention: a guide for healthcare professionals. Global Initiative for Chronic Obstructive Lung Disease; 2017.

2. Garvey C, Fullwood MD, Rigler J. Pulmonary rehabilitation exercise prescription in chronic obstructive lung disease: US survey and review of guidelines and clinical practices. J Cardiopulm Rehabil Prev 2013;33:314–22.
3. American Association of Cardiovascular and Pulmonary Rehabilitation. Guidelines for pulmonary rehabilitation programs. 4th edition. Champaign (IL): Human Kinetics; 2011.
4. Nici L, Donner C, Wouters E, et al. American Thoracic Society/European Respiratory Society statement on pulmonary rehabilitation. Am J Respir Crit Care Med 2006;173:1390–413.
5. Carlin BW. Pulmonary rehabilitation and chronic lung disease: opportunities for the respiratory therapist. Respir Care 2009;54:1091–9.
6. Gosselink R, Troosters T, Decramer M. Peripheral muscle weakness contributes to exercise limitation in COPD. Am J Respir Crit Care Med 1996;153:976–80.
7. Rochester CL, Vogiatzis I, Holland AE, et al. An Official American Thoracic Society/European Respiratory Society Policy Statement: enhancing implementation, use, and delivery of pulmonary rehabilitation. Am J Respir Crit Care Med 2015; 192:1373–86.
8. Spruit MA, Singh SJ, Garvey C, et al. An official American Thoracic Society/European Respiratory Society statement: key concepts and advances in pulmonary rehabilitation. Am J Respir Crit Care Med 2013;188:e13–64.
9. Roig M, Eng JJ, MacIntyre DL, et al. Falls in people with chronic obstructive pulmonary disease: an observational cohort study. Respir Med 2011;105:461–9.
10. Roig M, Eng JJ, MacIntyre DL, et al. Deficits in muscle strength, mass, quality, and mobility in people with chronic obstructive pulmonary disease. J Cardiopulm Rehabil Prev 2011;31:120–4.
11. Coventry PA, Hind D. Comprehensive pulmonary rehabilitation for anxiety and depression in adults with chronic obstructive pulmonary disease: Systematic review and meta-analysis. J Psychosom Res 2007;63:551–65.
12. Hill NS. Pulmonary rehabilitation. Proc Am Thorac Soc 2006;3:66–74.
13. Hui KP, Hewitt AB. A simple pulmonary rehabilitation program improves health outcomes and reduces hospital utilization in patients with COPD. Chest 2003; 124:94–7.
14. Williams S, Baxter N, Holmes S, et al. IMPRESS guide to the relative value of COPD interventions. In: British Thoracic Society Reports, 4. British Thoracic Society and the Primary Care Respiratory Society UK; 2012.
15. Sin DD, Anthonisen NR, Soriano JB, et al. Mortality in COPD: Role of comorbidities. Eur Respir J 2006;28:1245–57.
16. Rochester CL, Fairburn C, Crouch RH. Pulmonary rehabilitation for respiratory disorders other than chronic obstructive pulmonary disease. Clin Chest Med 2014;35:369–89.
17. Puhan MA, Gimeno-Santos E, Cates CJ, et al. Pulmonary rehabilitation following exacerbations of chronic obstructive pulmonary disease. Cochrane Database Syst Rev 2016;(12):CD005305.
18. Ram FS, Robinson SM, Black PN, et al. Physical training for asthma. Cochrane Database Syst Rev 2005;(9):CD001116.
19. Ong HK, Lee AL, Hill CJ, et al. Effects of pulmonary rehabilitation in bronchiectasis: a retrospective study. Chron Respir Dis 2011;8:21–30.
20. McCarthy B, Casey D, Devane D, et al. Pulmonary rehabilitation for chronic obstructive pulmonary disease. Cochrane Database Syst Rev 2015;(2):CD003793.
21. Bradley J, Moran F. Physical training for cystic fibrosis. Cochrane Database Syst Rev 2008;(1):CD002768.

22. Dowman L, Hill CJ, Holland AE. Pulmonary rehabilitation for interstitial lung disease. Cochrane Database Syst Rev 2014;(10):CD006322.
23. Cesario A, Ferri L, Galetta D, et al. Pre-operative pulmonary rehabilitation and surgery for lung cancer. Lung Cancer 2007;57:118–9.
24. Wickerson L, Mathur S, Brooks D. Exercise training after lung transplantation: a systematic review. J Heart Lung Transplant 2010;29:497–503.
25. Ries AL, Make BJ, Lee SM, et al. The effects of pulmonary rehabilitation in the national emphysema treatment trial. Chest 2005;128:3799–809.
26. Mainguy V, Maltais F, Saey D, et al. Effects of a rehabilitation program on skeletal muscle function in idiopathic pulmonary arterial hypertension. J Cardiopulm Rehabil Prev 2010;30:319–23.
27. Global Initiative for Chronic Obstructive Lung Disease. Global strategy for the diagnosis, management, and prevention of chronic obstructive pulmonary disease (2018 report). Global Initiative for Chronic Obstructive Lung Disease; 2018.
28. Anthonisen NR, Connett JE, Murray RP. Smoking and lung function of Lung Health Study participants after 11 years. Am J Respir Crit Care Med 2002;166: 675–9.
29. Gladysheva ES, Malhotra A, Owens RL. Influencing the decline of lung function in COPD: use of pharmacotherapy. Int J Chron Obstruct Pulmon Dis 2010;5:153–64.
30. Rice KL, Dewan N, Bloomfield HE, et al. Disease management program for chronic obstructive pulmonary disease: a randomized controlled trial. Am J Respir Crit Care Med 2010;182:890–6.
31. Coventry PA. Does pulmonary rehabilitation reduce anxiety and depression in chronic obstructive pulmonary disease? Curr Opin Pulm Med 2009;15:143–9.
32. Celli BR, Cote CG, Marin JM, et al. The body-mass index, airflow obstruction, dyspnea, and exercise capacity index in chronic obstructive pulmonary disease. N Engl J Med 2004;350:1005–12.
33. Green RH, Singh SJ, Williams J, et al. A randomised controlled trial of four weeks versus seven weeks of pulmonary rehabilitation in chronic obstructive pulmonary disease. Thorax 2001;56:143–5.
34. Lally P, van Jaarsveld CH, Potts HW, et al. How habits are formed: Modeling habit formation in the real world. Eur J Soc Psychol 2009;40:998–1009.
35. Beauchamp MK, Evans R, Janaudis-Ferreira T, et al. Systematic review of supervised exercise programs after pulmonary rehabilitation in individuals with COPD. Chest 2013;144:1124–33.
36. Guell R, Casan P, Belda J, et al. Long-term effects of outpatient rehabilitation of COPD: a randomized trial. Chest 2000;117:976–83.
37. Spencer LM, Alison JA, McKeough ZJ. Maintaining benefits following pulmonary rehabilitation: a randomised controlled trial. Eur Respir J 2010;35:571–7.

Preoperative Pulmonary Evaluation

Angela Selzer, MD[a], Mona Sarkiss, MD, PhD[b],*

KEYWORDS

- Preoperative evaluation • Preoperative testing • Pulmonary disease
- Preoperative risk assessment

KEY POINTS

- The preoperative assessment is a valuable opportunity to mitigate risk and optimize and educate patients.
- Preoperative risk assessment should include evaluation for risk of obstructive sleep apnea, pulmonary complications, cardiac complications, and venous thromboembolism.
- Routine preoperative testing is unnecessary. Preoperative testing should be triggered by findings on examination, patient history, and review of systems and should be appropriate for the scheduled surgery.
- Patients with pulmonary pathologies require thorough evaluation and planning for optimal outcomes.
- Smoking cessation should be encouraged and supported in all patients presenting for preoperative evaluation and is associated with higher success rates than cessation at other times.

INTRODUCTION

The preanesthesia evaluation is an opportunity to elucidate a patient's underlying medical disease, determine if the patient is optimized, treat modifiable conditions, screen for potentially unrecognized disorders, and present a clear picture of the patient's overall risk for perioperative complications. Relative to their nonevaluated peers, patients who have a thorough preoperative evaluation in a preanesthesia clinic

Disclosure Statement: The authors do not have any relationship with a commercial company that has a direct financial interest in subject matter or materials discussed in article or with a company making a competing product.
[a] Department of Anesthesiology, University of Colorado, 12401 East 17th Avenue, 7th floor, Aurora, CO 80045, USA; [b] Department of Anesthesiology and Perioperative Medicine, University of Texas MD Anderson Cancer Center, 1515 Holcombe Boulevard, Unit 409, Houston, TX 77030, USA
* Corresponding author.
E-mail address: msarkiss@mdanderson.org

Med Clin N Am 103 (2019) 585–599
https://doi.org/10.1016/j.mcna.2018.12.016
0025-7125/19/© 2019 Elsevier Inc. All rights reserved.

medical.theclinics.com

have been shown to have reduced same-day case delays and cancellations,[1,2] decreased hospital length of stays,[3] and a reduction in in-hospital mortality rates.[4]

In this article, the authors present the preoperative assessment of pulmonary patients in 2 sections. First, the components of a thorough assessment of patients presenting for preanesthesia evaluation, which should occur for all patients, regardless of the presence of pulmonary pathology, are discussed. Then, the considerations unique to patients with pulmonary diseases commonly encountered are described.

GENERAL PREANESTHESIA ASSESSMENT

According to the American Society of Anesthesiologists (ASA) Practice Advisory for Preanesthesia Evaluation,[5] the minimum component of a preanesthesia evaluation includes a history taking, evaluation of pertinent medical records, ordering and review of indicated testing, a patient interview, and a focused physical examination. This examination must include an airway evaluation and cardiopulmonary examination.

Testing

There are no routinely indicated laboratory tests or investigations, and patients without significant systemic disease undergoing low risk surgery should proceed to surgery without any testing, regardless of age. Reducing routine preoperative testing in these patients is a focus of the American Board of Internal Medicine Choosing Wisely campaign (www.choosingwisely.org).[6,7] Routine preoperative laboratory testing, cardiac testing, and chest radiographs have been identified as a significant source of unnecessary testing.

On the other hand, patients scheduled for high-risk surgeries (such as open vascular, lung resections, or major spine) should have their hemoglobin, platelet count, and electrolytes tested and a type and screen ordered. Patients with severe systemic disease may require testing even if scheduled for low-risk surgery, to assess whether a patient is optimized. For example, patients with liver disease may require liver function testing, a platelet count, and coagulation testing. Hypertensive patients should have a baseline creatinine measured.[8] A thorough review of systems also may lead to additional testing if, for example, a patient reports a significant bleeding history.

Routine chest radiography is not recommended by the American College of Radiology[9] but may be indicated in the presence of symptoms, findings on examination, or prior abnormal radiograph. The 2009 American Heart Association (AHA) Science Advisory on the Cardiovascular Evaluation and Management of Severely Obese Patients Undergoing Surgery advocates for a screening chest radiograph in severely obese patients (body mass index [BMI] >40).[10]

Routine ECG screening is not indicated in asymptomatic patients with low perioperative risk of death or myocardial infarction. In patients with risk factors for coronary artery disease, further testing should be obtained if indicated by the American College of Cardiology /AHA Guideline on Perioperative Cardiovascular Evaluation and Management of Patients Undergoing Noncardiac Surgery.[11] The algorithm for testing (**Fig. 1**) requires assessment of cardiac risk as well as assessment of the patient's functional status.

Functional Assessment

Patients who can achieve an activity level of greater than or equal to 4 metabolic equivalents of tasks (METs) without symptoms do not require further testing. One MET is equivalent to the resting oxygen uptake in an adult (3.5 mL O_2/kg/min). Functional status can be assessed by asking patients what is the most strenuous activity

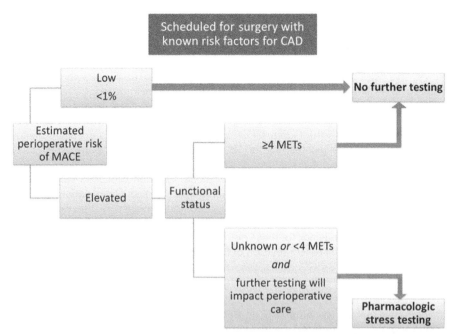

Fig. 1. Algorithm guiding preoperative cardiovascular testing. MACE, major adverse cardiac event. (*Data from* Fleisher LA, Fleischmann KE, Auerbach AD, et al. 2014 ACC/AHA guideline on perioperative cardiovascular evaluation and management of patients undergoing noncardiac surgery: executive summary: a report of the American College of Cardiology/American Heart Association Task Force on practice guidelines. Circulation 2014;130(24):2215–45.)

they participate in and then correlating that activity with a METs score according to the METs activity code table.[12] For example, strenuous housework, mowing the lawn, or walking up a flight of stairs are all activities that typically result in greater than or equal to 4 METs of energy expenditure. Patient surveys, such as the Duke Activity Status Index,[13] also are established and validated as accurate tools of assessment. Cardiopulmonary testing and oxygen consumption per unit time measurement are considered the gold standard for functional testing but uncommonly used in the United States due to cost, accessibility, and physical limitations.

Cardiac Risk Assessment

In addition to functional assessment, patients' relative cardiac risk also should be determined. There are several cardiac risk indices in use today, but the most widely used and validated is the Lee Revised Cardiac Risk Index (RCRI),[14] developed in 1999. This index is a modification of the original Goldman Cardiac Risk Index from 1977.[15] Given that the RCRI requires only yes-or-no answers to 6 questions, it is easy to use. It was developed, however, using a relatively small cohort of patients (4315) prior to the adoption of minimally invasive surgery techniques. Therefore, it tends to overestimate risk in the ambulatory surgery population.[8]

Newer-risk indices require the use of an online calculator to perform. The Gupta index, published in 2011, assesses risk for perioperative myocardial infarction and cardiac arrest (MICA).[16] It was developed from the 2007 National Surgical Quality Improvement Program (NSQIP) database and included 211,410 patients. It was validated from the 2008 NSQIP data set of 257,385 patients but was not externally validated. The Gupta MICA risk prediction model had a better C statistic than the RCRI score (0.884 vs 0.747, respectively).

The American College of Surgeons (ACS) developed an online Surgical Risk Calculator (SRC), which assesses individual risk for several adverse events, including cardiac.[17] This was also derived from the NSQIP database from 2009 to 2012 and included 1,414,006 patients. Use of the ACS-SRC requires knowledge of a patient's specific surgery (as designated by 1 of 1557 Current Procedural Terminology [CPT] codes) and entry of 19 specific patient factors (**Table 1**). Therefore, it is more cumbersome to use than both the Gupta MICA and RCRI indices. It is particularly useful, however, because it evaluates risk for 12 complications and compares these risks to those of the average patient having the same surgery, providing the patient a visual representation of the relative risk of complications. The complications included are serious complication, any complication, pneumonia, cardiac complication, surgical site infection, urinary tract infection, venous thromboembolism (VTE), renal failure, readmission, return to the operating room, death, and discharge to nursing or rehabilitation facility. The C statistics for these complications are high and range from 0.76 to 0.94, based on the most recent revision of the ACS-SRC.[18] The C statistic for cardiac risk is 0.884 in the ACS-SRC, statistically equivalent to the Gupta MICA.

Pulmonary Risk Assessment

Postoperative pulmonary complications (PPCs) occur as frequently as cardiac complications and result in increased costs, morbidity, and long-term mortality.[19] Therefore, it is important to assess pulmonary risk in all preoperative patients. The ACS-SRC calculates risk of pneumonia, but there are also 4 other risk calculators specific to

Table 1
American College of Surgeons Surgical Risk Calculator

Variable Included	Outcome Assessed
Surgical CPT code	Serious complication
Age	Any complication
Gender	Cardiac complication
Functional status	Surgical site infection
Emergency case	Urinary tract infection
ASA class	VTE
Use of steroids for a chronic condition	Renal failure
Ascites within 30 days prior to surgery	Readmission
Systemic sepsis within 48 hours of surgery	Return to the operating room
Ventilator dependent	Death
Disseminated cancer	Discharge to nursing or rehabilitation facility
Diabetes	
Hypertension requiring medication	
Congestive heart failure in 30 days prior to surgery	
Dyspnea	
Current smoker within 1 year	
History of severe COPD	
Dialysis	
Acute renal failure	
BMI	

Data from American College of Surgeons National Surgical Quality Improvement Program. Surgical risk calculator. Available at: https://riskcalculator.facs.org/RiskCalculator/. Accessed December 18, 2018.

pulmonary complications. Arozullah and colleagues[20] developed the first pulmonary-specific risk index in 2000. This index, which predicted relative risk of postoperative respiratory failure, was derived from a cohort of patients that included only men having major noncardiac surgery and, therefore, has an unknown applicability in other patient populations.

In the following decade, 2 Gupta indices were developed, 1 for respiratory failure and 1 for pneumonia, developed in 2011 and 2013, respectively.[21,22] Like the Gupta MICA calculator, the Gupta pulmonary risk calculators were derived and validated from 2007 and 2008 NSQIP data. Both indices found ASA status, dependent functional status, type of surgery, and the presence of preoperative sepsis significant risk factors for PPCs. Emergency surgery is included in the respiratory failure calculator. In the pneumonia calculator, age and diagnosis of chronic obstructive pulmonary disease (COPD) or a smoking history are included.

In 2010, Canet and colleagues[23] published the ARISCAT pulmonary risk calculator. This calculator was derived from a much smaller cohort of 2464 patients with an even gender distribution. An important feature of the ARISCAT (Assess Respiratory Risk in Surgical Patients in Catalonia) calculator is that it predicts the likelihood of any PPC, including pneumonia, respiratory failure, pleural effusion, atelectasis, pneumothorax, bronchospasm, and aspiration pneumonitis. Given the outcome included 7 PPCs, patients' relative risks of PPCs are much higher via the ARISCAT index than the Gupta and Arozullah indices. Patients in the highest risk group of this index have a 44% risk of PPCs. Age, preoperative oxygen saturation as measured by pulse oximetry, respiratory infection within 1 month, anemia, surgical incision site, duration of surgery, and emergency surgery are the predictors used in the model.

Venous Thromboembolism Risk Assessment

Patients are at an increased risk of VTE in the perioperative period due to venous stasis, inflammation, reduced mobility, and a hypercoagulable state.[24] The assessment of VTE risk should be performed in all patients to develop an appropriate plan of perioperative VTE risk reduction. The most commonly used tool is the Caprini Score (http://venousdisease.com/dvt-risk-assessment-online/).[25] Patients with the lowest risk score (0) need only early ambulation during their hospitalization. Patients with the highest risk scores (≥8), however, are recommended to have compression boots and prophylactic anticoagulation for 30 days total.[24]

Obstructive Sleep Apnea Risk Assessment

It is estimated that 9% to 24% of the general population has obstructive sleep apnea (OSA). Of these patients, 80% of men and 93% of women with moderate to severe OSA are undiagnosed.[26] Patients with OSA have a significantly higher rates of PPCs, overall complications, and mortality and longer hospital lengths of stay.[27,28] These complications can be reduced by implementation of positive airway pressure (PAP) therapy during the perioperative hospitalization.[28] The Society of Anesthesia and Sleep Medicine Guidelines on Preoperative Screening and Assessment of Adult Patients with Obstructive Sleep Apnea from 2016 state, however, that there is currently insufficient evidence to support delaying surgery to obtain OSA testing and implement PAP preoperatively in patients with a high probability of OSA unless there is evidence of severe systemic disease, such as severe pulmonary hypertension (PH), resting hypoxemia, or hypoventilation syndrome.[28]

The STOP-Bang assessment tool is highly sensitive for OSA. Positive STOP-Bang questionnaires identified patients with mild OSA (apnea-hypopnea index [AHI] >5) in 84% of cases, 93% of moderate OSA cases (AHI >15), and 100% of severe OSA cases (AHI >30).[29,30] The specificity of the questionnaire is fairly low (37%–56%) and is not diagnostic, so patients deemed at high risk for OSA via the STOP-Bang questionnaire should receive formal testing. Reported snoring, observed apnea, tiredness during the daytime, hypertension, BMI greater than 35 kg/m^2, male gender, and increased neck circumference (>41 cm in women and >43 cm in men) are associated with increased OSA risk (**Table 2**).

Patients with known OSA on PAP therapy at home should have continued use of that therapy at their prescribed settings during their hospitalization, unless contraindicated. According to institutional protocol, patients may bring their own PAP equipment or use the facility equipment. PAP may be administered continuously, autotitrated, or bilevel. The use of nonopioid analgesics and regional anesthesia techniques also helps mitigate risk of postoperative desaturation. Patients with known OSA may not be candidates for surgery in an outpatient center if they are noncompliant with PAP therapy, are unable to use PAP postoperatively, or have significant comorbidities.[31]

Smoking Cessation

Smoking cessation in the preoperative period has been shown to result in higher rates of long-term cessation than smoking cessation at other times.[32] It is well known that smoking results in widespread physiologic detriment. In the perioperative period, smokers are at an increased 30-day mortality and risks of major morbidity, including PPCs, surgical site infection, ICU admissions, wound complications, neurologic complications, and septic shock.[33,34]

A majority of smokers are motivated to quit and the preoperative assessment is an opportunity to support cessation. Cessation for 6 weeks to 8 weeks prior to scheduled

Table 2
STOP-Bang questionnaire to assess obstructive sleep apnea risk

STOP	Bang
Snore • Do you snore loudly (louder than talking or loud enough to be heard through closed doors)?	BMI >35 kg/m^2
Tired • Do you often feel tired, fatigued, or sleepy during daytime?	Age >50 y
Observed • Has anyone observed you stop breathing during your sleep?	Neck circumference: >41 cm (females), >43 cm (males)
Blood pressure • Do you have or are you being treated for high blood pressure	Gender: male
Risk stratification	
0–2 YES answers	Low risk
3–4 YES answers	Intermediate risk
5–8 YES answers	High risk
2 + STOP answers + BMI >35	High risk
2 + STOP answers + increased neck circumference	High risk
2 + STOP answers + male gender	High risk

Data from Chung F, Yegneswaran B, Liao P, et al. STOP questionnaire: a tool to screen patients for obstructive sleep apnea. Anesthesiology 2008;108(5):812–21.

surgery is ideal but rarely achievable. Cessation for shorter durations results in reduced circulating levels of carboxyhemoglobin, increased delivery of oxygen to the tissues, and improved ciliary clearance.

PREANESTHESIA ASSESSMENT FOR PATIENTS WITH PULMONARY PATHOLOGY

Preoperative assessment specific to patients with pulmonary pathology is addressed. There are several excellent review articles and book chapters that address this topic in detail.[35–44] OSA and pulmonary risk assessment are discussed previously and are particularly applicable to this patient population. Other common pulmonary conditions are discussed in this section. Many patients, however, have a combination of pulmonary comorbidities, such as asthma and COPD or OSA and PH.

In any patient managed for chronic disease by a pulmonologist, preoperative consultation with that pulmonologist should be sought. This is necessary to determine the extent, severity, and stability of the disease to determine if the patient is optimized, assess compliance with prescribed therapies, evaluate perioperative risk of PPCs, obtain recommendations for risk mitigation in the perioperative period, and gather results of recent pulmonary function tests (PFTs) or chest imaging. If time permits, a formal preoperative assessment with the pulmonologist could be obtained. Alternatively, a copy of the most recent office consult note along with a discussion between pulmonologist and preoperative provider or anesthesiologist may be adequate.

Referral to a pulmonologist may be considered in patients with unexplained dyspnea on exertion, hypoxemia, hemoptysis, PH, poorly controlled asthma or COPD, abnormal chest imaging, or recent hospitalizations or emergency room visits for acute pulmonary processes (**Table 3**). It is reasonable to delay elective surgery in patients with an acute exacerbation, recent infection, or worsening of symptoms for 4 weeks to 6 weeks from resolution of symptoms. All patients, especially patients with pulmonary disease, should receive smoking cessation counseling and support.

Asthma

Well-controlled asthma is not a risk factor for PPCs. Poorly controlled asthma and/or the presence of wheezing on examination, however, are risk factors.[38,45] Signs of poorly controlled asthma include presence of symptoms or the use of short-acting bronchodilators greater than 2 days per week, peak expiratory flow rate less than

Table 3
Reasons for and considerations of preoperative pulmonology referrals

Referral Reason	Considerations
Abnormal chest imaging	Evidence of nodules, ILD, COPD, airway obstruction
Dyspnea on exertion	Suspected pulmonary etiology. Consider: chest imaging, PFTs, CBC, BMP, BNP, albumin, echocardiogram
Emergency department visits/ hospitalizations for pulmonary processes	Poorly controlled or undiagnosed chronic pulmonary disease Consider: chest imaging, PFTs, ABG, BMP, BNP, echocardiogram, OSA testing
Hemoptysis	Consider: chest imaging and CBC
Hypoxemia	Desaturation at rest or with activity requiring oxygen Consider: chest imaging, PFTs, ABG, BMP, BNP, echocardiogram, OSA testing
PH	Detected on cardiac imaging: referral to PAH specialist

80% of personal best, weekly nighttime awakening, and 2 or more exacerbations requiring systemic corticosteroids in the past year.[38] Treatment is determined based on a stepwise approach.[46] Frequent symptoms or exacerbations despite compliance to treatment should elicit a pulmonology referral. Spirometry may be obtained to evaluate patient status relative to baseline. All medications should be continued preoperatively and taken on the day of surgery.

Chronic Obstructive Pulmonary Disease

COPD is a risk factor for PPCs. The Global Initiative for Chronic Obstructive Lung Disease (GOLD) classification system assesses severity of COPD based on forced expiratory volume in the first second of expiration (FEV_1) as a % of predicted.[47] Many patients with COPD do not have a formal diagnosis. Patients with risk factors for COPD, hypoxia on room air, or symptoms, such as cough, sputum, and dyspnea, should have testing and therapy prior to elective surgery. Patients with a recent exacerbation or poorly controlled COPD should not undergo elective surgery until further optimized.

Pulmonary rehabilitation has been shown in this patient population to reduce postoperative morbidity and mortality, specifically in patients undergoing pulmonary resection.[48–50] Routine testing in patients with chronic, stable COPD is not necessary. If symptoms are reported or there are physical findings on examination, however, a chest radiograph, spirometry, or arterial blood gases (ABG) may be helpful.

INTERSTITIAL LUNG DISEASE

Patients with interstitial lung disease (ILD) are at an increased risk for perioperative morbidity and mortality.[50,51] The highest-risk ILD patients have the following risk factors: preoperative hypoxemia, rapidly progressing ILD, emergency surgery, male gender, advanced age, newly diagnosed disease, and connective tissue disease–associated ILD.[40] Patients with long-standing hypoxemia require a through cardiovascular examination and should have a recent ECG. Abnormalities may lead to echocardiography to assess right heart function. Patients with connective tissue–related disease also should be assessed for the systemic sequelae of those diseases. Additional testing should be guided by the history and physical examination and may include basic metabolic panel (BMP), liver function tests (LFT), complete blood cell count (CBC), ABG, ECG, echocardiography, chest radiograph, and PFTs. All patients with a diagnosis of ILD should be under the care of a pulmonologist, consultation with whom should be sought.

PULMONARY HYPERTENSION

Perioperative morbidity and mortality for patients with PH is extremely high.[52,53] No patient with a new diagnosis of PH should proceed with elective surgery without a thorough work-up and evaluation with a PH specialist.[41] PH is classified into 5 groups based on etiology.[54] PH should be expected in patients with progressive dyspnea, signs of right ventricular failure, and chest pain or palpitations. Work-up includes bone natriuretic peptide (BNP), ECG, chest radiograph, an echocardiogram, and right heart catheterization (RHC).

Although severity of PH is determined by the extent of mean pulmonary artery pressure (mPAP) elevation, the mPAP should be taken in the context of the systemic pressures, and elevated mPAPs are most concerning in the setting of systemic hypotension. Likewise, RV dilation and/or reduced function are particularly concerning signs on echocardiography. Functional assessment via the World Health Organization

Class	Definition
Table 4 **World Health Organization functional classification of pulmonary hypertension**	
Class I	No limitation of physical activity No undue dyspnea or fatigue, chest pain, or near syncope with ordinary physical activity
Class II	Slight limitation of physical activity Comfortable at rest Undue dyspnea or fatigue, chest pain, or near syncope with ordinary physical activity
Class III	Marked limitation of physical activity Comfortable at rest Undue dyspnea or fatigue, chest pain, or near syncope with less than ordinary activity causes
Class IV	Signs of right heart failure Dyspnea and/or fatigue may be present at rest Inability to carry out any physical activity without symptoms

Adapted from Rich S. A new classification of pulmonary hypertension. Adv Pulm Hyper 2002;1(1):3–8; with permission.

(WHO) classification of PH should be assessed (**Table 4**). Patients who are WHO class III or IV should not undergo elective surgery, because they have a mortality risk as high as 40%.[55,56]

An RHC is necessary for definitive diagnosis and classification and is strongly recommended for patients with an estimated Pulmonary Artery Systolic Pressure (PASP) of greater than 45 mm Hg on echocardiogram. A vasodilator challenge of inhaled nitric oxide can be performed during the RHC to identify the small subgroup of patients with positive pulmonary vascular reactivity (approximately%). All medications for PH should be continued preoperatively and these patients are high risk for decompensation in the setting of PE, so VTE prophylaxis should take this in account.[57]

LUNG CANCER

Lung resection surgery confers the highest risk of complications of all noncardiac surgeries. The most common perioperative morbidities include arrhythmia, pneumonia, acute respiratory failure, and need for blood transfusion or reoperation.[42] It is not uncommon for patients presenting for lung cancer resection to have other pulmonary comorbidities. Research on outcomes for lung resection have shown a higher rate of complications in smokers[58] and in patients with concomitant COPD or ILD.[50,51] These surgeries are urgent but not emergent and it may be prudent to postpone surgery to better mitigate risk, especially in the setting of worsening pulmonary function.

Signs of spread of lung cancer may be found on examination or review of history and may lead to further imaging and evaluation prior to surgery. These include hoarseness, elevated hemidiaphragm, Horner syndrome, lymphadenopathy, localized chest pain, pleural effusion, and superior vena cava obstruction.[59]

These patients should have CBC, prothrombin time/partial thromboplastin time (PT/PTT), BMP, albumin, and liver function tests to assess baseline function and screen for metastatic disease.[59] They also should have blood typed and crossed prior to surgery. Most patients have CT-PET imaging ordered by their thoracic surgeon or pulmonologist. This is one group of patients for whom routine PFTs are warranted. Predicting the postoperative FEV_1 and diffusing capacity of lung for carbon monoxide is a component for determining surgical candidacy.[60] Short-term preoperative exercise therapy does not seem to improve long-term outcomes after lung cancer surgery but ability to perform exercise does impart a decreased morbidity in the short term.[61–64]

Patients with inadequate pulmonary function or widely metastatic disease may not be candidates for resection but can present in the preoperative clinic for evaluation prior to palliative surgeries or procedures. These patients are high risk for PPCs. All patients with cancer are at an increased risk of VTE, and a plan for adequate perioperative VTE prophylaxis should be established.

LUNG TRANSPLANTATION

Patients who are candidates for lung transplantation may present for evaluation prior to transplantation or may be seen in clinic after transplantation for another surgery. Because of superior outcomes, patients are most commonly candidates for double-lung transplant. Single-lung and heart-lung transplants, however, also are performed. Indications for lung transplantation include cystic fibrosis, chronic bronchiectasis, ILD, PH, COPD, congenital disease, and prior rejection.[64] The lung allocation scoring (LAS) system incorporates patient variables to determine organ allocation.[65] The LAS score is provided to the United Network for Organ Sharing (UNOS) and must be updated every 2 weeks to 6 months, depending on score.[66] As part of the LAS system, patients have PFTs, RHC, echocardiography, and exercise assessment.

Additional testing for these patients includes ECG, BNP, BMP, CBC, PT/PTT, and albumin. Packed red blood cells (pRBC), fresh frozen plasma (FFP), and platelets should be typed and crossed. Patients should be screened for comorbidities, such as cardiac disease, renal insufficiency, and VTE. Periodic re-evaluation is necessary to address recipient candidacy.

Patients with prior lung transplantation may present for follow-up biopsies or other nonpulmonary procedures or surgeries. These patients should be routinely monitored by their transplantation team and consultation with them should be sought as part of the thorough preoperative evaluation. The indication for and date of transplant should be noted as well as whether it was a single transplant, double transplant, or retransplant. Noting the location of anastomosis and presence of stents can assist the anesthesia team in selection of airway device. Patients frequently are surveilled with biopsies and PFTs. Chronic rejection may result in bronchiolitis obliterans syndrome and deterioration of pulmonary function.[64] Approximately 2% of transplants are retransplants due to rejection or graft failure.

Evaluating the most recent PFT report and a good functional assessment are important.[67] The presence of findings on physical examination may warrant further chest imaging with the input of the transplant team.

Patients with transplanted organs are on chronic immunosuppression, which they should continue perioperatively. Stress-dose steroids may be indicated. Signs and sequelae of chronic steroid use should be identified and risk modification undertaken when applicable. Treating hypertension, hyperlipidemia, or hyperglycemia may be warranted to reduce risk and improve outcomes.[67]

ANTERIOR MEDIASTINAL MASS

Patients with anterior mediastinal masses represent a great challenge due to the well-reported and feared complications of lost airway and cardiovascular collapse, either at induction of anesthesia or during the postoperative period. A thorough preoperative assessment of the compressive effect of the mass on vital mediastinal structure is essential for the planning of the anesthetic and surgical management as well as anticipating postprocedure complications.[68]

The severity of signs and symptoms varies depending on the structures compressed and the degree of compression. For example, compression of the recurrent laryngeal nerve can cause hoarseness or Inspiratory stridor. Tracheal compression can result in expiratory stridor, orthopnea, use of accessory muscles, hypoxemia, and the need for supplemental oxygen. Esophageal compression results in dysphagia, malnutrition, and dehydration. Superior vena cava compression can manifest as swelling of the face and upper extremity, enlarged neck veins, and engorged collateral venous plexus on the anterior chest wall. Patients can present in extremes with tachycardia, arrhythmias, hypertension due to anxiety, hypoxemia, and carbon dioxide retention.[69]

CT imaging with and without contrast is essential for assessment. Laboratory testing should include ABG, CBC, and BMP. Although PFT has been advocated to reflect the degree of airway obstruction, no significant correlation was found between peak expiratory flow rate and intraoperative airway collapse. Peak expiratory flow rate of less than 40%, however, was associated with a 10-fold increase in postoperative respiratory complications.

Predictors of perioperative complications are cardiorespiratory symptoms and signs, mixed obstructive and restrictive pulmonary disease on PFT, and the presence of pericardial effusion. Meanwhile, tracheal compression greater than 50% and mixed pulmonary syndrome on PFT are commonly associated with postoperative respiratory complications.

Pretreatment of patients with anterior mediastinal mass with chemotherapy and/or radiotherapy can decrease the size of the mass and its compressive effect but can pose another risk due to the side effects of such treatment, for example, bleomycin lung toxicity or doxorubicin cardiotoxicity.

SUMMARY

The preoperative evaluation is an important opportunity to improve patient outcomes during the perioperative period. PPCs can lead to long-term morbidity, increased health care costs, and even mortality. Therefore, it is crucial to mitigate the risk of these complications as much as possible. Patients with underlying pulmonary disease require careful attention and planning for optimal outcomes. In addition to ensuring that their underlying pulmonary diseases are optimized and stable, these patients benefit from standard risk reduction strategies as well. Cardiac, VTE, pulmonary, and OSA risk assessments should be performed in all patients. Preoperative testing should be appropriate for the invasiveness of surgery and guided by patient history and physical examination. It is the duty of the preoperative physician to encourage and support smoking cessation for optimal long-term health.

REFERENCES

1. Fischer SP. Development and effectiveness of an anesthesia preoperative evaluation clinic in a teaching hospital. Anesthesiology 1996;85:196–206.

2. Ferschl MB, Tung A, Sweitzer B, et al. Preoperative clinic visits reduce operating room cancellations and delays. Anesthesiology 2005;103:855–9.

3. van Klei WA, Moons KG, Rutten CL, et al. The effect of outpatient preoperative evaluation of hospital inpatients on cancellation of surgery and length of hospital stay. Anesth Analg 2002;94:644–9.

4. Blitz JD, Kendale SM, Jain SK, et al. Preoperative evaluation clinic visit is associated with decreased risk of in-hospital postoperative mortality. Anesthesiology 2016;125:280–94.
5. Pasternak LR, Arens JF, Caplan RA, et al. Practice advisory for preanesthesia evaluation: an updated report by the American Society of Anesthesiologists Task Force on preanesthesia evaluation. Anesthesiology 2012;116:522–38.
6. Things physicians and providers should question. Choosing wisely. American board of Internal Medicine Foundation; 2014. Available at: http://www.choosingwisely.org/doctor-patient-lists/.
7. Colla CH, Morden NE, Sequist TD, et al. Choosing wisely: prevalence and correlates of low-value health care services in the United States. J Gen Intern Med 2015;30(2):221–8.
8. Cohn SL. Preoperative evaluation for noncardiac surgery. Ann Intern Med 2016; 165(11):ITC81–96.
9. Expert Panel on Thoracic Imaging, McComb BL, Chung JH, et al. ACR appropriateness criteria routine chest radiography. J Thorac Imaging 2016;31(2):w13–5.
10. Pourier P, Alpert MA, Fleisher LA, et al. Cardiovascular evaluation and management of severely obese patients undergoing surgery: a science advisory from the American Heart Association. Circulation 2009;120:86–95.
11. Fleisher LA, Fleischmann KE, Auerbach AD, et al. 2014 ACC/AHA guideline on perioperative cardiovascular evaluation and management of patients undergoing noncardiac surgery: executive summary. A report of the American College of Cardiology/American Heart Association Task Force on practice guidelines. Circulation 2014;130:2215–45.
12. Ainsworth BE, Haskell WL, Whitt MC, et al. Compendium of physical activities: an update of activity codes and MET intensities. Med Sci Sports Exerc 2000;32: S498–516.
13. Hlatky MA, Boineau RE, Higginbotham MB, et al. A brief self-administered questionnaire to determine functional capacity (the Duke Activity Status Index). Am J Cardiol 1989;64(10):651–4.
14. Lee TH, Marcantonio ER, Mangione CM, et al. Derivation and prospective validation of a simple index for prediction of cardiac risk of major noncardiac surgery. Circulation 1999;100:1043–9.
15. Goldman L, Caldera DL, Nussbaum SR, et al. Multifactorial index of cardiac risk in noncardiac surgical procedures. N Engl J Med 1977;297:845–50.
16. Gupta PK, Gupta H, Sundaram A, et al. Development and validation of a risk calculator for prediction of cardiac risk after surgery. Circulation 2011;124:381–7.
17. Bilimoria KY, Liu Y, Paruch JL, et al. Development and evaluation of the universal ACS NSQIP surgical risk calculator: a decision aid and informed consent tool for patients and surgeons. J Am Coll Surg 2013;217(5):833–42.
18. Liu Y, Cohen ME, Hall BL, et al. Evaluation and enhancement of calibration in the American College of Surgeons NSQIP surgical risk calcolator. J Am Coll Surg 2016;223(2):231–9.
19. Lakshminarasimhachar A, Smetana GW. Preoperative evaluation: estimation of pulmonary risk. Anesthesiol Clin 2016;34:71–88.
20. Arozullah AM, Daley J, Henderson WG, et al. Multifactorial risk index for predicting postoperative respiratory failure in men after major noncardiac surgery. The National Veterans Administration Surgical Quality Improvement Program. Ann Surg 2000;232:242–53.
21. Gupta H, Gupta PK, Fang X, et al. Development and validation of a risk calculator predicting respiratory failure. Chest 2011;140:1207–15.

22. Gupta H, Gupta PK, Schuller D, et al. Development and validation of a risk calculator for predicting postoperative pneumonia. Mayo Clin Proc 2013;88:1241–9.
23. Canet J, Gallart L, Gomar C, et al. Prediction of postoperative pulmonary complications in a population-based surgical cohort. Anesthesiology 2010;113(6): 1338–50.
24. Guyatt GH, Akl EA, Crowhter M, et al. Antithrombotic therapy and prevention of thrombosis 9th ed: American College of Chest Physicians evidence-based clinical practice guidelines. Chest 2012;141:p7S–47S.
25. Falck-Ytter Y, Francis CW, Johanson NA, et al. American College of Chest Physicians. Prevention of VTE in orthopedic surgery patients: antithrombotic therapy and prevention of thrombosis, 9th ed: American College of Chest Physicians evidence-based clinical practice guidelines. Chest 2012;141:e278S–325S.
26. Singh M, Liao P, Kobah S, et al. Proportion of surgical patients with undiagnosed obstructive sleep apnea. Br J Anaesth 2013;110(4):629–36.
27. Memtsoudis SG. The impact of sleep apnea on postoperative utilization of resources and adverse outcomes. Anesth Analg 2014;118(2):407–18.
28. Chung F, Memtsoudis SG, Ramachandran SK, et al. Society of Anesethesia and Sleep Medicine guidelines on preoperative screening and assessment of adult patients with obstructive sleep apnea. Anesth Analg 2016;123(2):452–73.
29. Chung F, Yegneswaran B, Liao P, et al. STOP questionnaire: a tool to screen patients for obstructive sleep apnea. Anesthesiology 2008;108(5):812–21.
30. Chung F, Subramanyam R, Liao P, et al. STOP-Bang score indicates a high probability of obstructive sleep apnoea. Br J Anaesth 2012;108(5):768–75.
31. Joshi GP, Ankichetty SP, Gan TJ, et al. Society for Ambulatory Anesthesia consensus statement on preoperative selection of adult patients with obstructive sleep apnea scheduled for ambulatory surgery. Anesth Analg 2012;115(5): 1060–8.
32. Yu S, Warner DO. Surgery as a teachable moment for smoking cessation. Anesthesiology 2010;112:102–7.
33. Turan A, Mascha EJ, Roberman D, et al. Smoking and perioperative outcomes. Anesthesiology 2011;114:837–46.
34. Gronkjaer M, Eliasen M, Skov-Ettrup LS, et al. Preoperative smoking status and postoperative com.plications: a systematic review and meta-analysis. Ann Surg 2014;259(1):52–71.
35. Bapoje SR, Whitaker JF, Schulz T, et al. Preoperative evaluation of the patient with pulmonary disease. Chest 2007;132:1637–45.
36. Hong CM, Galvagno SM. Patients with chronic pulmonary disease. Med Clin 2013;97(6):1095–107.
37. Sweitzer BJ, Smetana GW. Identification and evaluation of the patient with lung disease. Anesthesiol Clin 2009;27(5):673–86.
38. Costescu F, Slinger P. Asthma. In: Sweitzer BJ, editor. Preoperative assessment and management. 3rd edition. Philadelphia: Wolters Kluwer; 2019. p. p171–4.
39. Costescu F, Slinger P. Chronic obstructive pulmonary disease. In: Sweitzer BJ, editor. Preoperative assessment and management. 3rd edition. Philadelphia: Wolters Kluwer; 2019. p. p166–71.
40. Costescu F, Slinger P. Restrictive and interstitial lung diseases. In: Sweitzer BJ, editor. Preoperative assessment and management. 3rd edition. Philadelphia: Wolters Kluwer; 2019. p. p174–8.
41. Gouvea F, Gouvea G. Pulmonary hypertension. In: Sweitzer BJ, editor. Preoperative assessment and management. 3rd edition. Philadelphia: Wolters Kluwer; 2019. p. p139–42.

42. Alfille PH, Bao X. Patients for lung resection. In: Sweitzer BJ, editor. Preoperative assessment and management. 3rd edition. Philadelphia: Wolters Kluwer; 2019. p. p211–6.

43. Costescu F, Slinger P. Cystic fibrosis. In: Sweitzer BJ, editor. Preoperative assessment and management. 3rd edition. Philadelphia: Wolters Kluwer; 2019. p. p178–80.

44. Alfille PH, Shapiro L. The patient for a lung transplant. In: Sweitzer BJ, editor. Preoperative assessment and management. 3rd edition. Philadelphia: Wolters Kluwer; 2019. p. p186–90.

45. Alfille PH, Shapiro L. The patient with a lung transplant for subsequent surgery. In: Sweitzer BJ, editor. Preoperative assessment and management. 3rd edition. Philadelphia: Wolters Kluwer; 2019. p. p190–3.

46. Woods BD, Sladen RN. Perioperative considerations for the patient with asthma and bronchospasm. Br J Anaesth 2009;103(suppl 1):i57–65.

47. Global initiative for Asthma—Global strategy for asthma management and prevention. Available at: www.ginasthma.org.

48. Global Initiative for Chronic Obstructive Lung Disease—Global strategy for the diagnosis, management and prevention of chronic obstructive pulmonary disease. Available at: www.goldcopd.org.

49. Erdich T, Sadovnikoff N. Anesthesia for patients with severe chronic obstructive pulmonary disease. Curr Opin Anaesthesiol 2010;23:18–24.

50. Mujovic N, Mujovic N, Subotic D, et al. Preoperative pulmonary rehabilitation in patients with non-small cell cancer and chronic obstructive pulmonary disease. Arch Med Sci 2014;10(1):68–75.

51. Minai OA, Yared YP, Kaw R, et al. Perioperative risk and management in patients with pulmonary hypertension. Chest 2013;144:329–40.

52. Memtsoudis SG, Ma Y, Chiu YL, et al. Perioperative mortality in patients with pulmonary hypertension undergoing major joint replacement. Anesth Analg 2010; 111(5):1110–6.

53. Simonneau G, Gatzoulis MA, Adatia I, et al. Updated clinical classification of pulmonary hypertension. J Am Coll Cardiol 2013;62:D34–41.

54. Rich S. A new classification of pulmonary hypertension. Adv Pulm Hyper 2002; 1(1):3–8.

55. Raina A, Humbert M. Risk assessment in pulmonary arterial hypertension. Eur Respir Rev 2016;25(142):390–8.

56. Pilkington SA, Taboada D, Martinez G. Pulmonary hypertension and its management in patients undergoing non-cardiac surgery. Anaesthesia 2015;70:56–70.

57. DeHoyos A, DeCamp M. Preoperative smoking cessation for lung resection patients. In: Ferguson MK, editor. Difficult decision in thoracic surgery: an evidence-based approach. 3rd edition. London: Springer-Verlag; 2014. p. 85–98.

58. Kumar P, Goldstraw P, Yamada K, et al. Pulmonary fibrosis and lung cancer: risk and benefit analysis of pulmonary resection. J Thorac Cardiovasc Surg 2003; 125(6):1321–7.

59. Spiro SG, Gould MK, Colice GL. Initial evaluation of patients with lung cancer: symptoms, signs, laboratory tests, and paraneoplastic syndromes: ACCP evidence-based clinical practice guidelines (2nd edition). Chest 2007;132: 149S–60S.

60. Ferguson MK, Watson S, Johnson E, et al. Predicted postoperative lung function is associated with all-cause long-term mortality after major lung resection for cancer. Eur J Cardiothorac Surg 2014;5(4):660–4.

61. Marjanski T, Wnuk W, Bosakowski D, et al. Patients who do not reach a distance of 500m during the 6-min walk test have an increased risk of post-operative complications and prolonged hospital stay after lobectomy. Eur J Cardiothorac Surg 2015;47(5):e213–9.
62. Karenovics W, Licker M, Ellenberger C, et al. Short-term preoperative exercise therapy does not improve long-term outcome after lung cancer surgery: a randomized controlled study. Eur J Cardiothorac Surg 2017;52(1):47–54.
63. Piraux E, Caty G, Reychler G. Effects of preoperative combined aerobic and resistance exercise training in cancer patients undergoing tumour resection surgery: a systematic review of randomized trials. Surg Oncol 2018;27(3):584–94.
64. Kreider M, Kotloff RM. Selection of candidates for lung transplantation. Proc Am Thorac Soc 2009;6(1):20–7.
65. LAS Calculator US Department of Health and Human Services. Available at: https://optn.transplant.hrsa.gov/resources/allocation-calculators/las-calculator/. Accessed September 30, 2018.
66. United Network for Organ Sharing. Questions and Answers about Lung Allocation. Available at: https://www.unos.org/wp-content/uploads/unos/Lung_Patient. pdf Accessed September 30, 2018.
67. Hartigan PM, Pedoto A. Anesthetic considerations for lung volume reduction surgery and lung transplantation. Thorac Surg Clin 2005;15(1):143–57.
68. Gothard J. Anesthetic Considerations for Patients with Anterior Mediastinal Masses. Anesthesiology Clin 2008;26:305–14.
69. Béchard P, Létourneau L, Lacasse Y, et al. Perioperative Cardiorespiratory Complications in Adults with Mediastinal Mass. Incidence and Risk Factors. Anesthesiology 2004;100:826–34.

Moving?

Make sure your subscription moves with you!

To notify us of your new address, find your **Clinics Account Number** (located on your mailing label above your name), and contact customer service at:

Email: journalscustomerservice-usa@elsevier.com

800-654-2452 (subscribers in the U.S. & Canada)
314-447-8871 (subscribers outside of the U.S. & Canada)

Fax number: 314-447-8029

Elsevier Health Sciences Division
Subscription Customer Service
3251 Riverport Lane
Maryland Heights, MO 63043

*To ensure uninterrupted delivery of your subscription, please notify us at least 4 weeks in advance of move.

Printed and bound by CPI Group (UK) Ltd, Croydon, CR0 4YY

03/10/2024

01040481-0002